T0332593

Insight in Psychiatry

Questions concerning the nature of insight in patients with mental illness have interested clinicians for a long time. To what extent can patients understand disorders which affect their mental function? Does insight carry a prognostic value? Is impaired insight determined by the illness or are other factors important? Despite considerable research examining insight in patients with psychoses, non-psychotic disorders and chronic organic brain syndromes, results are inconclusive and insight remains a source of some mystification.

Ivana S. Marková examines the problems involved in studying insight in patients with mental illness in order to provide a clearer understanding of the factors that determine its clinical manifestation. She puts forward a new model to illustrate the relationship between different components of insight in theoretical and clinical terms, and points to directions for future research.

Dr Ivana S. Marková is a Senior lecturer in psychiatry with an interest in insight, descriptive psychopathology, the epistemology of mental phenomena and neuropsychiatry. She holds further qualifications in history and philosophy of science. Her work in insight is widely published, both in journals and book chapters.

Insight in Psychiatry

IVANA S. MARKOVÁ

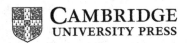

CAMBRIDGE
UNIVERSITY PRESS

CAMBRIDGE
UNIVERSITY PRESS

University Printing House, Cambridge CB2 8BS, United Kingdom

One Liberty Plaza, 20th Floor, New York, NY 10006, USA

477 Williamstown Road, Port Melbourne, VIC 3207, Australia

314-321, 3rd Floor, Plot 3, Splendor Forum, Jasola District Centre, New Delhi - 110025, India

103 Penang Road, #05-06/07, Visioncrest Commercial, Singapore 238467

Cambridge University Press is part of the University of Cambridge.

It furthers the University's mission by disseminating knowledge in the pursuit of education, learning and research at the highest international levels of excellence.

www.cambridge.org
Information on this title: www.cambridge.org/9780521825184

First published 2005

A catalogue record for this publication is available from the British Library

ISBN 978-0-521-82518-4 Hardback

Contents

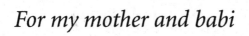

For my mother and babi

DRH

Preface

Throughout history, human beings have been variously occupied with enquiries into self-knowledge and self-understanding. In Western cultures these themes have persistently raised vital and profound questions not just for individuals but, particularly in the last two to three hundred years, for the sciences and humanities. Psychiatry has been no exception to this. However, although as we shall see in this book, interest in *insight* in psychiatry has a relatively long past, it is only in the last fifteen or twenty years that psychiatry has become engrossed with the empirical question concerning the presence and nature of insight in patients with mental disorders. It is a question that encompasses many facets. From one perspective, it addresses in a practical way the degree of understanding patients have about their conditions. In turn, this raises important issues relating to clinician-patient communication and carries implications for the management of the individual patient. From another perspective, however, the question of patients' insight reaches to the core of our understanding of mental disorders themselves. It forces us to consider, for example, how mental functions might act and interact in health and illness. Can mental disorders have selective effects on mental function? To what extent can mental dysfunction in one area affect mental function or capacity in another area? The question of insight from yet a different perspective is wider still and focuses enquiry on the nature of self in relation to mental illness. Here, questions arise concerning the sorts of factors that may contribute to self-knowledge and to what degree these might differ in the 'healthy' individual and the person with mental illness. To what extent can the self be considered independent of the mental illness that disturbs the very functions which are thought to constitute it? The question of insight in patients with mental disorders is clearly not simple. Moreover, the nature of the issues raised demands explorative processes which straddle medical, psychological, philosophical and historical approaches.

A great deal of research has been carried out in order to answer different aspects of the question of insight in psychiatry. Most such research has involved empirical studies exploring insight in different clinical populations and examining relationships between patients' insight and a variety of clinical and individual variables.

A range of innovative measures to assess insight have been devised and approaches to the study of insight have varied from one clinical area to another. Interestingly, outcomes of such studies both within a particular clinical area and between different clinical areas have been striking in their variability. Consequently, it remains difficult to arrive at consistent answers with respect to insight in psychiatry. Methodological issues aside, such variable study outcomes highlight the presence of complexities around the conceptualisation of insight and its ensuing translation into clinical forms amenable to empirical assessment. It follows that research is needed at a conceptual level to explore the notion of insight in depth, to identify and disentangle the complexities that contribute to many of the problems around the study of insight.

This book is specifically concerned with the complexities surrounding the study of insight in psychiatry. It sets out to examine the nature of these complexities in order to help clarify our understanding of insight, to detail the factors important in determining insight clinically and to specify assumptions underlying the clinical phenomena elicited. Thus, on the basis of historical, clinical and conceptual analyses, complexities inherent to the concept of insight are defined and localised at various theoretical and clinical levels. This allows for the formulation of a structure for insight which delineates constitutive components and their interrelationships. In addition, this enables the differentiation of phenomena of insight to be determined in the context of a particular clinical situation. In turn, this provides a basis on which future empirical research on insight can be systematically developed.

The study of insight itself is a major enterprise for it entails work not only in diverse areas, both clinical and non-clinical, but also on many levels. As such, this is beyond the scope of this book. Instead, the book attempts to preserve a fairly strict focus on unravelling the theoretical and practical difficulties faced by empirical research on insight. Why is insight so difficult to capture clinically? How can it be measured? Does it make sense to try to measure it in a quantitative form? What is it about insight that makes it complicated to define or, rather, to define in an operational way? These are the sorts of questions that are addressed by this book with the purpose of both furthering clinical understanding of insight and developing new directions for future empirical work. Whilst approaching these issues from an epistemological perspective, there is no appropriate room here for a wider philosophical enquiry that might explore the notion of insight in all its possible metaphysical dimensions.

The book concentrates on insight in psychiatry but even within this remit has had to be selective and to set boundaries to the amount and types of material examined. Thus, both for the maintaining of the book's focus and for reasons of space, there are areas that have not been covered and which are important in future work on the subject. In this regard, for example, insight into medical illness has not been included within the review section. Emphasis has been given to studies on insight in general psychiatric disorders and in dementia. Areas which have clearly contributed to the approaches taken to the exploration of insight in such disorders have also been included, namely, psychological and neurological approaches. Within general psychiatry, current studies on insight have focused predominantly on the psychoses and affective disorders and this material is therefore reviewed and analysed in the book. Less empirical research has been carried out on insight in other psychiatric disorders, notably, neurotic, stress-related, dissociative disorders or anxiety states and this is an area which again would be important to study in the future. In fact, much of the work that has examined insight in these particular clinical areas has come from the psychoanalytic psychological perspective and this is covered in Chapter 2. The clinical reviews themselves are not aimed to be fully comprehensive though the bulk of the work in the various areas has been covered. For the purposes of the book, however, the clinical reviews are intended primarily to illustrate and define the essential conceptual issues arising from the empirical studies of insight within the respective areas. The historical chapter is restricted to examining the concept of insight in Western cultures. It is further limited, for practical reasons, to literature in English, French and German languages.

The book is divided into two parts. The first part (Chapters 1–5) reviews and analyses insight into mental illness from its evolution as an independent concept to the ways in which insight has been conceptualised and explored in clinical psychiatry and related disciplines. Chapter 1 examines the concept of insight in mental illness from a historical perspective, concentrating predominantly on the views held by the late nineteenth century French alienists. This focus is the result of, firstly, the importance and influence of nineteenth century French psychopathology on Western psychiatry in general. Secondly, the French debates on this issue were particularly explicit in showing how ideas on awareness and insight developed in the context of the changing philosophical and medical-pathological views at the time. Chapter 2 explores insight from the psychological perspective and emphasises both the differences in conceptualisation of insight held by the Gestalt, cognitive and psychodynamic schools and the ways in which these perspectives have influenced approaches to insight in clinical psychiatry. Chapter 3 reviews the empirical work on insight in general psychiatry. It shows the wide range of definitions of insight employed by the studies, the different approaches taken to assess insight empirically and the mixed and inconclusive study outcomes. Chapter 4 examines work on insight and awareness carried out in neurological states and, as such, forms an introduction to Chapter 5. In comparison with the 'psychiatric' notion, impaired insight or unawareness is viewed as a much narrower concept and approaches taken to its assessment reflect this different conception. The importance of unawareness or anosognosia in this narrow sense is stressed in the light of its influence on approaches to the study of insight in dementia and in general psychiatry. Chapter 5 reviews the empirical studies on insight in dementia. As in general psychiatry, outcomes of such studies are variable and inconclusive. Likewise, a range of methods have been developed to assess insight and these have, more particularly, been influenced by approaches taken by various clinical disciplines.

The second part of the book (Chapters 6–9) addresses the conceptual issues raised from the earlier chapters and proposes a structure for insight that can provide a useful framework for understanding insight and its determinants. Chapter 6 focuses on the meaning and nature of insight. A distinction is made between the *concept* and *phenomenon* of insight and the problems related to each are specified. In turn, the implications such problems carry for the empirical study of insight are explored. Chapter 7 examines the relational aspects of insight. It shows how different 'objects' of insight assessment determine different clinical phenomena of insight and emphasises the implications of this for the structure of insight and its empirical assessment. Chapter 8 argues, on theoretical and empirical grounds, for a meaningful distinction to be made between *awareness* and *insight*. Distinguishing features between awareness and insight are described in terms of their quantitative and qualitative aspects. Chapter 9 presents a schematic representation of the structure of insight that is based on the distinction between awareness and insight. It shows how the phenomenon of insight can be placed within this structure, determined by it and also by the 'object' of insight assessment as well as the measures used for its elicitation. The implications for understanding insight and for future research are then discussed.

The book is based on thoughts that have developed and changed over a number of years. I have used and built on material presented in my doctoral thesis (Glasgow University, 1998) and on work already published. I would like to thank the publishers of the *British Journal of Psychiatry, Comprehensive Psychiatry, Journal of Nervous and Mental Disease, Neurology Psychiatry & Brain Research* and *Psychopathology* for allowing me to use materials from papers of mine which appeared in their pages. Special thanks are owed to Dr. German E. Berrios from the Department of Psychiatry, Cambridge University, with whom I have had countless discussions and explored many of the ideas presented here. His deep scholarly knowledge has stimulated and inspired my own thinking and much of the conceptual work developed here has been the result of a joint struggle. In addition, he has pointed me towards numerous invaluable bibliographical sources crucial for the historical section of the book. I would also like to thank members of the AWARE project group (Awareness in early-stage dementia: understanding, assessment and implications for early intervention) for useful comments and thoughts in relation to the work on insight in dementia: Dr. Linda Clare, University of Wales, Bangor;

Mrs. Geraldine Kenny, North Eastern Health Board, Dublin; Dr. Barbara Romero, Bad Aibling, Germany; Professor Frans Verhey, University of Maastricht, Netherlands; Professor Michael Wang, University of Leicester and Professor Bob Woods, University of Wales, Bangor. In particular, I am grateful to Dr. Linda Clare for discussions which helped to clarify some of the theoretical aspects of this book. I am grateful also to the University of Hull for their encouragement of this work. Finally, I would like to thank my family for their enormous support and also my friends and colleagues who have shown extreme patience.

Part I

Historical and clinical

Historical overview

Exploring the history of insight in mental disorders is complicated by a number of factors. Foremost amongst these is the question as to which definition of insight to examine. As will become evident in subsequent chapters, insight and related terms can refer to concepts which range considerably in meaning from the very narrow to much broader notions. For example, much of the work on insight in patients with organic brain syndromes uses a fairly narrow concept relating to awareness of specific problems/deficits (Marková & Berrios, 2000). On the other hand, insight studied in general psychiatry, particularly in patients with psychoses, has tended to be viewed in a more general sense of awareness of illness (McEvoy et al., 1989a, b, c; Young et al., 1993, Amador & David, 2004) and/or with broader elaborations incorporated within the concept such as additional interpretations (Greenfeld et al., 1989), attributions (Amador et al., 1991), re-labelling (David, 1990) and self-knowledge (Marková & Berrios, 1992a; Gillett, 1994). Then there is the notion of insight viewed in terms of specific problem solving as in Gestalt cognitive psychology (Sternberg & Davidson, 1995) or, different again, is the deeper notion of insight as psychodynamic 'comprehension' (Richfield, 1954) and indeed the cognitive view according to which insight is a function of some 'mind reading system' (Baron-Cohen, 1995).

It could be argued that such differences in meanings of insight are simply the result of different disciplinary perspectives (e.g. general psychiatry, clinical psychology, neurology, neuropsychiatry, psychotherapy, etc.) and hence it would make more sense to trace individual historical accounts in relation to each clinical discipline. Whilst this would be important in order to facilitate understanding of the respective meanings and structures underlying insight in each case, it would not address the problem of the general history of insight in psychiatry and the question of whether there is a common structure or derivative to ensuing concepts of insight or whether the commonality lies just in the usage of the term 'insight'. Moreover, attempting to chronicle a general history of insight in psychiatry allows for the broadest of bases in terms of mental disorders. This is important as the separation of clinical disciplines and increasing specialisation is dependent not only on changes in views about the nature and classification of clinical disorders but also on the perceived needs of different patient groups. Thus, by definition, specialisation places its own constraints on the types of patients and the sorts of disorders included within specific categories at a particular time. This in turn affects the perspective from which different concepts are held. Consequently, focusing solely on individual disciplinary historical narratives might obviate the important contribution of the individuation of clinical disorders themselves towards the conceptualisation of insight.

How then to attempt a general historical account of insight in psychiatry? Berrios (1994a; 1996) has suggested that one way of approaching the construction of a valid historical account of symptoms or illness is to make an explicit distinction between the histories of the *terms*, the *behaviours* and the *concepts* relating to the object of inquiry. Differentiating between the histories of these aspects of insight helps to illustrate and clarify how the meanings of insight may change not only in time but also in relation to different contexts, whether these are social, cultural, intellectual, etc. This approach shall thus be followed here. However, it has to be emphasised that such distinctions in relation to the histories of insight do not entail their independence. For example, when considering insight as a 'behaviour', then clearly this cannot be considered as an a-theoretical object. Instead, interpreting a behaviour as insightful or insightless is the result of both overt and covert conceptualisation. This, in turn, is dependent on a background of related concepts such as ideas about the self, about the workings of the mind, about illness and mental illness, etc. These themselves are determined in part by the views and knowledge held during the particular historical period of the subject. In addition, insight as a 'behaviour' does not directly reflect an ontological entity in the way that, for example, a paretic gait might reflect a specific paresis. This does not mean that there cannot be a neurobiological basis to insight but simply that at this stage, elicitation of insight as a behaviour depends much more on conceptualisation and interpretation.

This chapter thus first examines some of the historical contexts forming the background to insight and related notions. Then a brief overview of the history of the term 'insight' is given, followed by an account of the history of the concept and behaviour of insight. The histories of the concept and behaviour of insight are discussed together because of their particular interdependence.

1.1 Historical contexts

In medicine, the concept of insight into madness seems to have started appearing in a consistent manner in the early part of the nineteenth century when the clinical descriptions offered by alienists began to include observations concerning patients' awareness of their pathological state. In 1820, Georget, commenting on the received view of madness [*folie*] as intellectual disorders in which patients were unaware, remarked how whilst this was true for most patients, there was nevertheless a small number of patients 'who are well able to assess their mental state, who tell you: I have an ill head, a disturbed spirit, I can no longer think, I know that my thoughts are disordered, I am behaving badly – but I cannot do otherwise …' (Georget, 1820, p. 94, my translation). And by the middle and late nineteenth century, specific debates concerning the question of insight and its relationship to different aspects of mental illness were already taking place (Société Médico-Psychologique, 1869/1870).

In order to try to understand why insight into mental illness became an issue of interest at this particular time and what factors helped shape its emergence, it is necessary to look at the historical space in which this was happening. Two particular contexts will be considered here. Firstly, a brief look is given at the way in which insight and self-knowledge were conceived in terms of the general thinking around this time. Secondly, the changing views around the conceptualisation of madness itself helped to influence the way in which insight into madness was conceived and debated and, for the purposes of this chapter, more focus will be given to this area.

1.1.1 General contexts

The concept of insight in relation to the 'healthy' mind has been for a long time a source of much interest to philosophers, psychologists, theologians, writers and lay people. In Western cultures, for example, interest in self-examination is already evident in ancient Greek philosophy. 'Know Thyself' is inscribed on the temple of Apollo at Delphi and self-knowledge was a dominant feature of Socrates' teaching (Plato, Charmides, 164e). According to Socrates, caring for one's soul was the individual's main duty. However, only when one had self-knowledge could one care for oneself (Plato, Alcibiades, 129b).

With the decline of the Greek culture, the interest in self-examination appeared to diminish. Morris (1972) argued that concern about human individuality reappeared in the eleventh and twelfth centuries, but primarily in relation to Christianity. The emphasis in the Middle Ages on self-examination seemed to lie in the pursuit of moral virtues and the self was viewed as under constant supervision and judgement by God. During the Renaissance, the conception of self changed. Accompanying the expansion in science, technology and the economy, interest became more focused on the self as an individual and on his/her relationship with the world. Amongst the Renaissance writers, Pico della Mirandola (1965) placed the self at the centre of the universe. He maintained that the individual was capable of judging himself and thus should be in control of his own life. In other words, the emphasis was on the self as someone who could exert effects on himself and on the world and society.

In the seventeenth century interest in individuality continued to develop. Descartes identified consciousness or awareness with thinking: 'It is correct that to be aware is both to think and to reflect on one's thought … [the soul] has the power to reflect on its thoughts as often as it likes, and to be aware of its thought in this way …' (Descartes, 1648/1991, p. 335). He assumed, as did Locke later, that every experience of the individual was accompanied by self-awareness (Perkins, 1969). Indeed, Locke went further to say that the identity of the self was determined by consciousness (Locke, 1700/1979) though the notion of self throughout this time was also a changing concept exerting independent as well as interdependent influences on the conceptualisation of mental illness and psychopathology (Berrios, 1993; Berrios & Marková, 2003). Nevertheless, it can be understood that consciousness or awareness of self in this context was conceived as intrinsic to thinking, feeling and experiencing rather than as a separate system that could assess such mental operations independently.

It was later, in the eighteenth and nineteenth centuries, during the Enlightenment and the period known as Romanticism, that the self as a whole being became the real focus of thought. Self-awareness obtained the meaning of self-reflection and self-consciousness in a much wider sense. In contrast to Descartes who focused predominantly on the individual's self, the Romanticists and some of the philosophers at the time argued that self-consciousness develops mutually with the consciousness of others. By being aware of others as reflexive beings, one is able to look at oneself through the eyes of others. One becomes the object of one's own observation (Mead, 1934; 1936). As a result, *introspection* became a prevailing theme of that time (Boring, 1953). The importance of the subjectivity of inner experiences was carried over to the psychiatry of the nineteenth century and legitimised the elicitation of psychopathology based on patients' accounts (Berrios, 1996).

Another important psychological concept emerging in the nineteenth century, and influencing psychiatry and the conceptualisation of insight was that of comprehension (*Verstehen*), as developed in different ways by Brentano (1874/1973), Dilthey (1976) and eventually, Freud, Husserl and Jaspers, amongst others (Berrios, 1992). This concept encompassed more than 'understanding' and more than 'looking into one's mind' (as suggested by introspection). Instead, it aimed to capture the totality of one's mental and existential state including non-conscious aspects. The conceptualisation of insight caught within this frame thus demanded more than an intellectual awareness of being ill but called on deeper processes involving emotions and volitions, and that extended to a self that embraced a wider and richer concept. The way in which such a holistic notion of insight was envisaged depended on the particular school of thought. For example, Brentano related this to his concept of intentionality and invoked a 'third consciousness': 'Experience shows that there exist in us not only a presentation and a judgement, but frequently a third kind of consciousness of the mental act, namely a feeling which refers to this act, pleasure or displeasure which we feel towards this act' (Brentano, 1874/1973, p. 143). Dilthey, on the other hand, emphasised a different aspect of the self as the focus of '*verstehen*', namely, experience or '*Erlebnis*'. This latter concept was conceived as the entirety of an individual's experience, comprising internal and external experiences (and the relationship between them) in its full historical context (Dilthey, 1976; Apel, 1987; Makkreel, 1992). Again, this deeper view of the self and capacity of 'understanding' the self enriched the general conceptualisation of insight. Also relevant to the broad notion of self-understanding at this time was the concept of *apperception*. Introduced much earlier into philosophy by Leibnitz, to distinguish special perceptions of which man was distinctly conscious, the concept was adopted in nineteenth century psychology particularly in the work of Wundt. Associated directly with activity of the will, apperception was conceived as the foundation of self-consciousness itself (Lange, 1906).

1.1.2 Insanity and the conceptualisation of madness

Until the early nineteenth century, the notion of madness encompassed a wide variety of meanings predominantly from the social, cultural and political perspective and, as such, was not generally considered a medical category (Foucault, 1971; Porter, 1990). In this context, whilst descriptions of behaviours, viewed as insane, are plentiful and often rich in literary and artistic colour (Porter, 1987), there did not exist the language of descriptive psychopathology. That is to say, there was no clinical and systematic method of capturing and classifying signs, symptoms and behaviours of abnormal mental states (Berrios, 1996). As Berrios (1996) has shown, the latter did not develop until the middle of the nineteenth century with the professionalisation of psychiatry as a discipline and, *inter alia*, in the context of emerging views concerning subjectivity and introspection. Instead, the behaviour of madness was depicted in the language of the lay and literary public, and portrayed as an all-or-none phenomenon. Officially, the definition of insanity then, as offered by Hobbes and Locke in the seventeenth century, was based on the presence of delusions (Berrios, 1994b) so that being deluded meant being mad and vice versa. In turn, delusions by definition incorporated the notion of insightlessness. Hence, before the nineteenth century, it would have been a logical contradiction in terms to talk about insight or awareness of delusions. Condillac (1746/1924, §86, p. 55), following Locke and influential in the thinking of the French alienists of the early nineteenth century, defined madness in terms of a disordered imagination (referring to delusional thinking) '*which one is not capable of noticing*'. Thus, insightlessness was inherent to the concept of delusion and madness and could not, in the thinking of the time, be conceived of and examined separately.

The early nineteenth century saw significant changes in the views and management of madness. The rise in the numbers of asylums for the insane, the increased interest shown by the physicians into the nature and treatment of insanity as well as the development of 'psychiatry' as an independent profession all contributed to this (Goldstein, 1987). Important in the conceptualisation of insight as something that could be studied independently and in relation to madness were the changing views around the notion of insanity as an all-or-none phenomenon. Instead, the notion of such a total insanity was being challenged by the development of various concepts of partial insanity. The latter was not a unitary notion but referred to a number of different concepts and terms which seemed to evolve during the first half of the nineteenth century. Common to these various concepts was the view that madness could be accompanied, to a greater or lesser extent, by lucidity. This could take place either in time, i.e. madness interspersed by lucid or sane periods, or within the madness itself, i.e. madness could be restricted to one or a few regions of the psyche whilst sparing others (Trélat, 1861; Legrand du Saulle, 1864; Despine, 1875). The development of the notion that insanity could be partial in these ways was important. It opened up a space in which awareness or insight into madness could be conceived as possible, occurring either in relation to the unaffected *periods* in the course of the illness or in relation to the unaffected *faculties* of the mind. Furthermore, not only was space created in which insight into madness could be conceived, but the partial insanity debates themselves, because of their questions concerning the nature and manifestations of madness, and the relationship between divisions of the mind, were directly relevant to the conceptualisation of insight into madness, particularly, in the latter part of the nineteenth century. In view of this, it is useful to briefly look at some of the factors likely to have been influential in the development of the concepts of partial insanity.

Probably one of the most important factors in the conceptualisation of partial insanity relates to the empirical observations of the alienists at the time. Whilst psychiatry as a profession did not fully emerge until near the middle of the nineteenth century, there was, at the turn of the century, increasing interest shown by physicians in the treatment of the insane (Goldstein, 1987). Pinel and Esquirol in France and Prichard in England were amongst the earliest alienists to suggest that patients could appear to be mad in some areas of their psyche but not in others. On the basis of his clinical observations, Pinel (1801) proposed the category 'manie sans délire' to refer to insanity in patients who appeared to be afflicted by uncontrollable excitement and rage, and yet were able to reason and judge coherently. Whilst later retracting the category, he continued to maintain that patients could have 'reasoning madness' ('folie raisonnante') in which their madness was partial:

... the examples of manic patients with fury but without délire and without any incoherence in their ideas, are far from being rare in both women and men, and they go to show how much lesions of the will can be distinct from those of the understanding, even though they frequently occur together.

Pinel (1809, p. 102, my translation)

Questioning how such cases could be explained if the views held by Locke and Condillac were followed, he went on to note that patients could appear to have lesions of the affective faculties only, or even isolated lesions involving attention, memory, thoughts or judgement. Such observations were difficult to reconcile with the doctrine of indivisibility of human understanding (Pinel, 1801).

More explicit and distinctive still was the concept of partial insanity promoted by Pinel's disciple, Esquirol and his own followers, namely that of '*monomania*'. The monomanias comprised a range of partial insanities where the partial aspect referred mainly to the content of the ideas/affects/behaviours around which the madness was observed to be circumscribed. As a result, types of monomanias were identified and named such as erotic monomania, homicidal monomania, drunkenness monomania, etc. (Esquirol, 1838). The concept of monomania became extremely popular in the early nineteenth century both as a diagnosis made frequently by alienists and as a defence used by lawyers in criminal proceedings (Goldstein, 1987). In fact, challenges made by lawyers against the concept of total insanity (as well as the opposing arguments of the prosecutors) had been prominent for several hundred years beforehand (Orange, 1892). It was only when madness became the focus of more specific medical interest (rather than a social category) and converged with the legal interest that such debates became significant contributors to the questions posed around the existence of partial insanities. The term 'monomania', however, lost popularity and by the middle of the century was almost lost while related concepts were developed and replaced it. What is clear, however, in many debates about monomanias and partial insanity at that time (Guislain, 1852; Brierre de Boismont, 1853; Delasiauve, 1853; Falret, 1866), was that discussions seemed to be hampered by inconsistencies and sometimes contradictions concerning understanding of what the 'partial' aspect of insanity was referring to. Thus, in the case of monomania, Esquirol himself defined this variously from a partial délire, i.e. a délire concentrated on one or a few objects (giving rise to the types of monomanias named above), to disorders characterised by partial lesions of the intellect or affect or the will (giving rise to '*monomanie intellectuelle*', '*monomanie affective*' and '*monomanie instinctive*', respectively) (Esquirol, 1819; 1838). In addition, he distinguished between lypemania and monomania on the basis of exaltation of ideas, psychological and physical excitement in the latter (Esquirol, 1819), thereby, invoking yet another criterial form. In other words, clinical observations and their analyses were occurring at different levels and distinctions between different partial insanities were made simultaneously on the basis of different categories. Hence, some distinctions were made empirically, sometimes on the basis of the contents of patients' madness, and other times on the basis of the types of emotions or energy affecting the patients. Yet other distinctions were made theoretically on the basis of postulated lesions of the mind. A similar point is made by Kageyama (1984) in relation to Pinel's classification of madness and it is likely that these inconsistencies also played a part in the related debates around insight and awareness into illness (see below).

Another form of partial insanity was introduced by Prichard in England as 'moral insanity'. Influenced by Pinel, Esquirol and Georget, but based on his observations, he defined the category of 'moral insanity' as a partial insanity characterised by affective and behavioural disturbance. This particular insanity was, he qualified, 'without any illusion or erroneous conviction impressed upon the understanding: it sometimes co-exists with an apparently unimpaired state of the intellectual faculties' (Prichard, 1835, p. 12). The important issue here is that patients were observed as preserving some aspects of their mental function whilst being deranged in others. Irrespective of the confusion engendered by the different categories of distinctions made in relation to the partial insanities, the focused clinical observations of the alienists at this time made possible the concept of partial insanity itself. This in turn was necessary for the conceptualisation of insight as an independent phenomenon.

Apart from the empirical observations of alienists, there was another development important to the conceptualisation of partial insanity and hence insight that contributed to the debates around the distinctions between different insanities. This was the gradual emergence of different forms of faculty psychology. In broad terms, faculty psychology refers to the view that the mind consists of individual units or functions, actual or potential, which can conceivably operate, and be affected, to varying extents, independently. This view contrasted with the associationism of Locke and Condillac that had been prevalent and influential at the time of the early nineteenth century alienists and which held that the mind was indivisible. Faculty psychology was not a unified doctrine but simply reflected the changes in perspectives that were developing around the way in which the mind was conceived as working. Ideas from some of the eighteenth century Scottish philosophers, particularly Thomas Reid, provided a source of some forms of faculty psychology. These ideas appeared to be influential in the thinking of French philosophers and alienists during the early and middle part of the nineteenth century (Boutroux, 1908; Brooks, 1976). Reid focused explicitly on faculty psychology as the basis to his epistemology and conceived faculties as independent powers (albeit working together) driving the individual operations of the mind such as perception, memory, appetite, passions, etc. (Reid, 1785/1994). But, the nature of faculties themselves, their origin, development, numbers, extent of independence and relationship with other organic functions, etc. were issues that were unclear and debated amongst philosophers and alienists at the beginning of the nineteenth century (Rullier, 1815).

Another more extreme departure from associationism, in the early part of the nineteenth century, was the faculty psychology promoted by Gall and Spurzheim in the shape of the phrenology movement. Arguing explicitly against the prevailing sensationalism, Gall introduced his organic thesis of innate faculties which were localisable to specific organs in the brain. However, he rejected the notion that faculties comprised of understanding, will, memory, etc. and proposed instead the idea of specific fundamental faculties which enabled differentiation of characteristics between individuals. In other words, his concept of faculties was that of mental qualities, constitutive of both mind and character, e.g. pride/self-esteem, friendship/ attachment, sense of colours, music, verbal memory, memory for languages, etc. (Spoerl, 1936). Arousing debates and strong criticisms (Gordon, 1815; Lélut, 1837; 1843), the phrenology movement was nevertheless important. It influenced the views of alienists in early nineteenth century Britain (Cooter, 1979) and France where Gall and Spurzheim's courses were well attended by the alienists of the second decade e.g. Georget and Leuret (Goldstein, 1987).

Alongside the debates around faculties of the mind, ideas about partial insanity and the space in which insight into madness could become conceptualised were also shaped by changing views concerning the causes of insanity. These in turn related to changes in the notion of disease itself. An anonymous historian stated in 1840: 'all explanations of mental illness boil down to three options: they are localised in the brain ... or in the soul ... or in both' (Fabre, 1840, p. 118). Supporters of the anatomo-clinical view of disease, including madness (Ackerknecht, 1967), were thus more able to conceive and accept the notion of partial insanity and hence also the possibility of insight into the diseased mental faculties. In contrast, those who believed that insanity was exclusively sited in the mind or soul (*l'âme*) had difficulty in conceiving partial insanity and insight into illness since the soul was, in terms of the philosophy of the period, indivisible and could not become partially diseased.

The shift from the view that madness was as an all-or-none ontological entity to the possibility that madness could be partial in different ways carried major implications for the alienists in the nineteenth century. In the context of the factors described above, important discussions were taking place concerning the nature and classification of mental disorders. In particular, the different forms of faculty psychology permeating the thinking of the alienists, allowed for a more modular conception of the mind with more or less specific cerebral localisation. This in turn led to debates concerning the organisation and function of mental faculties, and their role in mental illness (Société Médico-Psychologique, 1866). Delasiauve (1853) argued that there was a categorical difference between the intellectual faculties and the instinctive/affective faculties. Whilst the former were interdependent, the latter, by contrast, could operate and be affected independently. Falret (1866), on the other hand, maintained that whilst it was useful to distinguish between independent mental faculties for study purposes, it could not be assumed that mental faculties operated independently in the healthy mind or could be injured independently in the ill mind. He believed, like Maudsley did some years later, that madness even when it affected predominantly one or a few faculties, had its effects on all. Others disagreed and held that insanity could be specific to different faculties (Delasiauve, 1866; Société Médico-Psychologique, 1866). In a different vein, Fournet (1870) focused on the importance of studying the relationship between mental events and events occurring at the cellular level of the brain. He emphasised, however, that mental activities should not be reduced to brain mechanisms and that psychological perspectives had to be preserved. It is within the context of such debates, in the spaces formed by the conceptualisation of partial insanities and the discussions around the independence/interdependence of mental faculties, that it became possible to conceive the existence of an insanity which could have awareness of itself. Thus, insight and insightlessness could become meaningful concepts, variables in their own right which could be examined in relation to and independent of insanity.

1.2 History of the word

It is interesting that the term 'insight' (and its equivalents) only exists in this unitary form in the North and West Germanic families of languages. The Latin languages (e.g. French, Spanish, Italian, Portuguese, etc.) do not have a corresponding unitary term and, hence, translation of insight into these languages depends on the specific meaning of the term intended in a particular context. For example, a well-known nineteenth century German–French dictionary translates the German word for 'insight' ('Einsicht'), as: 'inspection, examen, connaissance de cause, bon sens, jugement' (Rose, 1878). Individually, all these terms carry somewhat different meanings and hence the term chosen in a particular situation will vary according to the specific need of the speaker. It is of note that, within the countries of the Germanic languages, there has been more interest shown in the concept of insight in the general thinking. Whether or not having a unitary term (insight or Einsicht) carries implications for the conceptualisation of insight as an ontological entity has not, however, been determined.

For the German term 'Einsicht', Grimm and Grimm (1862) propose as equivalents the Latin terms 'intelligentia' and 'judicium', and suggest that the term gained wider usage in the work of Goethe and Kant (Pauleikhoff & Mester, 1973). Adelung, at the beginning of the nineteenth century, defined it as: 'Das sinneinsehen in eine Sache' [seeing into the meaning or sense of something] (Adelung, 1811, Vol. 1). Ritter claims that the Middle German term 'insehen' was present in Medieval mystical writings and meant 'hineinsehen' [looking into or inside], and that J.C. Günther at the beginning of the eighteenth century discarded the religious denotation and used 'Einsicht' as equivalent to personal evidence (Ritter, 1972, Vol. 2). In addition, Ritter suggests that the 'psychological' meaning introduced by Köhler (see Chapter 2) was a deviation in that it simply meant 'intelligence' and hence was closer to the old Aristotelian meaning of phronêsis ('thought or understanding').

As far as English is concerned, the *Oxford English Dictionary* (2002) states that the original notion of insight referred to 'internal sight', i.e. with the eyes of the mind or understanding and provides a set of definitions generally embracing the same metaphor, e.g. internal sight, mental vision or perception, discernment; the fact of penetrating with the eyes of the understanding into the inner character or hidden nature of things, a glimpse or view beneath the surface, the faculty or power of thus seeing.

In terms of the *clinical* usages of the term 'insight', i.e. its use in relation to mental illness, some early references to the terms can be seen in Pick (1882) as '*Krankheitseinsicht*' or insight into illness. Similarly, the term 'insightlessness' was used in Krafft-Ebing: 'in the later stages of insanity, where delusions have become organised or mental disintegration has ensued, the patient is completely insightless [*einsichtslos*] about his disease state' (Krafft-Ebing, 1893, p. 102, my translation).

1.3 History of the concept

Whilst there are some difficulties in arriving at a meaning that is common to the word 'insight' given the differences in historical roots and terminologies between the European countries as touched on above, there seems to be a more consistent conceptualisation of the notion as used in clinical practice. The history of the concept of insight into madness is necessarily embedded in the histories of related concepts such as reason, consciousness and self-knowledge as well as in the histories of views around the nature of disease and insanity. Having considered some of the historical contexts in which the concept of insight emerged, as a phenomenon that could be examined in relation to, and independent of, madness, this section will be concerned with the nature of the concept of insight itself and how this was conceived in the psychiatry of the nineteenth century until the present day.

1.3.1 French views

In the early and middle part of the nineteenth century, as noted earlier, alienists were already observing that some insane patients seemed to show awareness into their pathological states. However, from these early observations it is evident that, at that stage, the concept was not particularly clearly developed. Thus, descriptions were brief and various terms were used which seemed to touch on different aspects of awareness or insight but without these being further clarified or analysed. For example, Pinel (1801) variously referred to either a *judgement* made on the part of a patient, commenting on how sometimes a patient could, towards the end of his episode of madness, correctly assess his state (*apprécie avec justesse son état*) and himself request prolongation of admission (p. 32), or a *feeling* of impending illness (*sentent l'approche de leur invasion*) (p. 244). Similarly, Esquirol (1838) used different terms referring to a concept focusing either on *awareness*, e.g. 'some lypemanics have awareness of their state (*le sentiment de leur état*), they are aware (*la conscience*) of the falsity, of the absurdity of the fears which torment them; they can well perceive their disordered thinking ...' (Esquirol, 1838, Vol. 1, p. 420, my translation), or on more elaborate judgement when noting that patients could *reflect* on their state (p. 124). The Belgian alienist Guislain referred to awareness in patients (either *le sentiment de leur état* or *la conscience*), observing how some patients, particularly at the beginning of their illness, would tell others that they felt unwell, ill or that their illness was at the point of exacerbation. In his clinical descriptions of mental illnesses, Guislain further pointed out that 'awareness (*la conscience*) could remain intact and that the patient is able to say to himself: I am mad' (Guislain, 1852, p. 62, my translation).

More significant focus on the concept of awareness into madness seems to have been present by the middle of the nineteenth century. In the context of the debates around monomanias, Delasiauve (1861; 1863; 1865) specifically designated the term '*pseudo-monomanie*' for patients with monomania who had awareness of their morbid condition, though a similar concept had already been present in Esquirol when he suggested '*lypémanie raisonnante*' (Esquirol, 1838, p. 420). In the context of the discussions around what constituted partial madness, Baillarger (1853) drew special attention to the concept of awareness by explicitly arguing that this should be considered a criterion in distinguishing between patients who were and who were not insane. His conception of insight was specifically related to the cause that the patient attributed to the morbid symptoms. Thus, a patient with hallucinations, for example, who was convinced of the reality of his hallucinations in the outside world, based on persecutory ideas, had no insight (*la conscience*) and was truly mad. On the other hand, the patient with hallucinations who realised that these were caused by some derangement in himself, showed preservation of insight and should not be considered truly mad. According to Baillarger, partial madness could occur as a result of partial lesions of the understanding but insight or awareness itself could not, in the same way, be partial.

Falret (1866), who embraced a wider concept of insight as patients' awareness of their morbid states, disagreed with the notion that loss of awareness could be used as a criterion distinguishing between reason and insanity. He pointed out that individuals in healthy or rational states of mind sometimes could not recognise morbid changes in themselves, and would therefore accordingly lack insight. Nevertheless, these individuals would not be considered mad. Furthermore, he observed that many patients 'have perfect awareness of their states, which is in great conflict with their ill behaviours, ... with the delusional ideas imposed on them' (Falret, 1866,

p. 387, my translation). Hence, lack of awareness into one's state could not be used as a criterion of madness in all cases.

A major debate specifically concerning awareness of mental illness ('*la discussion sur les aliénés avec conscience de leur état*', Société Médico-Psychologique, 1870) was held by the Société Médico-Psychologique in 1869/1870, and again, to a lesser extent, in 1875. These discussions were held in the context of medico-legal concerns in relation to determining responsibility of patients/individuals for criminal and civil acts. In addition, however, the debates on awareness of mental illness extended into related areas including the nature of madness itself, the faculties of the mind, the notion of free will, the concept of self, and underlying brain lesions or processes. Awareness of mental illness was discussed in relation to all these areas and was, consequently, immersed and shaped by the problems that were being faced in trying to clarify the latter. It is difficult, therefore, to obtain a clear definition or conceptualisation of insight in isolation. However, the debates did begin to identify a possible structure to insight both in terms of clinical importance and in terms of possible components.

Concerning the question of legal responsibility for criminal acts, most alienists (Delasiauve, 1866; 1870; Falret, 1866; 1870; Billod, 1870; Girard de Gailleux, 1870; Maury, 1870; Morel, 1870) argued that patients could have awareness of their insane state and yet would be powerless against the urges/impulses arising from their madness that drove them to commit abnormal acts. Hence, they should not be held legally responsible for such behaviours. Insight or awareness was thus conceived as a form of passive observation made on the part of the sane aspects of the patient's mind, of the abnormal urges, feelings and thoughts produced by the insanity. The passivity of such observation was couched in terms such as 'spectator' (Morel, 1870) or 'witness' (Billod, 1870). Emphasising the importance of distinguishing between reason and awareness of illness, Morel (1870, p. 116) observed that some mad patients preserved their ability to reason and yet had no awareness of being insane. Other patients, however, could have a weakened reason which was unable to prevent them from committing criminal acts and, nevertheless, they had awareness of their insanity ('*aliénés irréponsables mais non des aliénés inconscients*'). In addition, the awareness of one's mental state and actions was explicitly distinguished from awareness of the right and wrong of one's actions (Morel, 1870). The main conclusion, however, was that the ability to observe one's madness did not confer the ability to resist its manifestations and consequences. This view was challenged by Fournet (1870) who claimed that awareness of illness actually implied the presence of some degree of reason and, hence, the amount of reason available to the patient would determine the amount of responsibility for his acts. In other words, he argued that the degree of responsibility for a criminal act was proportionate to the amount of the patient's reason. Fournet's position was based on his

Table 1.1 Prevalence of awareness in patients admitted to Vaucluse asylum between January and December 1869 (Billod, 1870)

Numbers of patients with awareness of mental illness	Admissions to asylum	
	Males ($n = 378$)	Females ($n = 350$)
Total numbers showing awareness	61 (in 55 of these, madness followed alcohol excess)	19 (in five of these, madness followed alcohol excess)
Numbers with complete awareness	49	12
Numbers with incomplete awareness	12	7

views about the central role of the self in the concept of insanity (see below) and his arguments were not generally upheld.

Discussions on awareness of mental states also raised questions concerning the nature of mental illness or insanity. Morel (1870) pointed out that patients ranged from having no awareness of their insanity to having full awareness and suggested that the extent of awareness held by patients depended on the site of the lesion causing the insanity. Thus, different insanities, with different aetiologies, not only showed different patterns of symptoms and manifestations but also were associated with different amounts of awareness (Girard de Gailleux, 1870; Morel, 1870). Billod (1870), reporting one of the earliest 'empirical' studies on awareness of illness, found that the number of patients with awareness of their pathological state was much lower than the number of patients who lacked awareness and that awareness was much commoner in patients whose insanity was the result of alcoholism. He presented his own figures (see Table 1.1) and divided patients into those with complete awareness and those with incomplete awareness of their morbid state.

His distinction between complete and incomplete awareness was interesting and raised again the issue of whether patients with awareness should be considered as truly insane. In essence, he first of all divided patients into two categories:

1 Those patients who were *not aware* of their pathological state, i.e. they were aware of strange experiences, hallucinations, disordered thoughts, etc. but attributed those wrongly.
2 Those who *were aware* of their pathological state, i.e. were aware of being insane.

He then subdivided this latter category into:

(i) Patients with *incomplete awareness*: They were aware of their pathological state but nevertheless believed in the reality of their delusions/abnormal experiences. Billod viewed this contradiction between their awareness of illness and at the same time their belief in their abnormal experiences as illogical and hence signifying a lesion of judgement. Consequently, he stated, this group of patients should be considered as truly insane.

(ii) Patients with *complete awareness*: They were aware of their pathological state and, in contrast to the first group, also recognised the falseness or unreality of their abnormal experiences even though they were still tormented by them. In this case, Billod maintained that their judgement was relatively intact and hence these patients should not be considered as truly insane ('*pseudo-aliénés*').

Exploring the concept of awareness further, Billod observed that following recovery, some patients had full awareness of the state of madness in which they had been and were able to give an exact account of what they had experienced and could judge this as having been the product of their madness. Following up patients longitudinally, he found that this retrospective insight was the best prognostic indicator in terms of illness recurrence. Thus, he reported that patients who had recovered from their madness but had no awareness of their previous state showed a 60% rate of relapse or recurrence. This contrasted with 10% of patients who relapsed after having recovered and who had shown good insight into their previous state. Indeed, Billod suggested that where patients lacked this awareness after recovery, then this could raise doubts concerning the completeness of their recovery.

Interestingly, as the concept of insight in these discussions became more clearly formed, particularly in Billod, different aspects of its structure were being tentatively raised such as the possibility that awareness itself could vary in extent and according to the particular insanity and the implications this carried for whether a patient had a true insanity. In turn, these issues led to more questions concerning the meaning of the underpinning mental and physiological structures (Delasiauve, 1870). Much debate focused on the emerging need for clarification of terms such as 'intelligence', 'reason', 'judgement' and even 'awareness' as distinctions were being proposed between them without consistency or clear rationale (Société Médico-Psychologique, 1870). Many of the arguments in the discussions at this time, however, related to the confusion engendered by the mixture of approaches taken by the alienists. These included perspectives from the organic or physiological together with the metaphysical and psychological, and heightened by the different languages of each. Fournet (1870), picked up on some of these problems and argued forcibly for the need to distinguish between the organic and the psychological in relation to reason and madness and to keep the approaches distinct without losing their individual legitimacy. It was on the grounds of his *psychological* conception of madness, as a removal of the soul's authority on the self, on personality and consequent failing or absence of free will, that he viewed awareness (and likewise responsibility for criminal acts) as something that could be reduced proportionately to the reduction in reason and free will. And because he conceived free will as being the sum of the constitutive faculties of the soul, then the loss of free will was not absolute but could occur in degrees. On this conception of madness, he distinguished between insanity (*l'insanité*) where some degree of reason and awareness were conserved, equating this with the concept of partial insanity (e.g. *folie raisonnante, folie lucide, Billod's pseudo-aliénés*), and insanity proper (*folie*) where there was no awareness or reason present. The importance of this distinction for him lay, once more, in the issue of legal responsibility for criminal acts which he believed was present and proportionate to the amount of awareness remaining in patients belonging to the former category. Thus, Fournet's notion of awareness was tightly embedded in his psychological conceptualisation of madness. He did not disavow the importance of brain pathology either as a primary source of the manifestations of madness or as a secondary complication of madness. However, the essence of madness itself, he claimed, lay in the disturbance of the activity of self as an autonomous agent, i.e. in the loss of free will. Similar views, again based on explicit distinctions between the brain and 'organic' language and explanations, and the mind (or soul) and 'psychological' language and explanations were shared by others, notably Despine (1875) (see below).

As was the case in the debates held in relation to partial insanities, debates on the concept of insight into madness were thus affected by the lack of clarity in the terms and concepts relating to the structures of the mind and disease that were necessary for such discussions. And, many of the disagreements evident in the debates (Société Médico-Psychologique, 1870) reflected the differences in perspectives and understanding of such structures. One specific problem in examining the concept of awareness or insight in nineteenth century French psychiatry, is the term '*conscience*' itself which refers to two rather different concepts. Prosper Despine (1875) pointed out that this was a source of confusion since psychologists and philosophers tended to use the concepts interchangeably. He suggested that the concepts needed to be distinguished explicitly and proposed that the term '*conscience morale*' should be used to refer to the English equivalent of 'conscience', i.e. knowledge of the right and wrong of things. On the other hand, the term '*conscience personelle*' (or '*conscienciosité*') should be used to refer to the English term 'consciousness'. Despine defined the latter concept as knowledge of one's mental faculties, i.e. knowledge of what is perceived, remembered, reflected, felt, feared, etc. and, like Locke earlier, he did not separate this from such activities themselves. Thus, he stated that *conscience personelle* 'is not a special faculty ... doing and knowing that one is doing, is the same thing' (Despine, 1875, p. 14, my translation).

Like Fournet, Despine defined madness in psychological terms. Similarly, not discounting the contribution of brain pathology to the manifestations of insanity, he nevertheless conceived madness as wider than just brain disease. Indeed patients could be afflicted by '*folie*' and yet be healthy. Thus, madness, he believed, lay in disturbance of the moral (i.e. instinctual/affective) faculties such that the self (*l'esprit*) was no longer in control but under the influence of the ensuing abnormal passions. Intellectual faculties (perception, memory and reflection) might be weakened but would continue to work, albeit under the influence of such passions. The crucial point for him was that it was not the actual abnormal passions, false ideas and irresistible urges that constituted the madness, but the blindness of the self (*l'aveuglement de l'esprit*), and hence unawareness, in relation to these pathological manifestations (Despine, 1875, p. 310). His conceptualisation of insight was necessarily bound up and determined by this same frame. Consequently, there is a fine distinction in the way he conceived insight or awareness in patients. Thus, he argued that, insight in the sense of consciousness ('*conscience personelle*'), because of its intrinsic link to the intellectual faculties themselves (i.e. knowledge of perception, memory, etc. as above), was preserved in madness. As he said: 'man always has *conscience personelle* of acts that he carries out, even when blinded by passion, he always knows what he is doing and can, subsequently recall it' (Despine, 1875, pp. 266–267, my translation). In this, he disagreed with Victor Cousin whom he cited as stating '… frequently the passions, removing our liberty, remove at the same time the consciousness of our actions and ourselves. Thus, to use common parlance, one doesn't know what one does' (Despine, 1875, p. 266, my translation). On the other hand, insight as awareness of madness itself (i.e. of the abnormal passions/impulses, false ideas, etc.) was not possible for Despine. By definition, madness was inherently unaware: 'the one afflicted by madness cannot judge it as madness because it is his own blindness that constitutes it' (Despine, 1875, p. 271, my translation).

Influenced by the debates on awareness into mental illness, there emerged a form of 'partial insanity with awareness' ('*folie avec conscience*' or '*monomanie avec conscience*') as a specific diagnostic category (Ritti, 1879). This was defined by two essential characteristics, namely: (i) awareness on the part of the patient of the disorder in thinking, feeling or behaving that affected him, i.e. recognition of the morbidity of his mental experiences and (ii) irresistibility of such morbid phenomena, i.e. despite the patient's awareness of his morbid state, he was powerless against it. This category, in fact, referred to rather mixed conditions including hypochondria, agoraphobia, a form of obsessional disorder and homicidal urges with awareness. In terms of the clinical descriptions, it reflected some of the already mentioned problems in classification of mental disorders in the middle of the nineteenth century. However, it is an important mark in that it highlights the recognition made at that time that different types of madness could be associated with different extents of awareness into madness. Furthermore, awareness into one's pathological state could itself be used as a classificatory criterion. Indeed, allowing for some anachronistic interpretation, this could be viewed as a point where awareness into mental illness was becoming pivotal in distinguishing between what were later to become the 'psychoses' and the 'neuroses'.

In a classic paper on 'Conscience et Aliénation mentale', Henri Dagonet (1881) focused specifically on the concept of awareness or consciousness (*conscience*) in mental illness. Eschewing existing psychological and anatomical perspectives, he was explicit in his aim to examine awareness or anomalies of awareness from a purely clinical viewpoint. He believed that in order to better understand mental illness and its relationship to brain changes, it was essential to examine mental symptoms themselves. And foremost amongst these, he argued, should be the study of anomalies of consciousness. His concept of awareness was broad and based on the ideas of Littré and Despine. The former had defined consciousness as 'the immediate, constant, intimate *feeling* of the activity of the self, that is within each phenomenon of moral and intellectual life' (Dagonet, 1881, p. 369, my translation and emphasis). Despine, as described above, had defined consciousness as 'the *knowledge* held by the psyche of its operations, its thoughts ...' (Dagonet, 1881, p. 369, my emphasis). Dagonet himself combined these ideas, holding that consciousness was 'the intimate (*intime*) knowledge of ourselves, of the moral and intellectual processes going on within us' (Dagonet, 1881, p. 370, my translation). However, he elaborated on this further and made two important points in his conceptualisation of awareness. Firstly, he gave awareness an active role, saying that not only did it capture the phenomena of our internal life and committed them to memory, but it was 'the *force* which enlightens the mind (*l'esprit*) and *directs* the reason' (Dagonet, 1881, p. 370, my emphases). Secondly, Dagonet included in his conception of awareness, 'the feeling of totality of the person (*le sentiment de la personnalité*), undergoing the same transformations experienced by the latter under the influence of illness' (Dagonet, 1881, p. 370, my translation). Thus, Dagonet was broadening the concept of awareness to include a deeper form of self-knowledge which was not only a recipient of individual experiences but an active determinant of their nature.

Dagonet examined anomalies of awareness from two perspectives, namely, situations where awareness was temporarily lost whilst patients appeared to think, act and feel normally, and situations where awareness or degrees of awareness were preserved in the light of various mental and brain disorders. He observed that in mental disorders, there existed a wide range of anomalies of awareness and illustrated these with examples of patients with absent or retained awareness. These were similar to the case descriptions from the earlier debates, e.g. patients with hallucinations, some showing no awareness of the morbidity of these experiences and others appreciating exactly the phenomena affecting them and searching for explanations. Interestingly, however, Dagonet also focused on the notion of modified awareness in mental illness. This related to his concept of awareness as the feeling of totality of a person and being subject, both passively and actively, to the changes produced by mental disorder. Thus, he remarked, that in a number of mad patients, this feeling of totality of the person is profoundly changed such that awareness can no longer perceive the external world in the same way as before. Where these changes are complete as in some cases of lypemania, hypochondria and various possession states, then the patient becomes another personality and his awareness, his ability to perceive and judge come under the auspices of that new personality. In other words, through its direct connection to the self, Dagonet viewed awareness as being capable of transformation by the same factors producing the madness or changes to the self. Furthermore, because of its active nature, the awareness in this new form 'contributes to the strengthening of the false convictions held by the individual' (Dagonet, 1881, p. 29).

In addition, Dagonet also identified patients who appeared to show different forms of doubling of personality ('Doubling of personality' was a common concept in late nineteenth century psychiatry which was often used to help explain contradictory mental states and behaviours (Berrios, 1996).) accompanied by what he termed 'double awareness' ('*double conscience*'). Such patients might exhibit impulsive and violent behaviours, and be dominated by fears, hallucinations and delusions but, at the same time, have 'intimate knowledge of what is happening to them. They judge correctly ... feel that their will is insufficient to resist against the terrible acts into which they are pushed' (Dagonet, 1881, p. 21, my translation). These patients would ask for help or admission to asylums. Dagonet viewed such double awareness as a state of splitting of the psyche, whereby one state of awareness was experiencing the bizarre phenomena of the ill personality and the other state of awareness was judging it, according to the well personality, in a correct manner. The resultant combination of experiences gave rise to perplexity and confusion. He presented an example of a patient suffering from persecutory delusions, believing that the whole world was concerned with him, that people were repeating what he was saying and thinking, and making obscene gestures at him. At the same time, the patient was analysing and studying his abnormal experiences and making correct judgements. As Dagonet (1881, p. 21) commented, 'he knows that the impressions he is experiencing are false interpretations'. Following Littré, Dagonet conceived different forms of double awareness. In one form, the awareness was concomitant in relation to the two personalities, i.e. both mental states had awareness and memory of each individual state. In another form, the awareness was successive, i.e. each mental state had awareness and memory only of their own individual state but not of the other. In a third form, the awareness was partial, i.e. when a mental state was aware of itself but not of the new mental state but the latter was aware of both.

Dagonet believed that the awareness of illness shown by some patients could be explained on the basis of Luys's hypothesis of pathological asymmetry of the cerebral hemispheres. Thus, he cited, 'the coexistence of lucidity and delusional illness [*délire*] can be rationally explained by the integrity of one cerebral hemisphere and pathological hypertrophy of the other' (Dagonet, 1881, p. 20, my translation). He claimed further support for this hypothesis on the grounds of an autopsy result on one of his mentally ill patients who had manifested clinically two distinct states of awareness. At postmortem, there was apparently considerable difference between the two hemispheres which suggested to Dagonet that each corresponded to the different mental states.

Finally, Dagonet also briefly considered the medico-legal implications of his observations. He stressed, as had the alienists in the debates some years earlier, that patients could retain self-awareness but nevertheless be 'forced' into unreasonable acts through the influence of delusional ideas. Specifically, he dissociated the notion of awareness of illness from that of legal responsibility:

awareness should not be considered [for the physician] as a thermometer measuring degree of responsibility ... more important are the pathological phenomena characterising the mental illness. The severity of these should be determined in order to ascertain the degree of resistance necessary for the patient to overcome dominating impulses.

Dagonet (1881, p. 32, my translation)

Seven years later, in a book examining the nature of reason in insanity and implications for legal responsibility, Victor Parant (1888) analysed the concept of awareness of self in mental illness (*conscience de soi*) in more depth. Like Morel and Falret, he emphasised that awareness should not be confused with reason and defined the former as a 'state [in mental illness] in which the patient can take account of his impressions, his actions, his internal experiences and their resultant effects'. In other words, awareness, 'implies not just knowledge of the mental state, but also the capacity, in varying degrees, to appreciate and judge this' (Parant, 1888, p. 174, my translation). Here, therefore, seems to be one of the earliest times when the concept of insight appears to have a more distinct form and is explicitly referring to two component but distinct aspects, namely, awareness or consciousness of mental experiences (as in Despine's sense) and some form of judgement of these. In contrast to Despine, Parant disagreed with Spurzheim's view, translated by Baillarger as 'madness is a misfortune which is unaware of itself' (Parant, 1888, p. 175) and concurred with Dagonet that patients could show a range of awareness and judgements with respect to the mental illness affecting them. Pointing out also that this varied according to the stage of the illness, i.e. whether early on in the illness, during the acute episode, or after recovery, Parant (1888, pp. 177–179, 188–218) classified mentally ill patients, during an episode of illness, into five groups on the basis of different types of awareness:

1 Those who were aware of their acts and who could judge if these were right or wrong, but who were unaware of their morbid state.

2 Those who were aware that they were in an abnormal state but who did not understand or would not admit that this state was insanity, e.g. patients recognising the abnormality of their experiences but interpreting them delusionally.

3 Those who were aware that their mental states, acts and ideas were the result of insanity but who, nevertheless, behaved as if they did not realise this, i.e. not fully accepting that they had a mental illness, e.g. patients with hallucinations and persecutory delusions, convinced by the reality of their delusional illness and yet, at the same time, believing that they were ill.

4 Those who were aware of their morbid states and understood that these were due to insanity but who were incapable of reacting or activating their will and hence were powerless to do anything about it.

5 Those who were aware of their morbid states and understood that these were due to insanity but who committed or were pushed into doing serious, dangerous acts.

The concept of awareness or insight that Parant held thus incorporated both awareness of mental phenomena and behaviours together with the judgement of these as being morbid or the result of mental illness. He maintained that whatever category of awareness the patients fell into, the presence of awareness implied a persistence of the faculty of judgement. Interestingly, his classification of awareness was based on both the subjective accounts given by patients as well as their observable behaviours, noting the range of discrepancies between the two, and emphasising the dissociation between patients' judgements and their manifest behaviours, particularly in relation to categories 3–5. Commenting on how some patients became extremely distressed the more accurate their understanding of reality was, he remarked that patients 'assist like helpless spectators of the collapse of what is most precious in themselves, that is their moral freedom as well as their intellectual faculties' (Parant, 1888, p. 223). Like Dagonet, he thus believed that preservation of awareness did not entail the preservation of free will and hence did not entail legal responsibility for criminal acts.

1.3.2 British views

In nineteenth century Britain, the concept of awareness or insight in mental illness was likewise a subject of debate. Interest, however, seemed to focus predominantly on the narrower notion of awareness or consciousness of mental operations (Mercier, 1892) (akin to Despine's 'conscience personelle'). In this context, discussions were concerned with examining the nature of conscious and unconscious mental processes from physiological and philosophical perspectives (Davies, 1873; Ireland, 1875). The wider concept of awareness of or insight into mental illness itself and the effects of this on mental faculties did not appear to figure as significantly in debates as it did in French psychiatry at that time. Instead, occasional reference to the concept can be found in the clinical observations of alienists in their descriptions of various forms of insanities (Bucknill & Tuke, 1858). Prichard (1835), for example, concurring with Georget whom he cited, noted that insane patients were fully convinced of their perfect sanity, 'yet, as the same author observes [Georget], there are some patients who are well aware of the disorder of their thoughts or of their affections, and who are deeply affected at not having sufficient strength of will to repress it' (Prichard, 1835, p. 121).

Some years later, Maudsley (1895) expressed considerable scepticism towards the importance and role placed on consciousness in relation to mental function. He stated:

it has been very difficult to persuade speculative psychologists who elaborate webs of philosophy out of their own consciousness that consciousness has nothing to do with the actual work of mental function; that it is the adjunct not the energy at work; not the agent in the process, but the light which lightens a small part of it ... we may put consciousness aside then when we are considering the nature of the mechanism and the manner of its work ...

Maudsley (1895, p. 8)

He reiterated this several years later: 'consciousness is the dependent phenomenon or so-called epiphenomena ...' (Maudsley, 1916, p. 7), a view stated earlier also by Mercier (1892).

Maudsley's conception of insanity precluded the possibility of insight or proper judgement concerning the nature of the mental derangement on the part of the patient. The insane patient, whose mental functions were deranged, became alienated from himself, and, 'he is now so self-regarding a self as to be incapable of right regard to the notself ...' (Maudsley, 1895, p. 1). Whilst clinically the line between sanity and insanity could not be well demarcated (Maudsley, 1885), in functional terms, Maudsley drew a strict line between the sane and insane aspects of the mind, with no real communication or exchange between them. According to him, the sane man was incapable of judging precisely the behaviours and experiences of an insane man (which carried implications for determining legal responsibility for criminal acts). In the same way, patients with partial insanity could not judge with their sane mental functions the phenomena produced by their insane mental functions. As he said: '... each self thinks its own *thinks* or *things* – that is, thinks its own world; the true self, or what remains of it, perceives the world as it looks to the sane persons, and the morbid self or double perceives it as a strange and hostile world' (Maudsley, 1895, p. 304). This conception of insanity very much echoes the views at that time on double consciousness in the narrow sense. This was the view that distinct mental states in the one individual, e.g. drunk versus sober, sleeping versus awake, insane versus sane, could, independently, be aware of, judge and remember such mental states but would have no recollection of, or communication with, the different states (Azam, 1892). Importantly, however, like Despine (1875) and antedating Lewis (1934) (see below), Maudsley did not believe it was possible for an insane mind to make a rational judgement concerning its derangement.

The question of the role and state of consciousness in insanity continued troubling writers well into the twentieth century. For example, Claye Shaw (1909), echoing many of Maudsley's views on consciousness, nevertheless, placed greater importance on the notion in relation to mental illness, particularly again with respect to determining legal responsibility. He suggested that the poor recall of events shown by patients with acute mental illness was due to altered consciousness or awareness at the time. Such changes in consciousness often may be subtle and difficult to discern, because, he argued, 'there are in reality as many forms of consciousness as there are different mental states' (Shaw, 1909, p. 408). However, linking consciousness to emotional tone he went on to postulate that one way of recognising altered consciousness in mental illness was by the dissonance or incongruence between patients' thoughts and their apparent emotional state: 'there is evidence that both in dream states and in insanity the emotional side of the idea may be wanting, and this must have great effect on both memory and consciousness … I have over and over again noticed that people with delusions of a very depressed type do not show the emotional tone which should co-exist with the delusions' (Shaw, 1909, pp. 406–407). Once again, the implication behind Shaw's views is that the disordered or deranged mind, unable to attend to either internal or external events, and hence unable to subsequently recall them, is unlikely to be capable of forming 'correct' or sane judgements concerning the nature of morbid pathology.

The notion of insight in its broader sense as awareness of mental illness rather than consciousness of mental processes was not, however, debated as widely and explicitly as in nineteenth century French psychiatry until Aubrey Lewis (1934) offered his exploration of the concept. Pointing to the confusion due to the different meanings given to 'insight' within and outwith psychiatry (including Gestalt and psychoanalytic psychology), he suggested his own definition of insight as 'a correct attitude to a morbid change in oneself'. He then proceeded to examine in turn the meaning of the individual terms within this definition and highlighted some of the problems inherent to the definition of underlying concepts such as 'normality', 'mental illness' and 'attitude'. Consequently, he pointed out, this made the meaning or understanding of insight itself complicated. Like some of the earlier alienists, notably Parant and Jaspers, in his conceptualisation of insight, Lewis distinguished between awareness of change and judgement of change, both being necessary components of insight. Thus, in order to have an 'attitude' to the change in oneself, the patient must first become aware of the change, before secondarily, forming a judgement of this. He considered the notion of awareness in more detail and went on to suggest that awareness itself could be further subdivided into: firstly, awareness based on primary or immediate perceptions, e.g. becoming aware of feeling different and unpleasant in depersonalisation, that is, the direct feeling that there is a change and secondly, awareness based on secondary data, e.g. becoming aware of a change in capacity to function, making mistakes, that is, the feeling that there must be a change. In other words, without elaborating on this explicitly, Lewis conceptualised insight as a complex of qualitatively different types of judgements, or rather, judgements based on different types of 'information'. The final judgement then referred to the patient's attribution of the experienced changes in terms of whether the patient believed they represented illness or some other explanations such as satanic possession, etc.

Like Maudsley, though on slightly different grounds, Lewis believed that it was not possible for patients with mental illness to attain complete insight, insofar as the definition of insight related to the attitude of a non-affected individual. He stated that:

In any mental disorder, whether mild or severe, continued or brief, alien or comprehensible, it is with his whole disordered mind that the patient contemplates his state or his individual symptoms and in this disorder there are disturbances which are different from the healthy function either in degree, combination or kind ... always there will be a disturbance which makes it impossible for the patient to look at his data and judge them as we, the dispassionate, presumably healthy outsiders do. His judgements and attitude can therefore never be the same as ours because his data are different, and his machine for judging is different in some respects.

Lewis (1934, p. 343)

Lewis based his argument on his conceptualisation of insight which by his definition, in terms of 'correct', included the comparison of view with a non-affected individual. Thus, there were two reasons why a mentally ill patient could not have full insight. Firstly, the mental illness itself caused disturbances in the subjective self which could not possibly be appreciated by an outsider (and therefore a concordance could not be achieved). Secondly, the tools with which the ill patient could make judgements ('disordered mind') were themselves affected by the mental illness and therefore could not make a just assessment. Interestingly, Lewis made it explicit, including in his explanation of 'correct attitude', that the clinical concept of insight related importantly to the judgement made by an unaffected observer and hence represented, to some extent, an interaction between the latter and the patient. The conceptualisation of insight in these terms, extending to a complex of judgements between individuals, was thus becoming yet more intricate.

1.3.3 German views

Early and middle nineteenth century German psychiatric writing likewise shows references to insight into madness in the form of clinical observations made by alienists (see review by Pick (1882)) and, as elsewhere at the time, the concept itself was not yet clearly formed. In the context of medico-legal perspectives, Hoffbauer's (1808/1827) influential book refers to mad patients being able to judge their behaviours without being able to suppress their passions or to resist the violent acts into which they are forced. Debates, however, examining specifically the concept of insight into madness were not prominent. This was pointed out by Arnold Pick who himself devoted a lengthy article to the subject in 1882. He focused predominantly on a historical account describing and quoting observations made by earlier alienists (French, German and English) on the presence of awareness or some degree of awareness in patients with different mental disorders and also included his own clinical observations. He did not provide a historical analysis of the conceptualisation of awareness or insight into mental illness but did make some interesting and important clinical and conceptual points.

In terms of the clinical, Pick emphasised that in most mental disorders (including mania, melancholia, obsessive compulsive disorders, psychoses, dementia, alcohol abuse, etc.) patients could show some awareness of their illness though this varied in extent and type according to the mental disorder affecting them. In addition, he noticed that in general, patients whose mental illnesses developed gradually over time seemed to show more awareness of their illness than those whose illnesses developed acutely. In terms of the conceptual, Pick explicitly defined his understanding of the notion of 'awareness of illness' which became influential in the conceptualisation of insight in later German psychiatry. Interestingly, he conceived awareness of illness ('*Krankheitsbewußtsein*') as the broad, general concept which encompassed all the phenomena relating to the feelings or recognition experienced by patients concerning the morbidity of their psychic events. He further subdivided this broad concept into two distinct components, namely, awareness of feeling ill ('*Krankheitsgefühl*') and insight into illness ('*Krankheitseinsicht*'). The former he viewed as an alteration in the *feeling* or sense of well-being. As such, he viewed this as a disturbance of the '*Gemeingefühl*'. This term referred to the old distinction made between skin senses, i.e. touch, temperature, pressure, etc. and the senses left after these were separated off [common feeling or Gemeingefühl] and hence included pain, well-being, pleasure, fatigue, etc. (Berrios, 1996). The latter, i.e. insight into illness, Pick defined as the product of reason or reflection. Thus, patients with some awareness of illness ('*Krankheitsbewußtsein*') could have either awareness of feeling ill, or insight into illness or they could have both. Pick further observed that the relationship between feeling of illness and insight into illness was not straightforward. Whilst many patients with awareness of feeling ill did progress to developing insight into their illness, other patients, notably those with hypochondriacal conditions, had marked feelings of being ill and yet had no insight into their illness (Pick, 1882).

Whilst agreeing with Pick's distinction between awareness of feeling ill and insight into illness, Arndt (1905) pointed out that awareness of feeling ill and the reflective insight into illness were, in fact, interdependent since the 'feeling' had to depend on some knowledge of bodily change. Likewise, the 'knowledge' of change had to depend on some feeling of change. He thus suggested that the distinction between 'awareness of feeling ill' and 'insight into illness' did not lie in the difference between 'feeling' in the former and 'reflection' in the latter but was based on the difference in clarity with which the insight is experienced. Patients whose awareness of illness was based on the feeling of being ill experienced insight into their illness with much greater clarity and self-involvement. On the other hand, patients whose awareness of illness was based on rational or reflective insight into their illness experienced this with less clarity and often clouded by suspicion. In other words, Arndt emphasised the importance of the *experiential* aspect of insight, which, interestingly, shares similarities with later psychoanalytic perspectives (Chapter 2). Arndt went on to analyse what he viewed as the necessary elements in the development of insight of illness, namely, the feeling of illness, reasonable judgement and past experience. Each of these elements could be disturbed, in different ways, in patients with mental illness. For example, he pointed out that in mental disorders the feeling of illness might not be present in the conventional sense. Patients could feel different and sometimes this feeling resonated with psychological states (e.g. guilt feelings and home sickness) but the feeling did not have to relate to 'illness' in the normal sense. Consequently, experienced changes could be attributed to other non-illness factors (e.g. external influences) and hence, almost by definition, patients with mental illness would lack this element constituting insight into their illness. Arndt (1905) also speculated on the underlying processes that might be disturbed in patients with mental illness who showed impaired insight. In this vein, he suggested a role for attention, memory, capacity for observation, judgement, conceptual thinking and education.

Following the distinction made and terminology used by Pick concerning awareness into illness ('*Krankheitsbewußtsein*'), Aschaffenburg (1915), concentrated from a purely clinical perspective, on examining each suggested component, namely, the feeling of illness ('*Krankheitsgefühl*') (defined as vague fears and uncertainties) and insight into illness ('*Krankheitseinsicht*') (defined as understanding the nature and severity of the illness) and the relationship between them. On the basis of clinical observations, he pointed out, as had Pick and Arndt earlier, that there was not a direct progression from awareness of feeling ill to insight into being ill and indeed there was often a discrepancy or mismatch between patients' subjective feeling of illness and their insight into illness. Thus, patients could have no feeling of illness and yet have good insight into the fact that they were ill, as in some cases of syphilis. Likewise, patients could have intense feelings of being ill and yet have little insight into their illness, e.g. patients with various neuroses or hypochondriacal illnesses. He distinguished between the awareness of feeling ill in patients with physical and with mental illnesses. In the former, this developed into awareness of illness when patients clarified and formulated such feelings into fears of the unknown, fears of pain, operations, etc. In the latter, i.e. awareness of feeling ill in patients with mental illness, this was often the first sign of their illness itself, such as depressive symptoms. In contrast to the case in physical illness, as such feelings were 'clarified' and judged, then the experience of feeling of illness itself tended to reduce as this was superseded by the pathological 'rationalisation' of the illness process itself (Aschaffenburg, 1915, pp. 367–369).

By extending his observations of these components of insight into patients with different mental disorders, he was able to suggest different possible mechanisms that could affect patients' judgements of their illness. Like Jaspers (see below), he emphasised the difficulties in clinically determining patients' insight and amongst reasons for this, included his observation that insight as a judgement evolved over time and that different morbid symptoms and features of the illness required different amounts of time to judge. In addition, he was clear about discrepancies between insight as expressed by patients and their behaviours which were counter to their utterances, for example, compulsions in a patient who had insight into his illness (Aschaffenburg, 1915, pp. 369–371).

The concept of insight in terms of its nature, its diagnostic and predictive significance, did not seem to interest Kraepelin (or Bleuler) a great deal. Kraepelin referred to the notion under 'judgement': 'what always surprises the observer anew is the quiet complacency with which the most nonsensical ideas can be uttered by them and the most incomprehensive actions carried out' (Kraepelin, 1913/1919, p. 25). He observed that some patients showed awareness of the morbidity of their state early in the disease, but that this left them as the disease progressed: 'the patients often have a distinct feeling of the profound change which has taken place in them. They complain that they are "dark in the head", not free, often in confusion, no longer clear, and that they have "cloud thoughts" … understanding of the disease disappears fairly rapidly as the malady progresses' (Kraepelin, 1913/1919, pp. 25–26). Beyond subsequently commenting that 'a certain insight into their diseased state is frequently present' in patients with the catatonic form of dementia praecox (Kraepelin, 1913/1919, p. 150), and that, in contrast to patients with dementia praecox, patients with manic-depressive psychosis had 'more tendency to, and ability for, the *observation of self*, to painful dissection of their psychic state' (Kraepelin, 1913/1919, p. 264), Kraepelin did not further elaborate on the concept.

It was Karl Jaspers who focused specifically on the concept of insight into mental illness and indeed the concept appeared to develop more in depth and detail with successive editions of his 'General Psychopathology' (1913 (1st edition) to 1959 (7th edition)). From a combination of both clinical and psychological/philosophical perspectives, he explored the concept of insight in several different ways, breaking this up in terms of awareness of mental processes (consciousness in the narrow sense), awareness of the sense and activities of the self and attitudes towards mental illness. His conception of insight in these component forms emphasised a close and bi-directional relationship between the personality judging the mental phenomena affecting him and the manifestation of the psychopathology itself. In other words, and crucially, it was not only that patients became aware and judged the mental symptoms and illness that affected them, but the expression of the mental symptoms themselves was affected by the awareness and judgements made by the patients. He thus believed that it was essential to study patients' understanding or insight into what was happening to them: 'Patients' self-observation, their attentiveness to their abnormal experience and the processing of their observations in the form of a psychological judgement that can communicate to us their inner life, is one of the most important sources of knowledge in regard to morbid psychic life' (Jaspers, 1948, p. 350, my translation). On the basis of his clinical observations, Jaspers described various stages in the manifestation of patients' awareness. He observed that, in the early stages of their psychotic illness, patients became bewildered, this being an understandable reaction to the new experiences they were undergoing. Awareness here, he contended, was related to the multitude of different sensations they were experiencing and as such was not really a judgement as a whole (akin to the awareness of immediate data in Lewis above). As the illness progressed, patients tried to make sense of their experiences, for example, by elaborating delusional systems. Thereafter, Jaspers described how, when the illness produced changes in personality, a patient's attitude to the illness became less understandable to others as he/she could appear indifferent or passive to the most frightening delusions.

Jaspers distinguished between these stages of changes which referred to awareness of the content of patients' experiences and insight itself which referred to judgements made by the patient concerning their illness and hence involved the relationship between such awareness and the self. Influenced by Pick, though conceptualising the structure of insight slightly differently, he made a distinction, in the latter judgements, between awareness of illness ('Krankheitsbewußtsein') and insight proper ('Krankheitseinsicht'). The former referred to the experience of feeling ill and changed but without this awareness reaching all symptoms or the illness as a whole. The latter, however, included an objectively correct assessment of the nature and severity of the illness affecting the individual both as a whole and of each individual symptom (Jaspers, 1948, pp. 349–350). Jaspers did qualify this requirement of objectively correct judgement as one that would be made by an average, healthy individual from the same cultural background as the patient. In fact, Jaspers emphasised that such judgements depended on the intelligence, background and culture of the individual. Indeed, because these judgements are inherently a part of the personality make-up, then in the case of patients with intelligence below a certain level, e.g. idiocy, it would be more appropriate to consider loss of personality rather than loss of awareness as the feature in their lack of knowledge of themselves.

Jaspers also observed that while transient insight may occur during acute psychoses, there was no lasting or complete insight. He insisted that where insight persisted, the patient was more likely to be suffering from a personality disorder (*Psychopathie*) than a psychosis. In patients who recovered from the psychotic state, Jaspers made a distinction between psychoses such as mania and alcoholic hallucinosis where the patients were able to look back on their experiences with 'complete' insight, and a psychosis such as schizophrenia where they did not show full insight. He reported the latter patients as being unable to talk freely about the contents of their experiences, becoming overtly affected when pressed to do so, and occasionally maintaining some features of their illnesses. He further described patients with chronic psychotic states who, from their verbal contents, often appeared to have full insight, yet in fact such verbal contents would turn out to be learnt phrases and meaningless to the patients themselves.

In terms of assessing patients' insight, Jaspers was clear that there were limits to the extent to which outsiders could hope to understand patients' attitudes to their illness. He formulated this by stating that it was easier to assess patients' objective knowledge ('*objektives Wissen*'), that is, their ability to understand and apply medical knowledge to themselves, than their comprehending appropriation ('*verstehendes Aneignen*') of it. The latter understanding, Jaspers claimed, was intrinsically linked with the patients' selves, and hence could not be divorced from the knowledge of self-existence itself.

In a similar vein to Jaspers, in terms of conceiving insight as a process of awareness of change in the self and the environment, albeit not using the term explicitly, Conrad (1958) depicted these experiential changes in patients in his long-term observations around the development and progression of the psychotic state. He named the early stage of the schizophrenic illness the 'trema'. During this stage, he noted that patients found it difficult to express their feelings and experiences; some would talk about fear, tension, anxiety and anticipation, while others would describe feelings of guilt and helplessness. Conrad believed that the common theme was a feeling of oppression, an awareness that something was not right, and a sense of restriction of one's freedom. During the next stage of illness, the 'apophany', patients attributed meaning to feelings and experiences; for example, when in the state of 'anastrophe', patients believed themselves to be the centre of the world.

Conrad described further stages during which destructive processes were followed by partial resolution as residual schizophrenic effects persisted, and postulated that schizophrenia was an illness affecting the higher mental functions which differentiate humans from animals. Thus, it affected the whole self-concept and, in particular, the ability of the individual to effect the normal transition from looking at oneself from *within* to looking at oneself from the *outside*, by the eyes of the world.

1.4 Conclusion

The concept of insight into mental illness emerged around the middle of the nineteenth century as an independent phenomenon that could be explored in patients. This can be understood in the contexts of: (i) general increased interest in individuality and self-reflection at this time, together with the development of concepts such as introspection, apperception and 'verstehen' legitimising subjectivity as an area of enquiry and (ii) changing views on the nature of mental illness and the conceptualisation of partial insanities, opening up a space in which it became possible to conceive insight into madness. The partial insanity debates were, in turn, influenced by the empirical observations of alienists, the medico-legal challenges of the courts and the development of faculty psychology including phrenology.

In the early part of the nineteenth century, the concept of insight into mental illness was not yet clearly formed and patients were simply observed as having or not having awareness of their illness. Awareness at this point seemed to refer variously to feelings or judgements. By the middle of the nineteenth century debates specifically addressed at the concept of insight were taking place, particularly in France. In the context of these discussions, where insight was explored in relation to mental disorders, to the notion of self, to mental faculties and to the issue of legal responsibility for criminal acts, the concept of insight began to develop a structure as attempts were made to define and distinguish between independent mental processes (Falret, 1866; Billod, 1870; Morel, 1870). Clinically, insight was also becoming more prominent as a feature to be examined in different clinical groups and mental disorders (Billod, 1870; Morel, 1870), as a criterion distinguishing between clinical disorders (Ritti, 1879) and as a prognostic variable (Billod, 1870).

Towards the end of the nineteenth century, insight into mental illness seemed to refer to two main concepts. Firstly, there was the narrower concept of awareness or consciousness of mental operations (Despine, 1875; Maudsley, 1895). Alienists holding this concept generally believed that whilst patients could have awareness of particular mental processes, this did not extend to an awareness of such processes being morbid. Secondly, there was the wider concept of insight which included both an awareness of mental phenomena together with some awareness of the self as an individual but, in addition, a judgement made by patients concerning the illness affecting them (Dagonet, 1881; Billod, 1882; Pick, 1882; Parant, 1888). Alienists conceiving insight in this broad way tended to believe that patients could have insight and even different degrees of insight into their illness. Part of the problem in attempting to define the emerging structure of insight, however, is the difficulty involved in trying to clarify the nature of the constituent components. Whilst some alienists could conceive clear distinctions between awareness, feeling and judgement, for others those demarcations were blurred or did not exist. In turn, such disparities seemed to be based on different understanding of the nature of, and relationship between, mental processes themselves and their connection or otherwise to brain processes. Nevertheless, a rough structure can begin to be identified with components based on distinctions between different types of awareness (Dagonet, 1881), between different types of judgements (Billod, 1882), between feelings and reason (Pick, 1882) and between subjective utterances and observed behaviours (Pick, 1882; Parant, 1888).

After the turn of the century, the broader conceptualisation of insight into mental illness seemed to hold. However, this became more complicated in terms of determining individual components, e.g. contribution of intelligence, culture, past experience, capacity for observation, memory, etc. (Arndt, 1905; Jaspers, 1913) as well as defining the boundaries of such a structure, e.g. extent of knowledge demanded, level of concordance needed with the unaffected individual (Lewis, 1934), both from a theoretical and the clinical perspective. In addition, qualitative differences in insight between patients with different types of mental disorders were beginning to be identified (Arndt, 1905; Aschaffenburg, 1915). This, together with the unresolved issues concerning the nature of the components of insight, further compounded the complexity of the insight structure. Nonetheless, insight conceived as an awareness of change together with some judgement made of this change has remained the core of the theoretical concept ever since.

2

The psychological perspective: Gestalt, cognitive and psychoanalytic

A significant influence on both the conceptualisation of insight in psychiatry as well as on its empirical assessment, particularly within the neurosciences (e.g. in specific neurological deficits, neuropsychological impairments, dementias, etc.), has come from psychology. Such influence has, in the main, arisen predominantly from two psychological schools of thought, namely, Gestalt psychology (and Gestalt-influenced cognitive psychology) and the psychoanalytic psychologies. Whilst it is not the place here to explore the history of psychology as a discipline, it may be useful to very briefly contextualise the origin of the above schools of thinking. Neuropsychological approaches to the conceptualisations of awareness will be dealt with in Chapters 4 and 5.

The previous chapter highlighted the contribution made to the conceptualisation of insight as a clinical phenomenon by, amongst other things, the emergence of or focus on various psychological concepts during the eighteenth and nineteenth centuries. Amongst these, the notions of *Verstehen, introspection, self-reflection, apperception,* etc. were particularly important and related in different ways to attempts at describing and understanding the subjectivity of inner experiences. Towards the end of the nineteenth century, psychology was concerned with the scientific study of the contents or 'facts' of consciousness. These facts of consciousness ranged from the most basic or 'atomic' units of analysis, such as sensation or attention to more complex units such as perceptions, apperceptions or memory, which were understood as being formed from the combination of the atomic units through the laws of associationism. All these facts of consciousness were accessible to the individual and scientist by means of introspection. Such facts of consciousness were viewed as reflecting in a direct way both the external world and the brain. In other words, there was envisaged a structural correspondence or relationship between the elements making up the external world and the elements forming the contents of consciousness. This structural relationship, furthermore, could be defined and studied by means of psychophysical laws. Wilhelm Wundt (1832–1920) was the major figure in the development of this scientific or physiological psychology and, together with the Würzburg School, was important in formulating such psychophysical laws (Wundt, 1886/1880).

At the turn of the century, there arose, independently, various challenges to this form of scientific psychology. Whilst all seemed to argue against the validity of thus analysing the contents of consciousness, the nature of their objections was very different. *Behaviourism* rejected completely the notion that consciousness could be a valid object of inquiry and turned instead to the study of relationships between events that could be 'objectively' observed and measured. Introspection was conceived as too subjective and hence 'inaccurate' and, consequently, consciousness was placed in a metaphorical black box whilst psychological studies focused on correlations between its inputs (experimental stimuli) and outputs (behavioural or physiological responses). *Gestalt* psychology, on the other hand, challenged the way in which the 'facts' of consciousness were analysed. Specifically, the Gestalt psychologists argued against the mechanistic structural correspondence that was conceived between the external world, the contents of consciousness and the brain itself. Instead, they put forward a functional correspondence that depended on the mind responding not just to the aggregated constituents of objects but also to the functional relations between such constituents in the formation of the object as a whole. In other words, the whole was viewed as different from the sum of its parts. Brain processes reflected this capacity to integrate functional interrelationships in order to produce the experience of the whole in the mind of the individual. From a different perspective again was the objection held by *psychoanalytic* psychologists. They claimed that the validity of using the contents of consciousness as the object of inquiry was compromised because such contents were inherently unstable and distorted by unconscious mental processes. It thus made more sense, the psychoanalysts argued, to focus instead, by means of interpretation and other strategies, on such unconscious mental processes as the objects of psychological inquiry.

For the purposes here, it is with the latter two schools of psychological thought that insight is explored. The chapter thus first looks at the notion of insight as developed by the Gestalt psychologists and by the Gestalt influenced but contemporary cognitive psychologists. Then, the notion of insight as conceived within the psychoanalytical framework is examined together with its perceived role in psychotherapeutic processes. The aim in briefly exploring these psychological perspectives on insight is two-fold. Firstly, as already mentioned, both schools of thought make an important contribution to the conceptualisation and assessment of insight in clinical psychiatry and neuropsychiatry. Secondly, there are also significant differences between the ways in which insight is conceptualised from these perspectives and from within psychiatry in general. Such differences are important to highlight in order to help clarify some of the confusion that is present around the terms and meanings relating to insight in empirical studies. The nature of these and other differences, evident in the conceptualisation of insight, together with the implications these carry for understanding results of empirical work and for determining a structure for insight will be discussed in the second part of this book.

2.1 The concept of insight in Gestalt psychology and cognitive psychology

One of the main principles underlying Gestalt theory was that the whole was greater than (and different from) the sum of its parts. This idea appeared to be originally articulated by Ehrenfels (1890), a member of the Würzburg School. Using the example of a melody (the whole) consisting of separate tones (individual elements), he argued that even when the tones were played in a different key, the melody could still be recognised as a particular melody but that when the same tones were played in a different sequence the melody was no longer recognisable. Thus, it was not just the sum of the individual elements (tones) that was important in the perception of the whole (melody) but the relations of such elements to each other (i.e. their organisation) that was important in the perception of the whole melody. He coined the term 'Gestaltsqualitäten' (qualities of the Gestalt (Gestalt is variously translated as 'form', 'shape' or 'configuration' and simply refers to a particular whole)) to specify that wholes had such qualities. These were not perceived simply in terms of the sum of their elements but it was the way in which the elements were organised, that gave the qualitative aspect to the whole and which helped to determine a particular experience or perception of the whole. This notion was taken up and developed by Max Wertheimer, the Principal Founder of Gestalt Psychology, and by Wolfgang Köhler and Kurt Koffka, his younger colleagues. Much of the early work in Gestalt psychology was focused on the area of perception but subsequently the Gestalt principles were extended to other areas of psychology, particularly to learning, problem-solving and developmental psychology.

Within Gestalt theory, the concept of insight has carried a very specific meaning which contrasts, both in terms of content and specificity, to the way in which insight has been conceptualised in general psychiatry (Chapter 3) and in neurological states (Chapters 4 and 5). Its essence lies in the grasp or understanding an individual (or animal) obtains of a specific situation in a particular way. Thus, it is not just understanding of a situation or problem but it is a 'genuine' or 'productive' understanding that is based on appreciation of the functional inner relatedness of the parts of the structure of a situation (Wertheimer, 1945/1961). Köhler applied this concept to the study of intelligent behaviour in chimpanzees. He asked the question whether chimpanzees were capable of behaving with insight, i.e. whether they could find solutions to certain problems that were based on insight rather than on chance or trial-and-error learning. In order to determine this, he devised various tasks for the apes whose solutions were not straightforward or direct but depended on the ape taking account of the task as a whole in terms of available components and their relationships with each other. For example, one such task involved placing fruit within sight but just out of reach of the chimpanzee. There was a small stick in the cage with the animal (at this stage the apes were familiar with using sticks to help them reach fruit) but this was not long enough to reach the fruit. Outside the cage there was placed a longer stick which was out of reach of the animal but could be pulled within reach by means of the smaller stick. In turn the longer stick could then be used to reach the fruit (Köhler, 1924/1957). These sorts of tasks thus, argued Köhler, contained components which, if considered individually, could be seen as meaningless or irrelevant, or even contradictory to the structure of the solution as a whole. The criterion of insight, he went on to specify, was 'the appearance of a complete solution with reference to the whole layout of the field' (Köhler, 1924/1957, p. 164). It was only by consideration of the structure of the situation that a solution could be viewed as insightful. He distinguished between animal behaviours that led to solutions by chance and behaviours that resulted in solutions by insight. In the former, the chimpanzee's actions would be haphazard and consist of a number of single separate fractions which after some time might lead to the solution. By contrast, tasks that were solved by insight were characterised by behaviours which showed a 'smooth, continuous course, sharply divided by an abrupt break from the preceding (non-insightful) behaviour … this process as a whole corresponds to the structure of the situation, to the relation of its parts to one another' (Köhler, 1924/1957, pp. 163–164). In psychological terms, Köhler interpreted such behaviours as indicating 'the sudden occurrence of perfectly clear and definite solutions' (Köhler, 1924/1957, p. 207), thereby, reflecting the presence of insight in the animal.

In Gestalt terms, the notion of insight was thus conceived as a reorganisation of a particular situation through an understanding of the functional relationships between relevant component parts. (For example, sticks could be perceived as immaterial or as playthings or as specific tools according to the demands of a particular situation.) Furthermore, again in line with some of the early Gestalt work, Köhler understood this reorganisation to involve a *perceptual* process. Hence:

insight of the chimpanzee shows itself to be principally determined by his optical apprehension of the situation; at times he even starts solving problems from a too visual point of view, and in many cases in which the chimpanzee *stops* acting with insight, it may have been simply that the structure of the situation was too much for his visual grasp.

Köhler (1924/1957, p. 228 original emphasis)

Koffka (1935/1963) maintained that Köhler was offering insight simply as a description rather than an explanation in itself. However, Köhler did attempt to provide some explanation based on a modification of associationism. Thus, rather than relations between things being perceived by means of a mechanical association (i.e. links understood when there was frequent following of each other or occurring together), they could be perceived by means of a functional association, i.e. 'based on the properties of these things themselves' (Köhler, 1924/1957, p. 189).

There have since been numerous criticisms directed at Köhler's interpretation of the animals' behaviours as 'insight' (see Koffka, 1925/1980 for a comprehensive review) and indeed many of the issues raised have been echoed in subsequent debates in relation to more sophisticated cognitive experiments (see below). Nevertheless, this definition of insight, as a form of intelligent behaviour or thought characterised by a sudden, rapid, smooth and directed process through which a particular objective is attained, has remained at the core of the Gestalt and cognitive psychological conceptualisations of insight.

In an important work, published posthumously, Wertheimer (1945/1961) applied similar Gestalt principles to the study of learning and problem-solving in human beings. He attempted to analyse the processes that took place during insightful or 'productive' thinking. Distinguishing between understanding that was based on such productive thinking and understanding based on blind repetition or learning by rote, he showed in a number of experiments that only the former could result in subjects applying their knowledge to a variety of different, albeit related, problems. Indeed, he criticised the teaching of children by drill which, he argued, was counterproductive to thinking and induced habits of sheer mechanised action rather than leading to a true grasp of problems. Like Köhler, he emphasised the need for the subject to grasp the structure of the whole problem in terms of the inner relatedness of its parts. In this sense, he described the process of attaining insight as a top-down rather than bottom-up procedure. Attempting to break down such operations, Wertheimer focused repeatedly on the demands made by the structure of the task/problem. He suggested a process which was:

> not just a sum of several steps, not an aggregate of several operations, but the growth of one line of thinking out of the gaps in the situation, out of the structural troubles ... it is not a process that moves from pieces to an aggregate, from below to above, but from above to below, from the nature of the structural trouble to the concrete steps.
>
> Wertheimer (1945/1961, pp. 49–50)

Like Köhler, Wertheimer suggested that the processes underlying productive or insightful thinking could be considered in terms of modified associationistic laws which relied on functional rather than mechanical relationships. He suggested that such processes involved operations of dividing the whole into sub-wholes (though continuing to perceive how the sub-wholes fit together) and described such operations as grouping, reorganisation and structurisation.

Wertheimer's studies with human beings (often children) allowed him to access subjective experiences during learning and problem-solving exercises (e.g. working out the area of a parallelogram) and these also helped to distinguish between solutions that were insightful and solutions that occurred by chance or trial and error. Thus, he described subjects expressing the process of 'seeing the light ... (the problem) suddenly became transparently clear, meaningful, in the realisation of the inner structure, the inner requirements of the process' (Wertheimer, 1945/1961, p. 67). This subjective sense of clarity and new understanding together with a feeling of satisfaction has continued to characterise the phenomenon of insight in this area of psychology.

Likewise concentrating on analysing processes underlying problem-solving, Karl Duncker (1945) further developed Wertheimer's ideas on restructuring as a necessary condition for insight. Whilst Gestalt thinking explicitly objected to the prevailing associationistic explanations underlying thinking and behaviours, the proposed alternative framed in terms of functional associations, restructuring and reorganising of perceptual or cognitive fields has been, and continues to be, criticised for its lack of a clear theoretical and explanatory basis (e.g. Osgood, 1964; Ohlsson, 1984a, b; Isaak & Just, 1995; Mayer, 1995). Nonetheless Duncker (1945), in his important work on insight and problem-solving, attempted to provide a clearer and more detailed account of possible processes or stages underlying insightful problem-solving. He proposed that insight into a problem depended crucially on *restructuring* of the problem. In turn, this restructuring could occur in two main ways. Firstly, the functional goal (i.e. the general purpose) of the problem could be redefined (he called this process a suggestion from above), and, secondly, the function of the components of the problem could be reformulated (suggestion from below) such that the original information presented was defined in a different way. He also examined possible processes underlying the reasons why subjects might not achieve a problem solution, i.e. why restructuring might not occur. He proposed that a subject's past experience could have a detrimental effect on such restructuring because this could force a particular mode of thinking and detract from considering novel approaches. Thus, past experience could become an actual block to the individual and Duncker termed this *functional fixedness*. Duncker's ideas, his experimental problems and proposed psychological processes have been extremely influential in the approaches taken by cognitive psychologists in more recent studies on insight (Sternberg & Davidson, 1995).

It is of interest that the concept of insight as developed by the early Gestalt psychologists and refined by later cognitive psychologists has been and continues to be, despite its specificity, an area of much debate and dispute. As is the case with the ways in which insight is dealt with by the more clinical disciplines (see later), differences in views concerning the meaning of insight, its nature, its elicitation and its likely underlying mechanisms/processes are also prevalent in the psychological disciplines. These differences serve to highlight some of the complexities present around the conceptualisation of insight and it is useful to examine briefly some of these issues in turn.

2.1.1 The meaning of insight

The meaning of insight, in terms of definition, characteristics and nature, has itself been the source of much variability and often contradictory views (Hartmann, 1931; Bulbrook, 1932; Schooler *et al.*, 1995). Most commonly, and following early Gestalt views (Köhler, 1924/1957; Hartmann, 1931; Hutchinson, 1941), researchers define insight very specifically, as '*the sudden unexpected solution to a problem*' (e.g. Schooler *et al.*, 1995). The specificity, which contrasts with the more general definitions of insight in psychiatric usage (see next chapter), lies in several aspects of this definition. Thus, the *suddenness* specifies an abrupt emergence of the solution event (relating to behaviour or thought); the *unexpectedness* refers to the surprise element of the event or change and the *solution to a problem* delineates the discreteness of the event, implying both a particular task accomplished and a time-limited episode. Differing views, however, have emerged in relation to these aspects of the definition. In general, suddenness has been a relatively consistent defining characteristic throughout as identified in early Gestalt psychology (e.g. Köhler, 1924/1957) and prominent in contemporary cognitive psychology (e.g. Davidson, 1995; Henley, 1999). Arguing against the concept of partial or gradual insight as proffered by Alpert, Hartmann (1931) explicitly emphasised the importance of suddenness, 'where insight is not immediate or at least sudden it has lost its essential character' (Hartmann, 1931, p. 248). (This definitional feature contrasts particularly with the general psychiatric notion of insight, the latter being conceived in terms of knowledge of problems that develops gradually over unspecified lengths of time.) On the other hand, amongst the cognitive psychologists there are some dissenting views. For example, Weisberg (1995) argues against the view that suddenness and unexpectedness, as manifestations of the Gestalt 'Aha' experience, should be considered definitional criteria of insight. Part of the problem here, however, relates to the fact that many of the offered definitions of insight incorporate, to various extents, mixtures of theoretical, phenomenological/experiential and explanatory notions. This then makes it difficult to tease out the specific referents of the individual components of definitions. Some definitions achieve partial clarification by making certain distinctions. Smith (1995, p. 232) thus distinguishes between *insight* as an 'understanding' and an *insight experience* as the 'sudden emergence of an idea into conscious awareness, the "Aha!" experience'. Gruber (1995) distinguishes between insight as 'problem-solving', which includes the suddenness criterion, and insight as 'understanding' which focuses on knowledge or self-knowledge (in the psychoanalytic sense) rather than the moment of its attainment. Gick and Lockhart (1995) specify that suddenness and surprise relate only to the affective and not to the cognitive component of insight. Others have used descriptions of putative stages in the development of insight which partially separate out possible underlying processes and experiential descriptions occurring at different stages (e.g. Hutchinson, 1941; Csikszentmihalyi & Sawyer, 1995; Seifert *et al.*, 1995, see below). The experiential aspects of insight, i.e. the subjective elements have also carried various emphases in different definitions. For many, it has not been particularly relevant (Köhler, 1924/1957; Weisberg, 1995) but others have specified accompanying subjective experiences such as elation (Hutchinson, 1941), satisfaction and triumph (Seifert *et al.*, 1995) and delight, humour or chagrin (Gick & Lockhart, 1995). Interestingly, the question of whether the experiential aspects, in terms of the sense of revelation and satisfaction, could occur independently of correct solutions does not seem to have been explored. In other words, is it possible for subjects to experience the sudden feeling of clarity and sense of enlightenment when incorrectly solving a problem albeit under the impression it was correct? Clearly the assumption is that the subjective experience of clarity and understanding has to correspond intrinsically to a 'correct' appraisal of the problem or situation.

The specificity of insight in terms of referring to some form of problem-solving has also tended to be held with relative consistency. (This level of specificity is markedly in contrast to the notion of insight as conceived in psychiatric disorders.) Nevertheless, some variability is found here as well. Seifert *et al.* (1995) state clearly that insight is not restricted to problem-solving but includes knowledge about the world and about oneself. They thus provide a broader theoretical definition though they do limit this to problem-solving for empirical purposes. Similarly Finke (1995), in discussions around creative insight, defines this as 'an essential process by which we come to make surprising discoveries and realisations, both about real-world issues and problems, and about ourselves' (Finke, 1995, p. 255). This is a much wider conception of insight. Gruber (1995) whilst defining insight as a moment or flash of enlightenment, at the same time, places this as 'part of coherent life'. Some view insight as a state of mind (e.g. Dominowski & Dallob, 1995) while others define it as a process made up of several stages (Davidson & Sternberg, 1986; Ippolito & Tweney, 1995; Mayer, 1995).

Apart from the issue of specificity in regards to problem-solving, relating insight to *problem-solving* itself is a fundamentally different approach to the meaning of insight compared with its meaning in the clinical disciplines. The crucial difference lies in the *external* focus of insight in the Gestalt and cognitive frameworks as opposed to the *internal* focus of insight in the clinical disciplines. In other words, in the case of the former, insight is directed at the solution of an external problem (i.e. insight is equivalent to awareness of understanding a particular set task *outside* of the individual). On the other hand, insight in the clinical conceptions is directed at the understanding of something happening within the subject (i.e. insight is equivalent to awareness and understanding of changes, such as illness or symptoms or disability, etc. happening *within* an individual). Later, this will be conceptualised and understood in terms of different 'objects' of insight assessment

(Chapter 7) but at this stage it is important to emphasise this as an important difference in meaning.

One of the main interesting and continual areas of dispute around insight, linked with different views on underlying mental processes, concerns the question of whether insight represents a *special* mental process or whether it can be understood in terms of *ordinary* mental processes. This is not a new debate and since the time of Köhler's experiments varying views have been expressed concerning his interpretation of the animals' behaviours (Koffka, 1925/1980). Behavioural and experimental approaches to studying learning and behaviour in animals were developing in parallel to the Gestalt approaches and explanations were framed in terms of trial-and-error learning, and conditioning responses, etc. In a series of experiments with human subjects designed to explore the nature and possible mechanisms underlying insight, Bulbrook (1932, p. 453) concluded that there was 'no characteristic process, operation, form of conditioning or mode of discovery, which we could with propriety distinguish as "insight"'. In the same year, Hartmann (1932) argued that it was the introspective component of insight that determined its special nature. Ogden (1932), however, disagreed and proposed that insight simply referred to intelligent as opposed to non-intelligent behaviour. Subsequently, others tried to unify the notion of insight within models of learning as a whole thus conceiving all theories of learning as based on 'ordinary' mental processes. Kellogg (1938), comparing insight with trial-and-error learning viewed insight as different in degree ('high' learning as opposed to 'low' learning) but not in kind. Similarly, Osgood (1964) considered the differences between insight and learning by other means as mainly terminological and hence, for him, no special processes were involved.

With the increasing focus on exploring cognitive processes underlying learning and problem-solving, there has been a general shift in emphasis from the Gestalt perception-like formulations to more strictly cognitive information-processing models. This has had an effect on the conceptualisation of insight both in terms of its nature and its likely underlying mechanisms. For example, Ohlsson (1984a, b) attempts to integrate aspects of Gestalt theory within information-processing models and redefines problem-solving in terms of *selective searching*, combining both behavioural (trial-and-error learning) and Gestalt (productive/good thinking) concepts in a specific cognitive system. As far as the nature of insight is concerned, there seems to be a clear polarity between views of insight as 'special', as involving qualitatively different psychological processes (e.g. Metcalfe, 1986a, b, 1998; Metcalfe & Wiebe, 1987; Schooler *et al.*, 1993; Dominowski & Dallob, 1995; Mayer, 1995) and views of insight as understandable in terms of 'ordinary' mental processes (e.g. Perkins, 1981; 1995; Keane, 1989; Kaplan & Simon, 1990; Weisberg, 1992; 1995; Gick & Lockhart, 1995). A few position themselves in between these poles, for example, arguing that insight is special but not mystical (Davidson & Sternberg,

1986) or that insight is mostly non-special but a few 'special' processes are involved (Seifert *et al.*, 1995). A major proponent of the 'special' view of insight, Metcalfe and her colleagues described a number of experiments which, they argued, provided empirical support for this view (Metcalfe, 1986a, b; Metcalfe & Wiebe, 1987). The principles behind this empirical work lay in focusing on subjects' 'metacognitions' (judgements based on self-monitoring of mental states) as predictions of success in solving so-called insight problems and non-insight problems (memory tasks, algebra sums, etc.). The metacognitions were elicited either as a 'feeling of knowing' and/or as a closeness to solution which Metcalfe calls 'feeling of warmth', which the subjects had to rate in conjunction with carrying out the various tasks. In summary, findings across the different studies indicated that, on the basis of these metacognitions, subjects were able to predict success only in non-insight problems but not in the insight problems. In other words, there seemed to be no correlation between the subject's experience of feeling close to a solution and actual solution in the insight-dependent tasks whereas in the memory tasks, for example, there was an incremental growth of feelings of warmth corresponding to subjects' approaching of the solutions. In addition, the solution to 'insight problems' was marked phenomenologically by a 'sudden flash of illumination'. This, the authors argued, indicated that insight involved a qualitative change in mental processing. There was no incremental process of getting closer to a solution but instead the solution occurred suddenly and unexpectedly implying a discontinuity in mental processing.

Proponents of the view that insight is not a special process have criticised such empirical work both on methodological and on tautological grounds. Weisberg (1992; 1995), for example, argues that the distinction between so-called insight problems and non-insight problems is false and suggests that it would be more useful to think of problems in a multidimensional way and conceive a continuum of solutions some of which depend on incremental steps and others on short and fast steps, etc. His view in relation to problem-solving was that rather than invoking a special notion of insight, 'problem-solving should be considered as a cyclical process, involving retrieval of information from memory and the attempt to apply this information to the problem. Failure provides new information, which initiates further memory search, and so on' (Weisberg, 1992, p. 427). In other words, solutions to problems are to be found within memory systems of subjects and depend on appropriate access and use made of these by the subject rather than on other special mental processes. In addition, Weisberg criticised the circularity involved in using 'patterns of warmth' both as a criterion of an insight problem (a problem is an insight problem because of the pattern of warmth) and as a support for the validity of the construct (pattern of warmth, indicating insight, elicited in relation to insight problem). Finally, the 'Aha' experience as a criterion of insight has also been disputed, in that subjects can experience the same phenomenon when solving 'non-insight' problems (Weisberg, 1995).

In subsequent work, Metcalfe (1998) developed the argument further. Responding to the opposing view that problem solving depended on memory explanations, she pointed out that amnesic patients accomplished problem-solving tasks (insight-like problems involving puzzle sentences to complete) almost as well as healthy individuals even after a week's delay (see McAndrews *et al.*, 1987). This, she claimed, contradicts the hypothesis that insight relies only on recollection. She further suggested that there was a common insight-like metacognitive dynamic involved in the unprimed word/picture fragment completion tasks in that subjects likewise show no correlation between feelings of closeness to solution and actual solutions. Thus, she proposed, 'insight-like tasks and implicit memory tasks are one and the same' (Metcalfe, 1998, p. 192). It is of interest how this becomes interpreted in relation to the empirical work on insight in patients with amnesic syndromes or dementias (see below and Chapters 4 and 5).

2.1.2 Determination of insight

In line with the specific concept of insight detailed above, its elicitation has generally depended on experiments in which subjects are given particular problems to solve. (Some researchers have also carried out 'naturalistic' studies in which scientists are observed working and arriving at problem solutions within laboratory situations (e.g. Dunbar, 1995)). This is in contrast to the elicitation of insight in general psychiatry which is dependent instead on subjective accounts of current mental states and conditions. Interestingly, however, assessment of insight in neurological states, particularly in amnesia in focal and generalised organic brain syndromes (Chapters 4 and 5), likewise has relied on patients carrying out specific tests. Some of these have clearly been influenced by the cognitive and information-processing approaches mentioned above. There is, nevertheless, a crucial difference between the approaches which relates to the issue mentioned earlier concerning the differences in focus of insight (i.e. external versus internal). Within the Gestalt and cognitive psychologies, insight is determined as present when a particular task is successfully solved with or without the sense of enlightenment demanded by some of the definitions. Judgements made by subjects concerning their likelihood of success in such tasks (i.e. metacognitions) are deemed as irrelevant to insight in the sense that subjects' predictions have no correlation with successful solutions (Metcalfe, 1998). In contrast to this, within neuropsychological approaches to assessment of insight in patients with amnesia or dementia, insight is determined not on the basis of the solution to particular problems (in this case memory tasks, therefore 'non-insight' problems) but on the discrepancies between patients' judgements of performance (prediction or postdiction) and actual performance. In other words, here it is the metacognitions that are at the core of the assessment since these represent subjects' own judgements of their mental states, the latter being the foci (or 'objects') of insight assessment. Thus, for example, the 'feeling-of-knowing' metacognition has been used as an indirect assessment of awareness or insight in such patients (Shimamura & Squire, 1986; Shimamura, 1994, see Chapter 4). What this shows, and will be highlighted in more detail later (Chapter 7), is that similar terminology (metacognition and insight) used in the different contexts (clinical and non-clinical) can have different and even contradictory meanings and applications. Later, it will be demonstrated that the 'object' of insight assessment (solution to a problem, mental/physical symptoms, illness, etc.) is crucially important in determining the phenomenon of insight elicited.

As evident from the question concerning whether insight be considered as a special or non-special process, the nature of the particular problems given to subjects to solve for the purpose of eliciting insight has also been a source of some disagreement. In his experiments, Köhler explicitly devised problems for the chimpanzees that could not be solved directly but involved roundabout ('Umwege') or indirect methods of solution. Duncker, likewise, devised problems that, following Gestalt principles, depended on utilising given components in novel ways so that the subject would have to 'restructure' the situation in order to get to a solution. Subsequent 'insight problems' have been modelled along the same lines, i.e. as problems which are non-routine (Mayer, 1995), demanding some sort of restructuring, a new way of looking at the components and their relationships. This distinction between insight and non-insight problems is held by many (Sternberg & Davidson, 1995). One difficulty, however, as pointed out by Weisberg (1995), is that there is no system of classifying problems into those in which insight occurs and those in which it does not. He argues that many of the classical 'insight problems' are not, in fact, solved through insight and hence should not be considered as 'insight problems'. Others have qualified views. For example, Smith (1995) defines insight problems as problems whose solution is *more likely* to be reached by an insight experience, thus, allowing for other possible means of solution though not specifying any criteria for this. Schooler *et al.* (1995) distinguish between insight problems, non-insight problems and hybrid problems, the latter involving solutions through a mixture of both insight and non-insight means. Once again though the criteria for determining such distinctions are difficult to set and tend to depend on the manner in which problems appear to be solved, thus giving rise to some circularity.

2.1.3   Stages and mechanisms underlying insight

As mentioned earlier, views on the stages and possible mechanisms underlying insight have also been influenced by the shift from the original Gestalt conceptions to the more cognitively orientated information-processing models of mental processes. The conceptualisation of insight in terms of its nature and likely underlying processes has reflected this shift particularly in the move away from perceptual models (e.g. Köhler, 1924/1957; Hutchinson, 1941) to more 'cognitive' models of understanding insight (Sternberg & Davidson, 1995). Nevertheless, the perceptual metaphor is still evident in many of the processes proposed to underlie insight and this, amongst other things, helps to subdivide views in this area. Some explanatory mechanisms underlying insight are thus framed in perceptual terms, such as 'new perceptual organisation' (Ellen & Pate, 1986) or 'locus of explanation in the perceptual world' (Ippolito & Tweney, 1995).

In general though, insight is conceived as developing following some sort of restructuring of the problem. The nature of this 'restructuring' process, however, has been a source of difficulty in terms of agreement concerning what precisely this process involves. Duncker (1945) referred to an analysis of the problem situation and removal of blocks which impeded such analysis. Similarly, the Russian Psychologist Rubinštejn (1960) emphasised the importance of reformulation of the problem and the interactional relationship between reformulation and analysis. Clearly, some researchers view the restructuring process as perceptual, e.g. a perceptual reorganisation (Ellen & Pate, 1986) or pattern recognition (Schooler *et al.*, 1995). In more information-processing terms, the restructuring has been described as a change in the representation of the problem, i.e. finding the right problem representation (Ohlsson, 1984a, b; Kaplan & Simon, 1990; Gick & Lockhart, 1995). Other suggestions involving methods of restructuring have included: use of analogue, i.e. solving a problem on the basis of its similarity to a different problem (Gick & Holyoak, 1980; 1983), completing a schema, i.e. the addition of missing pieces to an incomplete though appropriate mental representation (Mayer, 1995; Seifert *et al.*, 1995), as a search of memory and working with the information accrued (Weisberg & Alba, 1982; Weisberg, 1992; 1995), apprehension of relations and fluency of thought (Ansburg, 2000), and many more (Sternberg & Davidson, 1995). Davidson and Sternberg (1986) suggest three distinct processes consisting of: (i) selective encoding (i.e. relevant information is sifted out from the irrelevant), (ii) selective combination (i.e. the assembling of seemingly unrelated facts or ideas into a coherent whole) and (iii) selective comparison (i.e. relating newly acquired or proposed concepts to the older concepts, analogies).

One of the more consistent findings in the descriptions of processes underlying insight has related to the postulated stages involved. Such stages had already been described in the early Gestalt work (Wallas, 1926 (cited in Mayer, 1995); Hutchinson, 1941) and have persisted, with modifications, within the cognitive literature (Sternberg & Davidson, 1995). In brief, the stages are described as follows:

1 *A mental preparation*: where the problem or situation is first confronted and where unsuccessful attempts at solving take place.

2 *Incubation*: where the problem is put aside temporarily. Various mechanisms have been proposed to underlie this stage such as unconscious processing (Csikszentmihalyi & Sawyer, 1995; Seifert *et al.*, 1995), or contextual change, i.e. being away from the problem situation can help remove the block to solution (Smith, 1995). Perkins (1995), on the other hand, rejects the need for an incubation stage and unconscious mental processing. Instead, he focuses on the problem space metaphor (i.e. the notion of thought moving through physical space) suggesting that the subject is simply engaged in a continual search through 'possibility' spaces.

3 *Illumination*: when suddenly and unexpectedly the solution is found, not preceded by the 'feeling-of-knowing' characteristic of non-insight problem-solving (Metcalfe, 1998). This is accompanied by the subjective feeling of satisfaction ('Aha' experience) and some even specify an increase in physiological arousal (Seifert *et al.*, 1995).

4 *Verification*: where details of the problem solution are worked out and tested.

It is evident that there is a wide range of descriptions and analyses of possible processes underlying insight. Indeed, and in contrast to studies of insight in clinical areas, much more emphasis has been placed on empirical investigation of such processes than on relating insight to other variables or attributes. In terms of the latter, there is little research in this field. Davidson (1995), on the basis of empirical work exploring insight in subjects with high IQ and those with lower IQ reported that insight solving was associated with greater intelligence. Perkins (1995), on the other hand, states categorically that insight has little to do with intelligence or cognition. In the area of creative insight, some studies have explored the relationship between affect and creative problem-solving, and suggest that positive affect, as opposed to neutral or negative affect, enhances insightful problem-solving (see Friedman & Förster, 2000, for review and experimental evidence). Finally, some suggestions have also been put forward linking insight problem-solving with cognitive processes associated with right hemispheric function (Fiore & Schooler, 1998) and, in this context, Pierce (1999) has proposed a possible evolutionary basis to the phenomenon of insight.

2.1.4 Summary

In summary, the concept of insight in Gestalt psychology is viewed in a very specific sense. Bound up in the theory of perception that is central to Gestalt thinking, insight results from the reorganisation or restructuring of a particular situation or problem, based on some form of perceptual shift ('things falling into place'). With the development of cognitive approaches, the perceptual analogy has largely been superseded by information-processing-like models though the behavioural aspect of the Gestalt notion remains. Insight has been studied both as an 'intelligent behaviour' through the solving of specific tasks and as a 'creative process' through retrospective and prospective research into scientific methods (Dunbar, 1995).

In contrast to the broader and more general meanings of insight in relation to mental illness (see next chapter), the specificity of the concept of insight in Gestalt and cognitive psychology is striking and manifest in several ways. Firstly, the experience of insight (whether conceived as a state or process) is characterised by certain features, namely, *suddenness, spontaneity, unexpectedness* and *satisfaction* (Seifert *et al.*, 1995). In other words, there is the sense of 'enlightenment' or 'revelation' that can be observed both in behavioural (the sudden smooth solving of a task) and in subjective (the 'Aha' experience) terms. Secondly, insight so conceived is a discrete event with determinable boundaries. Thirdly, insight is directed specifically at the solution of a particular task which, in contrast to the clinical perspective, lies external to the individual.

Partly as a result of changes in theoretical approaches and partly because of some circularity involved in studying the phenomenon of insight in so-called insight problems, opposing views have emerged concerning the validity of both the insight construct as such and the problems used to determine insight.

2.2 Insight in psychoanalytic psychology

In contrast to general psychiatry, the concept of insight within psychoanalytic psychology has, from the very beginning, held a central position as an integral component of psychoanalysis and, to a variable extent, of psychoanalytic psychotherapies. In other words, at the very core of psychoanalytic theory, as developed by Freud, was the search for a deep self-knowledge which was both inherent to the method of psychoanalysis itself and essential to any consequent personality or therapeutic change that ensued (Strachey, 1934; Fenichel, 1945; Freud, 1973a, b). Insight or self-knowledge as conceived in this psychoanalytic sense shares some similarities with insight as understood by Gestalt and cognitive psychology, and with insight as recognised in general psychiatry but it also shows important differences. An obvious and fundamental difference lies in the 'depth' of self-knowledge contained within the concept. In psychoanalytic terms, the depth refers to a level of understanding that an individual can develop in relation to his/her mental processes (and consequent behaviours) and these, in turn, are directly connected to the tripartite models of the mind as elaborated by Freud. Accordingly, in relation to the earlier topographical model of the mind, self-knowledge can thus relate to *conscious*, *preconscious* and/or *unconscious* mental processes. Within this metaphor, the deepest level of knowledge refers to knowledge of unconscious mental processes. As Freud clearly stated, 'our therapy works by transforming what is unconscious into what is conscious' (Freud, 1973a, p. 321). Later, as Freud's views changed and he developed the structural model of the mind, self-knowledge was conceived in a similarly deep but more active and integrative way ('where id was there ego shall be' (Freud, 1973b, p. 112)). Likewise, emphasising the depth of self-knowledge required for therapeutic benefit, Segal points out that insight '... must be deep enough. It must reach to the deep layers of the unconscious and illuminate those early processes in which the pattern of internal and external relationships is laid down, and in which the ego is structured' (Segal, 1962, p. 212).

Interestingly, whilst the *concept* of insight as a form of deep self-knowledge can be discerned in the earliest psychoanalytic writings, the *term* 'insight' only began to be used in this context around the early 1950s. Freud used the term 'insight' (*'Einsicht'* or *'Einblick'*) predominantly in the generic sense to denote knowledge or awareness of being ill. According to Anna Freud (1981), there was only one instance where Freud used the term 'insight' in the deeper sense of revelation as in the much quoted line from the 1931 preface to the 3rd English edition of *The Interpretation of Dreams*: 'insight such as this comes to one's lot but once in a lifetime' (Freud, 1900, p. xxxii). Nevertheless, the concept of insight in the sense of a self-understanding that reaches the unconscious levels of the mind has been implied in both the psychoanalytic aim and in the psychoanalytic treatment ('that here understanding and cure almost coincide, that a traversable road leads from one to the other' (Freud, 1973b, p. 180)). This conceptualisation of insight was subsequently made explicit by the convergent use of the term 'insight' in later psychoanalytic writings (e.g. Martin, 1952; Zilboorg, 1952; Kris, 1956) and, since then, has continued to be the source of much debate. In this regard, two main areas will be explored in this section. Firstly, the concept of insight itself will be reviewed and, secondly, the role of insight in psychoanalysis and psychoanalytic therapies will be examined in terms of its perceived contribution to promoting change or 'cure'. Whilst a division between these areas is being made here for the purpose of analysis, it has to be understood that this is something of an artificial division and the two areas considerably overlap. Indeed there is, as will be seen, a degree of circularity involved when exploring the relationship between insight and change in a situation where the conceptualisation of insight itself incorporates the notion of psychic or personality change within its definition.

2.2.1 The concept of insight

As with exploration of insight in other disciplines, conceptualisation of insight within the psychoanalytic field likewise shows variability in views held. Differences emerge, for example, in definitions and characteristics of insight, its essential components and classification, its likely mechanisms of development and the possible processes involved, etc. Nonetheless, the consistent core to the psychoanalytic concept of insight, referring to the knowledge or understanding of one's unconscious (or only partly conscious) mental processes, has persisted. The latter, in the psychoanalytic framework, encompass the instinctual drives, resistances and defence mechanisms such as repression, identification, introjection, denial, etc. thought to underlie personality structure and mental disorders, particularly neurotic manifestations (Fenichel, 1945). With the increasing use of the term 'insight' in this context, it was quickly recognised that the concept needed clarification (Zilboorg, 1952; Roback, 1974). Questions were thus asked about the meaning and nature of insight in terms of the *content* of knowledge involved, the *way* in which the knowledge was attained and the *consequences* of such knowledge. In turn, such questions raised various viewpoints and perspectives, and Freud's early implicit conceptualisation of insight simply as an awareness of unconscious mental processes was both elaborated and challenged. Loewenstein (1956) formulated this explicitly when he pointed out that insight was a more comprehensive concept than 'bringing to consciousness' (in the Freudian sense) but comprised also of 'the re-establishment of connexion'. This was echoed by Shengold (1981) and Blum (1979) who stated 'insight does more than make conscious; it establishes causes, meanings and connections' (p. 51). Content of the knowledge thus constituting insight became conceived in more involved and complex terms, and resulted in offers of a range of definitions of insight capturing or emphasising different aspects of such knowledge. For example, some definitions are wide and general as in Myerson (1960) who stresses the newness of knowledge relating to oneself and to one's interaction with the world, or Glucksman (1993) who suggests that insight refers to 'knowledge or some type of rationale that helps the patient explain his/her symptoms or problems' (p. 163). Other definitions are more technical and specific. For example, Neubauer (1979) defines insight during psychoanalysis as 'the expansion of the ego by self-observation, memory recovery, cognitive participation and reconstruction in the context of affective reliving' (p. 29). In contrast, Joyce and Stoker (2000) refer to an individual's 'self-knowledge (which) gradually leads to modification of his internal representations' (p. 1139), and many other examples can be found.

A number of attempts have been made to organise the complex conceptualisation of insight underlying such definitions and, here again, a range of distinctions have been suggested to differentiate between various types of insight. One of the earliest distinctions proposed has been that between *intellectual* and *emotional* insight. In broad terms, this refers to the difference between knowledge that is understood and accepted at an intellectual or theoretical level and knowledge that is grasped at a deeper level in the sense that the individual feels or experiences it in a direct way. However, this is a fairly general distinction for it is apparent in the psychoanalytic literature that it is interpreted in many different ways giving rise to some confusion (Zilboorg, 1952). Hatcher (1973) argues that this distinction was already present in Freud when the latter differentiated between 'knowing but not knowing' – as the intellectual understanding of the repressed (i.e. distant, non-involvement of the self with the unconscious) – and emotional understanding which was attained through the direct (experiential) struggle with the repressed in the transference reaction. In a similar vein, without referring to insight specifically, Strachey (1934) distinguishes between descriptive interpretations which can lead to intellectual understanding and 'mutative' interpretations which lead to modification of the patient's superego (i.e. to sustained change). The mutative interpretation, he specifies, 'must be emotionally immediate; the patient must experience it as something actual' (Strachey, 1934, p. 150). In general terms, it is this emotional or experiential aspect of insight that is considered one of the crucial aspects of psychoanalytic insight, one that is frequently equated with the definition of psychoanalytic insight itself, helping to differentiate it from insight as used in other areas (lay usage, general psychiatric usage, etc.) and often considered as the main factor in promoting change (Segal, 1962; 1991).

Other more specific approaches have been taken to distinguish between different types of insight. For example, Reid and Finesinger (1952) differentiated between *neutral*, *emotional* and *dynamic* insight. Objecting to the term 'intellectual' insight on the grounds of claiming that all insight was by definition intellectual (or cognitive), they proposed distinctions based on the level at which patients could understand the relationship between antecedents and manifested symptoms or behaviours. They defined *neutral* insight as occurring when patients were able to understand and accept superficial links between antecedents (e.g. quarrelling with spouse) and symptoms (e.g. indigestion). They further specified that at this level, emotions were not involved either in the act of understanding or as a release resulting from the understanding. *Emotional* insight, on the other hand, occurred when patients' understanding of the association between antecedents and symptoms included either an emotional component in the understanding process itself (e.g. anxiety/hostility underlying the quarrelling with spouse) or if emotion was experienced as a result of that understanding. Finally, *dynamic* insight was defined as the deepest form of insight when patients were able to understand the relationships between antecedents and symptoms in the Freudian sense of 'penetrating the repressive barrier and making the ego aware of certain hypercathected wishes that were previously unconscious' (Reid & Finesinger, 1952, p. 731). In other words, here the connection between antecedents and symptoms was based on knowledge of unconscious motivations and defences thought to underlie the emotional component of the antecedent. Of these three kinds of insight, dynamic insight was conceived as producing the most extensive changes in the personality of the subject and the most lasting therapeutic benefits.

Whilst agreeing that insight had to involve the patients' understanding of their unconscious mental processes in order to achieve therapeutic benefit, Richfield

(1954), argued that recognition of such unconscious processes on the part of the patient did not necessarily lead to a change in 'neurotic' behaviour. He proposed that it was not the *content* of the knowledge that was essential to the therapeutic effect of insight but the *form* in which this knowledge was experienced. Thus, on the basis of Bertrand Russell's classification of knowledge, Richfield distinguished between insight gained by description and insight gained by acquaintance. When patients attained *descriptive insight*, they became aware of the 'truths' about themselves by acknowledging the words of the analyst. When, however, they attained *ostensive insight*, they became 'personally acquainted' with the 'truths', for example, through transference when particular emotions and their significance were brought directly to patients' awareness. In other words, it is the method of gaining knowledge by direct experience that is considered the crucial component of insight irrespective of the content of such knowledge.

Bibring (1954), in contrast, focuses on the content of knowledge as a distinguishing factor between two forms of insight. Specifying also that different techniques are needed to achieve these insights he differentiates between insight through *clarification* and insight through *interpretation*. The former is based on working with conscious and/or preconscious processes of which the patient is not sufficiently aware and the latter is based on working exclusively with unconscious mental processes. Consequently, he argues, the two forms of insight are 'dynamically' different. Insight through *clarification*, because it deals only with conscious material, does not encounter resistance and patients are able to develop a more 'objective, realistic perspective' on problems and thereby achieve greater control over them. In that sense, the ego becomes 'detached'. Problems are not resolved but are viewed from a different perspective. Insight through *interpretation*, on the other hand, results in direct involvement of the ego in the process of dealing with the unconscious material but results in better solutions to underlying pathogenic conflicts. Somewhat differently, Myerson (1965) differentiates between *psychoanalytic* insight and *reality-oriented* insight on the basis of what seems to be a deeper form of understanding in the former. Here again, the focus is on knowledge of unconscious mental forces and, in particular, of these being directly experienced in the mental state. In reality-oriented insight a more superficial knowledge is defined with focus on realistic appraisals of relationships and environment rather than on underlying instinctual conflicts.

Describing some of the attempts at classifying the various modes of insight as *ad hoc* and intuitive rather than systematic or analytical, Lindén (1984; 1985) sets out a comprehensive but complicated framework for classifying insight using a developmental approach. She stresses the need for an adequate theory of cognition and for this purpose uses Nilsson's genetic-hierarchical theory which itself is based on an integration of Piaget's developmental theories and Freud's topographical representation of the mind. Insight, she proposes, can be hierarchically (i.e. structurally) localised in relation to sensorimotor, perceptual or conceptual levels of cognitive activity and along conscious–unconscious and intellectual–emotional dimensions. In recognition of the confusion arising from the general use of the term 'insight' she argues for the need to specify (within her proposed framework) the particular insight manifested within an analytic situation.

Apart from seeking to clarify and define various modes of insight, psychoanalytic approaches have also explored the possible processes and components involved. In contrast to the Gestalt notion, there is a much greater emphasis on conceptualisation of insight as a long gradual process in which insight is gained in slow increments (Strachey, 1934; Kris, 1956; Hatcher, 1973; Abrams, 1981; Mangham, 1981; Poland, 1988; Segal, 1991). Zilboorg (1952) argues that it has to be an affective process, in that insight can only develop through successive affective reconstructive experiences (thus arguing for the emotional/experiential component of insight as the crucial constitutive factor). Conceived as an ongoing process, there is the additional implication that insight can never be complete, that it is indefinite, and applies to the whole life of an individual and, indeed, some have stated this explicitly (Blum, 1979; 1992; Poland, 1988; Segal, 1991). Only a few authors refer to insight as an 'immediate' or sudden illumination as used in the Gestalt sense (Rhee, 1990; Elliott *et al.*, 1994) though some writers allow for the possibility of sudden flashes of insight occurring within the ongoing process as a whole (Martin, 1952; Blum, 1979; Olmos-de Paz, 1990; Wilson, 1998; Joyce & Stoker, 2000). Most views seem to agree that the process of insight is an active and creative one (Blum, 1979; Freud, 1981; Pollock, 1981; Shengold, 1981; Sternbach, 1989). Thus, it is *active* in the sense that the individual has to be him/herself directly involved in the process. Freud recognised this in his later work when dealing with the phenomenon of resistance. For this reason also, some writers have argued specifically against the notion of the analyst 'giving' insight to the subject (Zilboorg, 1952; Poland, 1988). The process is seen as a *creative* one in that attaining insight or understanding of unconscious mental processes is viewed as involving a restructuring or reintegration of aspects of the subject's ego to form something *new* rather than a restoration or clarification of the old (Segal, 1962; 1991; Freud, 1981; Sternbach, 1989). Abrams (1981, p. 261) puts this very clearly:

Insight-producing activity entails taking things apart and putting them together differently. It is the highly specialized expression of fundamental differentiating and integrating capacities, the operation of a relatively intact higher level of mental organisation. The new assemblage of drive and defence, desexualized and/or restructured, is an entirely different product from what has preceded it.

Interestingly, this conception of restructuring shares strong similarities with the Gestalt notion of insight. This is often reflected in the terminology used, e.g. 'each part of a meaningful whole' (Hatcher, 1973, p. 395) or, more explicitly in Myerson (1965, p. 791) when referring to stages of insight development which, 'become integrated into a Gestalt through the psychoanalytic process'. Similarly, in Neubauer (1979, p. 34), '[a] new Gestalt is established, a reorganised ego structure'. At the same time, however, the concept of restructuring in the psychoanalytic sense refers in a much more direct sense to the deeper connotation of psychic or personality change.

Mechanisms and possible components underlying psychoanalytic insight tend to be difficult to disentangle, reflecting the conception of insight as an ongoing restructuring process. In the main, the experience and interpretation of the transference situation has generally been considered as the most effective source of gaining insight (Strachey, 1934; Zilboorg, 1952; Segal, 1962; 1991; Sternbach, 1989). In other words, whilst interpretations of other aspects of the patient's mental life are viewed as important in the development or creation of insight within the individual, it is the interpretations relating to the transference relationship itself that are seen as the most significant in promoting change. This view probably relates to the conception of insight in the deeper sense of something that is experienced directly or emotionally. Thus, in the analysis of the transference relationship, the individual is confronted with emotions/thoughts which, on resonating with earlier experienced feelings, gain a direct or immediate quality thereby achieving a deeper personal understanding.

Some authors have emphasised self-observation on the part of the subject as an important prerequisite or component of the process of insight (e.g. Hatcher, 1973; Kennedy, 1979; Neubauer, 1979; Abrams, 1981). A few authors have tried to break up the process of attaining insight into separate components or stages. For example, on the basis of an analysis of two case reports, Abrams (1981) proposed several empirical components to 'insight-producing activity' that were common to both cases. These included the following: (1) attention, initially diffuse but becoming more focused, (2) distinct emotional tone, appropriate to the ideas, (3) recognition of link between different components (e.g. dreams or memories), (4) free movements within time periods, due to awareness of the meaningful relationship between past and present, (5) a sense of inner unity within the patient and, (6) at moment of discovery, a recognition that something new has happened. On the other hand, Elliot *et al.* (1994) based their model on a study comparing 'insight-events' in patients undergoing either psychodynamic interpersonal psychotherapy or cognitive-behavioural therapy. They proposed a five-stage model of insight comprising of: (1) contextual priming, (2) novel information, (3) initial distantiated processing, (4) 'insight' and (5) elaboration. This latter model shares many similarities with the Gestalt and cognitive models described earlier. This is perhaps influenced by the fact that these researchers were using a much narrower definition of insight as a discrete event thus running counter to the general conception of insight in the psychoanalytic sense. The difficulties in empirically defining and assessing insight in such situations, however, is made apparent in this study and raises questions concerning the validity of extending the model and the methods used to other areas, particularly, as clearly the content of 'insight-events' (as determined by qualitative analysis) in the two patient groups was very different.

Others have suggested that the ability to empathise was crucial to the development of insight, viewing the interactive process between subject and analyst as the mechanism underlying insight acquisition (Dymond, 1948). In fact, the contribution of the analyst, in terms of relationship to, and interaction with, the analysand, towards the attainment of insight, has been the subject of much discussion and of a variety of disparate views. Part of the problem, however, in trying to clarify some of the different perspectives is that there is confusing overlap with different aspects of the relationship between analyst and insight. These aspects can be broadly divided into three areas: (i) the meaning of analyst insight, (ii) the role of the analyst in the insight process and (iii) the role of the analyst in therapeutic change. This last area will be dealt with in the next section (see below). Concerning the analyst's insight, whilst there is general agreement that this has to be differentiated from the patient/subject insight, it is also apparent that there are opposing views as regards its meaning. Thus, some authors regard it as the understanding (intellectual and/or emotional) the analyst has of the patient's mental life and processes (Richfield, 1954; Blum, 1979; 1992; Pollock, 1981; Levenson, 1998). Indeed, Pollock (1981), focusing specifically on the nature of analyst's insight in relation to understanding elderly patients with cognitive impairment, proposes a distinction between *inductive* insight and *deductive* insight based on the type of knowledge held by the analyst. Thus, he defines the former as referring to the understanding of antecedent–consequent linkages as gained from transference repetition and the latter as referring to the understanding of meaning in relation to personal phenomena as gained from reconstruction. On the other hand, others argue that the analyst's insight cannot refer to the analyst's understanding of the patient's mental life but must refer to self-understanding, i.e. the analyst's understanding of own mental processes (Shengold, 1981; Poland, 1988; Joyce & Stoker, 2000). In other words, there is a polarity between those who do and those who do not hold that knowledge of the self is crucially different from knowledge of others. Thus, Anna Freud (1981) differentiated between knowledge of one's inner world (termed 'insight') and knowledge of one's external world (termed 'understanding'). Similarly, Shengold (1981) suggested that the analyst's insight into the patient's mind is called 'outlook' and should be distinguished from the analyst's insight into his/her own mind ('insight'). Lindén's (1984; 1985) distinction between insight and outsight is based on a similar principle.

The role of the analyst in the *insight process* has likewise been the subject of mixed views. Here the views range from those who focus on the insight process as something that is happening predominantly within and by the patient, albeit with guidance provided by the analyst (e.g. Bibring, 1954; Segal, 1962; 1991; Blum, 1979; 1992) to those who see the insight process as intrinsically interactive between the patient and analyst (Loewald, 1960; Shengold, 1981; Poland, 1988; Pulver, 1992; Etchegoyen, 1993; Levine, 1994; Steiner, 1994; Currin, 2000). Loewald (1960) argues against the traditional conception of the analyst as neutral and objective, a 'reflecting mirror' whose role is to observe and reflect back to the patient the latter's conscious and unconscious processes through verbal communication. Instead, he contends, in order for the patient to gain insight and attain structural personality changes, significant interactions between the patient and analyst must take place in which the analyst has a specific and active role. The analyst, he maintains, has to function as a 'co-actor on the analytic stage' and in order to do that, must be actively empathic and be able to regress within himself to the level of organisation of the patient. Insight attainment is thus viewed as an actively interactive process between the patient and analyst. Some differences emerge, however, between views concerning the nature or levels of interaction underlying the insight process. For example, Poland (1988) stresses the deep collaborative aspect of the patient–analyst interaction and the emotional engagement of the analyst in this process, 'the struggle towards insight is a shared task, actualised in the transference–countertransference process' (p. 355). At the same time, he is clear that within this interaction, the analyst remains 'an outsider', his mind interacting, but not merging, with that of the patient and, hence, not becoming part of the patient's mind. On the other hand, others suggest a more integrative model where there is direct incorporation of the analyst within the patient's mind by means of introjection (Strachey, 1934; Olmos-de-Paz, 1990). Some authors stress the interdependency of insight as self-knowledge and the empathic interactive relationship with the analyst, pointing out that one could not happen without the other (Pulver, 1992; Etchegoyen, 1993; Carveth, 1998; Currin, 2000). Others have focused more on the analyst in the interactive process. For example, Levine (1994) and Steiner (1994) both emphasise the lack of 'objectivity' within the analyst, arguing that the analyst's interventions were inevitably affected by personal values, desires, as well as by unconscious influences which were reactivated during the analytic session. Thus, they stress the need for analysts to have insight into themselves in order to be effective. Similarly, Currin (2000) emphasises the need to include the analyst's insight into him/herself as crucial to the integrative process of insight development in the patient. Sternbach (1989) and Sampson (1991) pointed out that it was possible for patients to develop insights without the necessity of the presence of the analyst (although based on previous analytic work).

2.2.2 The role of insight in psychoanalytic therapy

Closely linked, and sometimes difficult to separate from, the conceptual debate around insight is the other main area giving rise to mixed views, namely the role of insight within psychoanalytic therapy. The problem is, moreover, beset by the complexities of identifying goals of psychoanalysis and psychoanalytic psychother-apies in general (McGlashan & Miller, 1982). Nevertheless, how important is the attainment of insight for the therapeutic benefit of the patient? Fisher and Greenberg (1977) suggest that Freud's own concept of insight in relation to therapy and cure changed. They point out that while initially Freud maintained the existence of a direct relationship between the attainment of insight and behavioural change or cure, he later acknowledged the equal importance of time, working through and inner resistances. However, Freud's work can be interpreted rather as a change in the conceptualisation of insight from a passive (making unconscious conscious) to an active (confronting forces of resistance) form with both being essential to per-sonality or therapeutic change (see also Hatcher, 1973). Since Freud's time, there have been disparate views on the relationship between insight and change.

As already mentioned, one problem here is differentiating between personality or psychic or structural change which, in most conceptualisations of psychoana-lytic insight, is intrinsic to the definition of insight itself and actual therapeutic change or improvement from symptoms. Often this is not made explicit and is dif-ficult to infer. Some authors have alluded to this distinction when pointing out that the development of insight does not entail therapeutic improvement (e.g. Zilboorg, 1952; Neubauer, 1979). More overtly, Lehmkuhl (1989) argues for the need to sep-arate the concept of emotional insight from the concept of cure and that the for-mer does not necessarily lead to the latter. Views concerning the role of insight in contributing to the development of specific therapeutic improvement fall broadly into three main groups. Firstly, for many, insight remains the crucial factor in achieving symptomatic relief or cure (Strachey, 1934; Loewenstein, 1956; Segal, 1962; 1991; Blum, 1979; 1992; Schmukler, 1999). Thus, Blum (1979) states that 'analytic "cure" is primarily effected through insight and not through empathy, acceptance, tolerance, etc.' (p. 47) and similarly, a few years later, he reiterates that insight is the 'unique critical agent of psychic change in clinical psychoanalysis' (Blum, 1992, p. 257). His views are echoed strongly by Segal (1962; 1991) who maintains that insight is central to therapeutic change. Interestingly, she suggests a number of conditions (e.g. stable analytic environment, right attitude on the part of the analyst, favourable countertransference, analyst's correct understanding/ interpretation, correct timing and depth of interpretation) which are also import- · ant in promoting cure but only by providing the right background for the devel-opment of insight itself. The conditions themselves clearly refer to factors relating to the analyst. However, these are presented very much as extrinsic to the develop-ment of insight in contrast to the intrinsic, integrative way such analyst's factors are considered when the insight process is conceived as more explicitly inter-actional (see above). Others qualify the type of insight likely to promote the greatest curative effect, e.g. dynamic insight (Reid & Finesinger, 1952), insight through interpretation (Bibring, 1954) or ostensive insight (Richfield, 1954). On the other hand, Valenstein (1981) suggests that rather than having a direct curative effect, insight, through its effect on restoration of ego function, facilitates the conscious dealing of problems at a secondary process level.

Secondly, many authors in this area express doubts concerning the central role given to insight in the curative process and suggest that other factors may be more important in determining therapeutic effect (Kohut, 1977; Carveth, 1998). For example, Alexander and French (1946) emphasise the role of the 'corrective emotional experience', i.e. the curative effect of re-experiencing earlier conflicts within the transference relationship but in a context of the analyst assuming a different (and hence therapeutic) attitude from the original person of the past. The analyst in general has been given a more prominent role in helping to achieve therapeutic benefit by various means including providing a supportive environment and through the patient's relationship with both the analytic/transference personality and the 'real' personality of the analyst (Blum, 1992; De Jonghe et al., 1992; Glucksman, 1993). Some suggest that insight is not the cause but the consequence of therapeutic change. For example, Cautela (1965), reporting on three patients undergoing desensitisation for anxiety problems, found that they showed increased insight with improvement. He proposed the possibility that some insight-oriented therapies might be analogous to desensitisation procedures and that as patients relived their anxieties in the analytic situation, these represented successive re-exposures and it was this process that resulted in insight. Frank (1993) in a similar though more integrative vein also suggests that behavioural change (e.g. as achieved through cognitive-behavioural techniques) could help promote insight. This in turn could promote further behavioural change and thus it was this cycle between behaviour and analytic processes that could lead to the positive clinical outcome.

Thirdly, and probably most prevalent, is the view that insight and non-insight factors are equally important in promoting therapeutic change, particularly where factors such as interaction with the analyst are viewed as intrinsic to, or interdependent with, the insight process itself (De Jonghe et al., 1992; Pulver, 1992; Etchegoyen, 1993; Carveth, 1998; Currin, 2000). De Jonghe et al. (1992) provide a two-factor model in which both insight and 'support' are seen as important factors to therapeutic change based on different schools of psychoanalytic thought. Thus, insight, as a curative factor, is embedded within the classical Freudian background of ego psychology and addressing the intrapsychic conflicts thought to be responsible for pathology. On the other hand, 'support', as a curative factor, is contextualised against the postclassical analytic period (Anna Freud, Klein, Winnicott, etc.) of a psychology focusing on developmental arrest. Support in this case addresses the trauma thought to be the original pathogenic factor. Adopting the term 'mutative' to refer to the structural (and clinical) change that can occur with both 'insight' and 'support', De Jonghe *et al.* (1992) stress that both processes are important and occur simultaneously during analysis.

One of the problems in trying to answer the question of the relative contribution of insight and other factors to symptomatic improvement is the difficulty faced by empirical research in this area. Whilst the need for systematic research in this area has been well recognised (Roback, 1971; 1974; Hatcher, 1973; Wallerstein, 1983), in practical terms this does pose numerous problems and consequently empirical research has been relatively limited. Reviewing empirical studies in this area, Roback (1971) concludes on the basis of identified methodological limitations that there is a need for future studies to: firstly, adequately define insight in empirical studies; secondly, employ measures that can capture the degree of insight produced; thirdly, report on the specific operations carried out by the therapists in bringing about the development of insight and fourthly, provide validating material showing that insight has been developed. Such issues remain valid and have been reiterated in subsequent reviews (Crits-Christoph *et al.*, 1993). Clearly, however, one of the major difficulties identified concerns the translation of what is obviously a complex concept into an operational definition of insight that can capture and measure at least some of its constituents. As in other clinical areas, a number of different approaches have been taken and, correspondingly, this is likely to have contributed to the mixed ensuing results. Some of the early studies, for example, define insight in terms of the *congruence* between patient views of themselves and views held by others, with the assumption that 'others' hold the 'correct' views (Dymond, 1948; Feldman & Bullock, 1955; Mann & Mann, 1959). Similar methods have been adopted in the assessment of insight in patients with organic brain disorders (Chapters 4 and 5) but, in the psychodynamic field, this raises particular questions concerning the 'depth' of self-knowledge that can be assessed in this way.

Another approach to assess insight has been the use of patients' appraisals of specific vignettes (Sargent, 1953; Tolor & Reznikoff, 1960). In the method developed by Tolor and Reznikoff (1960), for example, 27 hypothetical situations depicting the use of common defence mechanisms were constructed. For each situation, four possible explanatory statements were provided and ranked according to the degree of 'insight' they were thought to represent. The test was given to a sample of 68 inpatients with various psychiatric diagnoses (schizophrenia, neurosis, personality disorder, etc.) and validated by comparing with independent insight ratings of patients taken by psychiatrists/psychologists involved in the patients' care. The authors subsequently reported that patients showed less insight on this test than untrained nurses who in turn showed less insight than trained nurses. The test was also used by Roback and Abramowitz (1979), who found that schizophrenic patients scoring higher, were rated by hospital staff as better adjusted behaviourally though more distressed subjectively. Interestingly, the use of 'vignettes' involving patients making judgements on hypothetical scenes has been used more recently as an approach to assess insight in general psychiatry (McEvoy *et al.*, 1993b; Chung *et al.*, 1997; Startup, 1997). The main problem with such an approach, however, rests with its assumption that the ability to understand a clinical picture presented, or the motivations of others as depicted by it, is equivalent or dependent on insight into one's self. As was seen above, many writers make an explicit distinction between knowledge of self and knowledge of others.

The most common systematic approach taken to assessing insight, particularly more recently, has been the use of observer ratings generally in the form of judgements based on patients' statements within psychoanalytic sessions which have been taped and transcribed. Various measures have been developed (Roback, 1972; Morgan *et al.*, 1982; Gedo & Schaffer, 1989; O'Connor *et al.*, 1994; Grenyer & Luborsky, 1996). Crits-Christoph *et al.* (1993) reviewing some of these methods point out that although in general inter-rater reliability is much better, the frequent lack of an operationalised definition of insight on which raters can base their judgements raises questions concerning validity. The main problem with these approaches is practical in that they tend to be cumbersome and time consuming as they depend on transcription of taped analytic sessions, and the coding and interpreting of individual statements. In addition, as Kivlighan *et al.* (2000) point out, insight may develop over a longer time frame than that captured by single client utterances. Some researchers have used ratings of insight provided by the therapists themselves (Gelso *et al.*, 1991; 1997) which has been more practically convenient but raises problems of reliability (as well as biases) since therapists only rate their own patients. In addition, the global ratings of such methods make it difficult to specify which aspects of patients' utterances or behaviours have contributed to the rating. Interestingly, Grenyer and Luborsky (1996) found no association between insight as assessed by a global judgement on the part of an observer (and by the therapist) and their Mastery Scale which incorporated assessment of insight within its complex rating system. They suggested that it was the difference between assessing a complex concept such as insight on the basis of a global judgement compared with its assessment in a specific structured way with reference to individual statements. The Insight Rating Scale as used by Morgan *et al.* (1982) is based on the definition of emotional insight as proposed by Reid and Finesinger (1952). It includes nine categories of behaviours (e.g. patient is able to relate present events to past events, patient recognises particular behaviours as indications of defensiveness or resistance, etc.) each of which are rated on a 10-point Likert scale and judged from transcripts of analytic sessions. The scale was found to have good inter-rater reliability and internal consistency. Increasingly sophisticated methods in terms of systematically assessing insight (and other factors important in psychoanalytic and cognitive-behavioural therapies) on the basis of transcribed statements (and their contexts) with specific guidance for clinical judgement have since been developed, e.g. Core Conflictual Relationship Theme (CCRT) (Crits-Christoph et al., 1993) or the Therapeutic Focus on Action and Insight (TFAI) (Samoilov et al., 2000).

Results of studies exploring the role of insight in psychoanalytic therapies including comparative studies with other 'curative' factors as well as with other psychotherapies have been mixed. Earlier studies reported very little role for insight as a therapeutic factor. For example, no relationship was found between levels of insight and outcome (in terms of individual adjustment) in subjects engaged in three different group experiences (Mann & Mann, 1959). Another study found that interaction group therapy (i.e. group treatment focused on inter-patient verbal communication and relations with no reference to psychological problems or personal difficulties) was more effective in producing improvement than insight-oriented group therapy in 'mostly schizophrenic' hospital in-patients (Coons, 1957). Individual systematic desensitisation was reported as determining more significant and lasting reduction in maladaptive anxiety than individual insight-oriented psychotherapy in undergraduate students with interpersonal performance anxiety (Paul, 1967). Reinforcement therapy (i.e. adaptive behaviours reinforced by various rewards) resulted in more significant improvement (hospital adjustment scale) in chronic schizophrenic patients than therapy promoting insight-interpretative statements and fostering of transference (Hartlage, 1970). Bogetto and Ladu (1989) reported symptomatic improvement both in patients receiving psychoanalytic psychotherapy and in those receiving psychopharmacological treatment although patients undergoing psychotherapy exhibited more insight. None of these studies, therefore, showed any significant role for insight in determining clinical outcome. However, all these studies are limited by the sorts of methodological problems as detailed above by Roback (1971; 1974). Thus, insight tends not to be well defined and it is not clear from the reports if patients receiving the different forms of insight-oriented therapy actually attained insight nor how insight was measured, etc.

Some studies have suggested that insight-oriented psychotherapies are likely to benefit only some individuals and sought to determine factors which might predict good response (Abramowitz & Abramowitz, 1974; Persson & Alström, 1983; 1984) but again findings are mixed and similar methodological problems apply. Reviewing outcomes between insight-oriented and other forms of psychotherapies, Luborsky et al. (1993) conclude that whilst insight-oriented psychotherapy seems to result in significant change in most patients, other treatments appear to obtain similar effects in relation to outcome. In other words, the specific role of insight remains unclear.

More recently, studies employing specifically defined and systematic methods of assessing insight have also yielded variable results. Some studies suggest that patients' insight seems to develop linearly as therapy proceeds (Gedo & Schaffer, 1989; Grenyer & Luborsky, 1996; Kivlighan *et al.*, 2000). Others report that patients' insight seems to follow a quadratic curve during the course of therapy, i.e. higher insight found at the beginning and end of treatment with a reduction in insight apparent during the middle of treatment (O'Connor *et al.*, 1994). The Kivlighan *et al.* (2000) study also found an association between higher insight and a greater reduction of complaints in 12 clients undergoing psychoanalytic psychotherapy. Other studies, however, have not found such a specific relationship between insight and outcome. In fact, most studies seem to suggest that it is the combination or interaction of insight and other factors that seems to determine positive outcome. For example, in the study by Morgan *et al.* (1982), patients' perceptions of the therapeutic relationship with their analysts were predictive of positive outcome. Although patients' insight correlated with the measures of therapeutic alliance, insight on its own did not predict outcome. Similarly, other studies have specified the combination of insight with other factors such as interaction (Roback, 1972), transference (Gelso *et al.*, 1991; 1997) or 'mastery' (i.e. emotional self-control as well as self-understanding) (Grenyer & Luborsky, 1996) as being associated with improved outcome.

2.2.3 Summary

It can be seen that a range of views are held concerning the definition of insight and approaches taken to its classification and to its empirical assessment. What is apparent from the various conceptualisations, however, is that psychoanalytic insight, in its broad sense, and particularly in comparison with conceptualisations of insight in other disciplines, emerges as a specially complex phenomenon. This complexity stands out because it relates not only to the content of the concept itself but also to its singular position within the structure of the psychoanalytic discipline. Furthermore, these two aspects of psychoanalytic insight are inextricably linked. As far as the content of the concept is concerned, its striking feature relates to the depth of knowledge that is invoked. This depth is apparent in two aspects relating to the concept. Firstly, it refers to a self-knowledge that is beyond 'normal' awareness or self-observation but reaches preconscious and unconscious mental states. This immediately raises complex problems relating to the epistemology of such unconscious mental processes. Thus, insight in the Gestalt and cognitive fields involves knowledge of problem solutions that are more or less directly verifiable. Insight in general psychiatry (Chapter 3) and in neurological states (Chapters 4 and 5) involves knowledge of illness/disability that is inferred from patients' verbal utterances which are subsequently matched with professionals' judgements of illness. In these other conceptualisations of insight, the validity of the knowledge that can be determined, in terms of its extent, its limitations and underlying assumptions, is more easily delineated (at least in theory). Knowledge of unconscious mental processes, in contrast, presents special difficulties in this regard. The most obvious one concerns the question of validity or truth, i.e. to what extent can knowledge of unconscious mental processes as presented in the understanding and acceptance of interpretations be considered correct? And, what does 'correct' mean in this context? Some writers, for example, insist that interpretations must be 'correct' (Bibring, 1954; Blum, 1979; 1992; Segal, 1991) and others claim that this is not necessary (Reid & Finesinger, 1952; Roback, 1974). At any rate, this issue raises major difficulties and has to some extent contributed to the circularity alluded to previously with respect to the relationship between insight and change. In other words, it is generally assumed that when an individual attains some degree of insight, this knowledge becomes integrated within the person's ego or personality such that the individual experiences some form of change – variously described in terms of subjective, intrapsychic, clinical, etc. At the same time, however, it is on the basis of the change itself that the individual is said to have attained insight.

Secondly, the depth characterising psychoanalytic insight is also apparent in the way in which the knowledge is attained. As writers have attempted to define in various ways, whether termed mutative, emotional, interpretative or ostensive insight, the emphasis has been on the individual somehow experiencing directly within him/herself this knowledge. This experience is clearly more than the 'Aha' experience described in the Gestalt literature for it refers to an experience that involves understanding of unconscious material that can be related to the present and hence the resulting reorganisation/restructuring reaches depths or dimensions that are not considered in Gestalt psychology.

In addition, the concept of psychoanalytic insight occupies a central and integral position within the psychoanalytic discipline which contributes to the special complexity surrounding psychoanalytic insight. This is evident from the role insight has played in the development of, the goals set, and the methods employed by the discipline. In particular, in the case of the latter, the unique dialectic within the patient–analyst relationship stands out as the distinctive element that serves to both deepen the concept of insight and at the same time intrinsically relates to the structure of the psychoanalytic discipline itself.

This complexity surrounding the conceptualisation of psychoanalytic insight has undoubtedly contributed to the limited empirical research in this area. Major difficulties arise in attempting to operationalise a concept that contains such elusive components as unconscious material and experiential elements. In addition, attempting to separate insight from other analytic concepts including the 'real' and the 'analytic' attitudes/actions of the analyst and the interaction itself between patient and analyst raise further empirical problems. Hence, results of empirical studies exploring the role of insight in promoting change are variable and the specific role of insight remains to be determined.

2.3 Conclusion

The conceptualisations of insight from the particular perspectives of Gestalt, cognitive and psychoanalytic psychological schools of thought, whilst sharing several similarities, are also profoundly different. Superficial similarities can be recognised from some of the terminology used in common such as 'restructuring' or 'reorganisation', albeit, that these terms refer predominantly to external events in the case of the Gestalt and cognitive psychologies, and to internal events in the case of psychoanalytic psychologies. In addition, some similarities have also been identified in a few empirical approaches based on a shared conception of insight as an 'event' culminating from various postulated stages (framed either in terms of mental preparation/incubation or 'working through').

Crucial differences emerge, however, between the conceptualisations of insight as developed from the various psychological perspectives. As was seen, the Gestalt and cognitive notion of insight as a specific discrete and sudden phenomenon contrasts strongly from the ongoing, limitless process conceived by the psychoanalytic school. The most obvious difference, however, concerns the relational aspect of insight in the two broad schools of thought. Thus, insight, in Gestalt and cognitive psychology refers to a specific form of knowledge or understanding in relation to a particular problem *outside* the individual. The problem may be restructured such that a solution is understood and experienced by the individual, but that understanding refers to the outside problem. Insight in psychoanalytic psychology, on the other hand, refers to a specific form of knowledge or understanding in relation to a particular state or problem *within* the individual. Understanding the self, i.e. one's conscious and unconscious mental processes, results in the restructuring of the psyche. Whatever way knowledge or understanding is framed, clearly, there are significant differences between the sorts of knowledge involved in relation to the external world and the sorts of knowledge involved in relation to the self. These differences are likewise reflected in the empirical evaluation (and determination) of insight in relation to the different disciplines.

In addition to differences in conceptualisations of insight between the psychological disciplines, there are differences apparent within the individual disciplines, in terms of views on specific definitions, underlying processes, importance of insight in the context of other mental processes, empirical approaches taken to its assessment and relationship to external factors. As in other areas, such differences are likely to reflect the inherent complexities surrounding the concept of insight as a form of knowledge irrespective of the framework in which this is embedded.

The psychological perspectives on insight are important to consider because they have been and continue to be influential in conceptualisations of insight in clinical psychiatry. The Gestalt and cognitive psychology views have been particularly important in relation to much of the work on insight and awareness in organic brain syndromes such as dementias especially in terms of some of the empirical approaches taken to assess awareness and implicit awareness (Chapters 4 and 5). Crucially, the role of metacognitions in determining insight is different when applied to cognitive psychology problems than when applied to clinical practice, i.e. in eliciting insight in neurological conditions. This carries implications for how insight is understood and differentiated in these areas. Psychoanalytic psychology views were inherent to some of the earlier empirical studies on insight in psychiatry at a time when this school of psychology was particularly dominant within clinical psychiatry as a discipline. As the disciplines diverged, psychoanalytic views on the nature of insight as a deep knowledge of unconscious mental processes have persisted in various forms. The usage of the concept of denial, for example, prevalent in studies on insight both in general psychiatry and in organic brain syndromes, refers specifically to the activity of unconscious mental processes to which an individual has no access.

3

Insight in clinical psychiatry: empirical studies

Until relatively recently, there has been little interest in the empirical exploration of insight in clinical psychiatry. However, over the last 10–15 years, increasing numbers of studies have focused on this area. Such studies have, predominantly, set out to examine the relationship between patients' insight and clinical variables, such as prognosis (McEvoy et al., 1989a; Amador et al., 1993), treatment compliance (e.g. Bartkó et al., 1988; Buchanan, 1992; Cuffel et al., 1996; Mutsatsa et al., 2003) and severity of psychopathology (e.g. McEvoy et al., 1989b; Amador et al., 1993; 1994; Carroll et al., 1999; Goldberg et al., 2001; Drake et al., 2004), and have concentrated mainly on examining this in patients with psychoses (Amador & David, 1998). More recently, a number of studies have explored the relationship between patients' insight and neuropsychological impairment (e.g. Young et al., 1993; 1998; Cuesta & Peralta, 1994; Lysaker et al., 1994; 1998a; 2002; Marks et al., 2000; McCabe et al., 2002; Mintz et al., 2004) and, indeed, structural brain lesions as assessed, e.g. by magnetic resonance imaging (MRI) (Takai et al., 1992; Flashman et al., 2001; Rossell et al., 2003). Much of this work has yielded, as will be shown in this chapter, somewhat mixed and inconsistent results. Consequently, the relationship between patients' insight and various clinical variables remains unclear (Marková & Berrios, 1995a, b). Various measures to assess insight have been developed (e.g. McEvoy et al., 1989b; David, 1990; Amador et al., 1991; Marková et al., 2003), suggesting that perhaps they capture different aspects of insight and this might contribute to some of the variability in results.

This chapter reviews the empirical work carried out in this area and focuses on identifying and defining some of the general and specific difficulties inherent to the clinical exploration of insight. Firstly, the different definitions of and approaches to assess insight in the various studies will be examined. Secondly, the results of studies exploring the relationship between patients' insight, and clinical and socio-demographic variables will be reviewed and discussed in the context of the conceptual and methodological problems of exploring patients' insight empirically.

3.1 Definitions of insight and methods of assessment

One of the most striking issues emerging from review of empirical work on insight is the absence of a consistent definition of insight and means by which it is assessed. In fact, there are two separate problems inherent to this issue. First, and obvious, is the variability itself in definitions of insight and methods of insight assessment, which clearly carries implications for making meaningful comparisons between studies. However, second is also the question of the extent to which a particular insight measure reflects the definition or concept of insight on which it is based. This problem more specifically has to do with the difficulties in translating from a complex concept to a measure that can capture the identified components in a clinical form and hence raises different sorts of issues. In general, methods of assessing insight can be broadly divided into those involving (i) categorical, and (ii) continuous approaches.

3.1.1 Categorical approaches to exploring insight

Most of the earlier empirical studies assessing the insight in patients with mental illness use categorical approaches, dividing patients into those with and without insight, and those with some or partial insight. The numbers of categories vary from a simple insight/no insight division (e.g. Van Putten *et al.*, 1976) to several categories designed to capture a hypothetically determined progressively graded amount of insight (e.g. Linn, 1965). Categorical measures are useful in allowing comparisons to be made between individuals on broadly defined characteristics but there are two main disadvantages with such approaches. Firstly, the distinctions between different categories are often difficult to determine (Eskey, 1958; Heinrichs *et al.*, 1985; Bartkó *et al.*, 1988, Dittman & Schüttler, 1990) hence casting some doubt on their reliability. On the other hand, some categorical approaches to insight assessment, as well as to general psychopathology evaluation, try to counter this problem by providing relatively specific criteria to help determine the appropriate category (e.g. insight items 104 and 105 on the Present State Examination, PSE (Wing *et al.*, 1974)). Secondly, there is the problem concerning the meaning that can be inferred from categorical descriptions. This incorporates a number of separate issues ranging from the general problems of categorisation and the relationship between categories when these are given ratings (e.g. is the 'distance' between categories 1 and 2 the same as between categories 2 and 3?) to the specific problems concerning how much of the underlying concept is actually captured by the categories. Examining some of the studies on insight illustrates a number of these problems.

The studies by Van Putten *et al.* (1976) and Heinrichs *et al.* (1985) both categorised patients into those with and without insight. The former study used a definition of insight according to which the patient acknowledged some degree of awareness of emotional illness. The latter defined insight as a recognition on the part of the patients that they were beginning to suffer a relapse of their psychotic illness. In both the studies, the fairly broad notions of insight are in fact reduced by the categorisation into all-or-none concepts and any detail concerning the type or degree of awareness or recognition is inevitably lost. Whitman and Duffey (1961) refer to the patient's 'perception of illness,' which again implies a fairly broad concept. Their translation of this into two categories, namely, patients expressing a functional reason for hospitalisation (e.g. feeling mixed up, having no control over thinking), and patients expressing a non-functional reason for hospitalisation (e.g. due to physical problem, being punished, etc.), however, suggests a narrower concept focused selectively on the attributed cause of hospitalisation rather than on subjective feelings of illness. Lin *et al.* (1979) defined insight as the patients' recognition of problems and the need for medical help. The authors translated this concept into a structured assessment based on three questions concerning whether patients thought they had (1) to be in hospital, (2) to see a doctor or (3) to see a psychiatrist. Patients were categorised as having insight if they answered affirmatively to any one of the questions. Again the relationship between the definition of insight and the assessment of insight is not straightforward here. Firstly, there is the assumption that recognition of existence of problems is equivalent to recognition of needing help. Secondly, affirmative answers to needing hospitalisation/doctors (without further exploration) may not necessarily reflect recognition of either having problems or needing medical help as they may include delusional ideas or motivational factors contributing to the responses. Clearly, there are difficulties in trying to capture the full content of definitions of insight into limited numbers of categories.

The concepts of insight held in these earlier studies vary in focus. Some define insight on the basis of acknowledged change in intellectual (Eskey, 1958) or emotional (Van Putten *et al.*, 1976) problems. Insight is thus conceived broadly and it is sufficient for patients to appreciate some disturbance in their mental states. Dittman and Schüttler (1990), using the term 'disease-consciousness', hold a similar concept of insight though slightly more focused in defining it in terms of some awareness of the existence of psychotic behaviour. They conceive this as a first step in gaining control over psychotic symptoms, thus contrasting with the more 'passive' conceptions of insight held by the early alienists (Chapter 1), and giving this a more active role in coping strategies employed by patients. Other definitions of insight demand more specifically the recognition of illness (Hankoff *et al.*, 1960; Wing *et al.*, 1974; Heinrichs *et al.*, 1985). In other words, patients need to not only acknowledge mental problems but also to interpret these as being the result of mental illness. More specificity still is required by definitions of insight which incorporate, in addition, the recognition by patients that they need medical intervention whether this is hospitalisation (Linn, 1965; Lin *et al.*, 1979) or treatment (Bartkó *et al.*, 1988) or both (Small *et al.*, 1964; 1965). Thus, a more precisely delineated conception of insight is held in these latter definitions, selectively focusing on the judgements of mental illness and the need for treatment.

From a different perspective, and based on Mayer-Gross' classification of patients' reactions to psychoses, Soskis and Bowers (1969) categorised patients into those with negative and positive attitudes towards their illness. In fact, they were conceiving a much wider notion, which contained attitudes towards insight (itself defined as understanding of problems) within a broader framework of patients' feelings about what was happening to them. However, it illustrates some of the difficulties inherent in the terminology itself when examining the meanings of insight and related notions. Thus, whilst e.g. Lewis (1934, (see Chapter 1)) used the term 'attitude' to refer to awareness and judgement made of the experience by the patient, Soskis and Bowers (1969), on the other hand, use this term to refer to value judgements; i.e. personal reactions to their judgements of their experiences. A similar approach (and likewise influenced by Mayer-Gross) was taken by Wciórka (1988) who categorised schizophrenic patients according to the type of attitude they held towards their illness. He conceptualised such attitudes broadly and distinguished between three types of composite attitudes: (1) *isolating*: where patients did not identify their illness with themselves, they evaluated it negatively and reacted in a non-reflective way; (2) *integrating*: where patients identified the illness with themselves, evaluated it positively and showed a reflective way of reacting to it and (3) *undecided*: where patients responded in a vague and incoherent fashion. Thus, these attitudes captured a wider complex of judgements and reactions to patients' experiences than some of the other notions relating to insight. Other different conceptualisations of insight, also emerging particularly in some of the earlier studies, relate to the psychoanalytic concept of denial, framed either in Freudian terms (O'Mahoney, 1982) or following Weinstein and Kahn's (1955) influential work (see Chapter 4) (Kahn & Fink, 1959). However, this clearly represents yet another conceptualisation of insight, incorporating the notion that understanding or knowledge is actively withheld from the self. Various empirical measures of denial following this line of thinking were devised and patients were generally categorised on the basis of scores on the rating scales (e.g. Kahn & Fink, 1959).

3.1.2 Continuous approaches to exploring insight

More recently, the other main approach to studying insight empirically has involved the conceptualisation of insight as a continuous process rather than the all-or-none or partial concept described above. Attempts have focused on assessing insight in a graded manner and using structured schedules in order to capture quantitatively in more detail some of the explicitly defined components of insight. However, some of the problems arising in relation to the categorical approaches to studying insight are equally pertinent here. Thus, there are differences in the definitions of insight between studies and likewise between the measures used to capture these; and, similarly, the extent to which such measures reflect the concept of insight held varies between the different studies.

McEvoy *et al.* (1989a, b, c) were amongst the first to develop a standardised questionnaire to assess insight in psychotic patients as a continuous process and defined it in terms of a correlation between the judgements made by patients and those made by clinicians. They maintained that, 'patients with insight judge some of their perceptual experiences, cognitive processes, emotions or behaviors to be pathological in a manner that is congruent with the judgement of involved mental health professionals, and that these patients believe that they need mental health treatment, at times including hospitalization and pharmacotherapy' (McEvoy *et al.*, 1989b, p. 43). Translating from this concept to an empirical measure, the '*Insight and Treatment Attitude Questionnaire*' (ITAQ), they focused on two aspects of their definition. Firstly, the questions in the measure relate specifically to patients' attitudes towards the need for hospital admission, for medication and for future follow-up. Secondly, the ratings of insight are based explicitly on the extent to which the patient is in agreement with the mental health professional concerning such attitudes. As a result, the empirical concept of insight captured by this measure emphasises more the (concordant) views patients have concerning their management rather than any detailed understanding they have concerning specific morbid experiences. The ITAQ (11 questions: score range from 0 (no insight) to 22 (maximum insight)) was validated against taped open interviews and was shown to correlate well with clinicians' judgements of patients' insight but it clearly reflects this specific and narrower empirical perspective borne out also by its single factor structure.

A broader conceptualisation of insight is offered by Greenfeld *et al.* (1989) following an exploratory study of patients' views concerning their psychotic experiences. They propose a model of insight consisting of five distinct and independent dimensions relating to: (1) views about symptoms, (2) views about the existence of an illness, (3) speculations about aetiology, (4) views about vulnerability to recurrence and (5) opinions about the value of treatment. Their semi-structured interview addresses each of these areas and insight is described qualitatively and separately in each domain. Thus, the conception of insight here, both in definitional terms and in its empirical evaluation, is focused more on patients' understanding of what is happening to them and what individual sense they are making of their experiences. As such, this represents a wider structure of insight. In empirical terms the qualitative capture of these components makes it difficult for 'ratings' of insight to be determined and hence comparisons between patients or patient groups are more cumbersome.

Other multidimensional models of insight have been proposed by David (1990) and Amador *et al.* (1991; 1993) and, in both, the emphasis lies in the translation from the models to structured empirical measures that rate insight quantitatively.

David (1990) conceives insight in psychotic patients as composed of three distinct though overlapping dimensions, namely: (1) recognition that one has a mental illness, (2) compliance with treatment and (3) the ability to relabel psychotic events (delusions and hallucinations) as pathological. Thus, the predominant focus in this definition lies in the acknowledgement of illness and needing treatment as well as a judgement concerning the morbid nature of delusions and hallucinations. This narrower and specific conception of insight lends itself to a more direct and quantifiable translation into an empirical measure. Hence, David's *Schedule for Assessing Insight* (SAI) reflects very closely the defined dimensions and patients are rated according to the extent to and/or frequency with which they accept they are ill, need treatment and judge their psychotic phenomena as real (total score range 0–14; (David, 1990)). Similarly, the *Insight Scale* (IS) devised by Birchwood *et al.* (1994) is an alternative direct translation from David's three-dimensional model of insight but in this case the empirical form is presented as a self-report measure (scoring 0–4 on each dimension, maximum: 12).

A more complex multidimensional model of insight is proposed by Amador *et al.* (1991). Based on an analysis of the variety of ways in which insight and related terms are used within the psychiatric literature, they conceive insight as comprising of (1) awareness of the signs, symptoms and consequences of illness, (2) general attribution about illness and specific attribution about symptoms and their consequences, (3) self-concept formation and (4) psychological defensiveness. Clearly, this represents a wider and more detailed structure of insight which incorporates comprehensively views on individual experiences and being ill, as well as including additional components relating to judgements about effects of such experiences and views relating more broadly to understanding of the self and the self's psychological processes. Recognising the practical difficulties in translating from such a wide and complex construct to an empirical measure of insight, Amador and Strauss (1993) narrowed this concept further to one comprising two salient components: (1) awareness of illness and (2) attribution regarding the illness. This concept thus picks up on the same dimensions or components identified by many of the earlier alienists and psychiatrists (e.g. Billod, 1870; Parant, 1888; Jaspers, 1948; see Chapter 1). The empirical measure based on this concept, the *Scale to Assess Unawareness of Mental Disorder* (SUMD) (Amador *et al.*, 1993) teases out in detail these components and this is reflected in the instrument consisting of 6 general items and 4 subscales from which 10 summary scores can be calculated (scores ranging from 1 to 5 on each item). The general items rate current and retrospective views around global awareness of mental disorder, awareness of achieved effects of medication and awareness of the social consequences of having a mental disorder. The four subscales (consisting of 17 items each) rate awareness and attribution of specific symptoms, signs and deficits (e.g. thought disorder, alogia and anhedonia, etc.), and again include separately both current and retrospective views. Thus, this is a comprehensive clinician-rated measure and, when used in its full form, places emphasis on the judgements made by patients concerning the nature of their individual symptoms. In turn, this is dependent on patients experiencing or showing the symptoms/signs in question. However, the authors make it clear that the items and scales can be used independently according to the need of investigators and in that sense the phenomena of insight elicited will necessarily vary depending on the scale/item employed. This is because the emphasis can change from rating a general awareness of being ill, and needing treatment to a more specific awareness and attribution of particular signs. For example, in their large study examining insight in 412 patients, Amador *et al.* (1994) used an abridged version of this instrument in which items relating to retrospective awareness and attribution regarding illness and symptoms were removed. Clearly, from a practical perspective it is not always possible to evaluate insight in the full detailed and comprehensive way demanded by the instrument but at the same time it is important to acknowledge that when the different components of the instrument are used independently they do not in themselves reflect the overall broad conceptualisation of insight that was the source of the empirical instrument but, instead, elicit different aspects of insight as originally defined. However, the structured nature of the measure allows for the different aspects of insight as captured by the independent components to be clearly defined and demarcated.

Partly to avoid some of the complexities involved in measuring insight with the above multidimensional models much of the empirical work on insight in psychiatry has used insight ratings taken from specific insight items within more general psychopathological assessments, such as the PSE (Wing *et al.*, 1974), the Manual for the Assessment and Documentation of Psychopathology (AMDP) (Guy & Ban, 1982) and particularly, the insight item from the Positive and Negative Syndrome Scale (PANSS) (Kay *et al.*, 1987). Within these structured psychopathological measures, insight is assessed along the same scales of increasing/decreasing severity as the other 'symptoms' or 'signs'. Thus, the 'lack of insight and judgement' item in the PANSS is rated from 1 (absent: no lack of judgement) to 7 (extreme: emphatic denial of past and present psychiatric illness), with intermediate ratings in between, in the same way that other 'symptoms' are rated as absent to extreme. Similarly, the insight item in the PSE is rated along a 4-point scale of severity (0 = full insight, 3 = denies condition entirely) in line with other 'symptoms' in the schedule. Such measures are useful in that they are practical and simpler to score but they lack the capacity to capture details of insight content and, despite the scoring systems, are basically categorical assessments of severity.

A different approach to evaluating patients' views about their illness was taken by Carsky *et al.* (1992) who devised a self-report scale. Rather than concentrating

on insight as such, they based their instrument on a concept spanning acknowledgement and denial of illness in hospitalised psychiatric patients. In this context,
they focused on a narrow definition of denial, specifically limiting this to a failure
to acknowledge: (1) having an illness or that the illness has a name or a cause,
(2) any need for hospitalisation and (3) that the illness has personal impact (Carsky
et al., 1992, p. 459). Their *Patient's Experience of Hospitalization* (PEH) is an
18-item (each item rated on a 4-point scale of severity or level of agreement with a
higher total score indicating greater denial) self-report scale which reflects predominantly views about being in hospital (e.g. whether this is necessary, whether
there can be gain from hospitalisation, etc.) and the degree to which the patient
worries about his/her condition. Thus, the focus of the concept, and reflected in
the empirical measure used, is less on the actual understanding patients have concerning their individual experiences and the sense they make of these but more on
their general responses or reactions to their situations, as well as their views on the
benefits of being in hospital.

Using the same concept but broadening it to some extent, Marks *et al.* (2000)
devised their *Self-Appraisal of Illness Questionnaire* (SAIQ) based closely on the
PEH but designed for use in community settings. Thus, again focusing on attitudes
towards illness rather than perception of experienced changes, the SAIQ is a
17-item self-report scale following the format of the PEH but substituting items
about hospitalisation with similar items relating to the need for treatment. A factor analysis of the SAIQ yielded three factors reflecting the specific foci of the concepts used, namely: (1) need for treatment, (2) worry about condition and (3)
presence/outcome of illness. Predictably, the authors found correlations between
the need for treatment and presence/outcome of illness subscales with specific
clinician-rated measures of insight including the abridged form of the SUMD
(Amador *et al.*, 1994). Interestingly, they found no correlation between their worry
subscale (items relating to patients worries about their condition) and clinician-
rated measures of insight indicating that perhaps different aspects of the concept
were being elicited. The authors themselves speculated that perhaps the worry
items, by picking up on patients' reactions or coping mechanisms, were addressing
components of insight that were not being captured by the other (clinician-rated)
measures of insight.

Our own work, also following a continuous approach to assessing insight,
developed a self-rating insight questionnaire designed to evaluate insight in
patients with psychoses (Marková & Berrios, 1992b; Marková *et al.*, 2003). Based
on Hamlyn's (1977) ideas on self-knowledge, as well as conceptual analysis of the
way in which insight was understood in the psychiatric literature, a broad concept
of insight was proposed as a sub-category of self-knowledge patients hold not only
about the disorder affecting them but also how the disorder affects their interaction

with the world (Marková & Berrios, 1992a, b; Marková & Berrios, 1995a, b). In other words, the concept here focuses on awareness of changes to the self (and how this affects perceptions of and interactions with one's world) in relation to the pathological state affecting the patient. In terms of conceiving insight as a continuous process, the issues behind this particular concept of insight were, firstly, to capture the intermediate stages of experienced change in the patient, i.e. before the judgement was reached (if ever) that the changes represented a particular mental illness and, secondly, to focus more on changes in perceptions of altered self. The empirical measure, the *Insight in Psychosis Questionnaire* (IPQ), translated from this broad concept of insight, consists of 30 items chosen on face validity grounds (clinical observation together with clinical descriptions (e.g. Conrad, 1958)), to reflect awareness of possible changes that individuals might experience during the course of a psychotic episode. Following piloting of the IPQ (Marková & Berrios, 1992b), some items were re-phrased, some were deleted (those relating to views about hospitalisation and taking medication) and the scoring was simplified to a dichotomous (agree/disagree) form, and the resultant measure was subsequently re-standardised (Marková *et al.*, 2003). Clearly, this measure is thus eliciting very different aspects of insight compared to most of the previous assessments where the focus was specifically on judgements of mental illness and judgements concerning the need for medication/treatment.

Finally, interesting approaches to assess insight have included the use of vignettes describing various pathological states (e.g. McEvoy *et al.*, 1993b; Chung *et al.*, 1997) and discrepancy measures, i.e. the difference in ratings made by patients and their relatives (e.g. Exner & Murillo, 1975; Taylor & Perkins, 1991; Dixon *et al.*, 1998). The latter are much less often used generally in psychiatry compared with empirical studies on insight in patients with neurological states (Chapters 4 and 5). In the case of vignettes, insight is determined according to views expressed by patients in relation to the content of the vignettes, e.g. the extent to which patients feel the vignettes resemble their own clinical states (McEvoy *et al.*, 1993b) or whether the contents represent mental disorders (Startup, 1997) or both (Chung *et al.*, 1997). Insight is thus assessed indirectly in that the phenomenon that is elicited is construed of judgements made in relation to third-person scenarios with or without further judgements made concerning any resemblance between such scenarios and patients' own subjective experiences. Similar issues to those raised in the review of insight measures used in psychoanalytic studies (Chapter 2) apply here. Thus, the aspects of insight captured by this type of assessment, where patients' judgements are demanded of external events, will necessarily be different from insight that focuses on judgements made concerning patients' views of themselves. The use of a vignette depicting an individual with psychotic symptoms given to a sample of the general population (Lam *et al.*,

1996) as well as in schizophrenic patients, relatives and the general public (Chung et al., 1997) raised another important issue in terms of conceptualising insight. Both the above studies reported a low recognition of mental illness and the need for treatment in general public subjects who were given the vignette. Indeed, recognition of illness and need for treatment was slightly higher (and hence insight in those terms better) in patients and relatives compared with the general public (Chung et al., 1997). This led the authors to highlight the need to consider patients' insight in the context of the background knowledge or understanding of the society and culture they lived in before attributing any impairment of insight to the psychotic process. Startup (1997) found no association between schizophrenic patients' insight as assessed by the ITAQ and their judgements' of others' mental disorder on the basis of vignettes suggesting that these different methods of assessing insight involved independent judgements. This is an important complicating factor in terms of conceptualising insight and illustrates the need to view insight as a multidimensional structure rather than solely as a symptom that can be related to a disease process (see Part II).

3.1.3 Summary of empirical assessments of insight

It has been shown that empirical studies in clinical psychiatry employ diverse methods to assess patients' insight, based on a range of definitions. It is worth reiterating some of these differences, which affect definitions, assessment methods and the relationship between them.

3.1.3.1 Definitions

As is evident, definitions of insight vary in terms of specificity, breadth, focus and complexity. Some studies define insight very specifically e.g. as the recognition of being mentally ill (Wing et al., 1974; Heinrichs et al., 1985) whereas other studies use more general definitions such as the recognition of some mental disturbance (Eskey, 1958; Van Putten et al., 1976). Some studies conceive insight narrowly in terms of considering views only about illness (Heinrichs et al., 1985; Dittman & Schüttler, 1990) whilst others broaden the concept to include a range of views about any experienced changes and about effects of the disturbance on the self and functioning (Greenfeld et al., 1989; Amador et al., 1991; Marková & Berrios, 1992a). The emphasis in the definitions varies in the studies with some focusing primarily on the acknowledgement of illness and/or the need for medical treatment (Lin et al., 1979; Bartkó et al., 1988; McEvoy et al., 1989b), and others focusing more on the sense patients are making of their experiences and the effects of these on themselves (Greenfeld et al., 1989; Marková & Berrios, 1992a; Marková et al., 2003). And, the complexity of the concepts varies in studies with some defining insight in fairly simple terms such as a judgement concerning what is happening to patients (Eskey, 1958; Wing *et al.*, 1974) whilst other studies propose more complex concepts which include a number of judgements or components relating to different aspects of their experiences (Greenfeld *et al.*, 1989; David, 1990; Amador *et al.*, 1991). Moreover, in all these respects, the level to which such definitions are delineated is also variable. For example, the individual components of the concept of insight in David (1990) and Amador *et al.* (1991) are clearly defined and demarcated. On the other hand, the broad concept of insight proposed in our work (Marková & Berrios, 1992a) lacks defined boundaries and, hence, the extent of knowledge or understanding patients are required to have concerning their condition and its effects in order to be deemed insightful is less clear.

3.1.3.2 Assessments

Assessment methods differ in a number of ways as well. Firstly, they differ in how closely they reflect the researchers' concept of insight. Where there does seem to be a close match between the original definition and the measure itself, then the same differences as described above, between the ways in which insight is defined, apply to the assessment methods themselves. Additionally, differences can be identified between the ways in which insight is captured and rated. Thus, the main difference lies between methods using a categorical approach to rate insight (Eskey, 1958; Small *et al.*, 1965; Van Putten *et al.*, 1976; Heinrichs *et al.*, 1985) and those using a continuous approach (McEvoy *et al.*, 1989; David, 1990; Marková and Berrios 1992b; Amador *et al.*, 1993). Categorical assessments are simpler to use and generally patients can be rated as having insight, not having insight or having partial insight according to the particular criteria employed. However, judgements are necessarily cruder in content and the anchor points between categories are often not clear. Continuous measures on the other hand tend to capture more specific information but vary in terms of the different components included in the measures as well as the particular focus (e.g. acknowledgement of illness or need for medication or awareness of effects, etc.). In addition, further differences exist between the methods using clinician rating of patients' insight (Greenfeld *et al.*, 1989; McEvoy *et al.*, 1989; David *et al.*, 1992; Amador *et al.*, 1993) and those using self-rating measures (Birchwood *et al.*, 1994; Marks *et al.*, 2000; Marková *et al.*, 2003). Thus the clinician ratings necessarily incorporate additional factors, which shape the clinician's judgements concerning patients' insight. The self-rating measures are more direct expressions of patients' views but do not allow for elaboration or explanation of answers. Similarly, methods using discrepancy measures involve assumptions concerning the judgements made by non-affected individuals and incorporate additional factors relevant to those whilst assessments using vignettes demand different types of judgements. These issues are explored in detail in Part II.

3.1.3.3 Implications

The differences in the conceptualisation of insight and in the measures devised to assess insight, that are clearly present in the studies detailed above, have important consequences. Firstly, they serve to highlight the difficulties in attempting to define in a practical sense what is a complex concept. Both the content and the limits or boundaries of the concept remain ill defined. Secondly, it is likely that, given such differences in definitions and approaches used to assess insight, different aspects of insight are elicited and rated in the various studies. This is an essential point as it means that comparisons between results of the studies will be problematic as it cannot be assumed that they are all capturing the same insight phenomenon. This is not to say that the insight measures are all eliciting completely different phenomena. Indeed, most of the studies, which have sought to correlate some of the insight measures have found generally modestly significant correlations between different insight assessments (e.g. David *et al.*, 1992; Sanz *et al.*, 1998; Francis & Penn, 2001) or different subscales/dimensions of the same insight measure (David *et al.*, 1992; Larøi *et al.*, 2000). However, some studies report more mixed results with modest correlations between only some subscales/dimensions of insight measures either with each other (Amador *et al.*, 1993; McCabe *et al.*, 2000) or with other insight assessments (Marks *et al.*, 2000). It is likely that whilst the various insight measures may be capturing something that is common to most of them, there will be, nevertheless, differences between them in the detail of the phenomena elicited. Further support for this claim comes from the finding that in a same study, different insight measures yield different results as far as relationship to clinical variables are concerned (David *et al.*, 1992; Cuesta *et al.*, 1998; Sanz *et al.*, 1998; Cuesta *et al.*, 2000). Furthermore, because, as was reviewed, differences between the insight assessments occur at more than the content level, then comparisons and generalisations between studies in terms of outcomes become more problematic and it is questionable whether stringent statistical methods such as meta-analysis (Mintz *et al.*, 2003) may be applied to summarise such studies in a meaningful way.

3.2 Relationship between insight and clinical and socio-demographic variables

The question then is what can the empirical studies on insight tell us about the nature of insight in patients with psychiatric disorders? The increased interest evident in exploring insight clinically seems to have arisen, in part, following observations that lack of insight is extremely prevalent in patients with psychiatric illnesses. Indeed, 'lack of insight' was described as the most frequent symptom of schizophrenia in the *Report of the International Pilot Study of Schizophrenia* (World Health

Organization, 1973). However, the basic question underpinning the empirical studies exploring insight in relation to patients' symptoms, illnesses and various socio-cultural and demographic variables, whether or not this is stated explicitly, is one concerning the *nature* of insight as a clinical phenomenon. This question can be reduced to some primary issues, namely: (i) is lack of insight in mental illness inherent to the mental disorder, i.e. a product of the disease process and hence to be considered as a 'symptom' in the same way as other illness features or (ii) can insight be considered a separate or independent mental phenomenon, one that can be affected by having a mental or other disorder, but also open to the internal and external influences that determine individual knowledge/beliefs. In effect, this basic issue is simply a reformulation of the question with which psychiatry has struggled since the notion of insight was conceived as an independent phenomenon (Chapter 1). In other words, is it possible for someone with a 'disordered' mind to have full awareness/insight of the disorder itself? In spite of numerous studies examining the relationship between insight and severity of the mental disorder or insight and cognitive impairment, it remains difficult to answer this basic question. As has already been seen, complexities around the definition and assessment of insight are an important factor in this. However, consequently, the relationship between insight and other clinical variables, such as prognosis, severity of psychopathology, treatment compliance, cognitive impairment, etc. remains unclear.

3.2.1 Insight and socio-demographic variables

Is the degree of insight held by an individual related to age, gender or education? To what extent might social and cultural factors contribute to the manifestation and indeed the elicitation of insight? Does the duration of mental illness, the age at which it developed have any relationship with the level of insight shown? These sorts of questions may be important to address when trying to explore the nature and determinants of insight into mental disorders. Whilst numerous studies have reported on the relationship between insight and socio-demographic variables, for most, this has not been the primary focus or aim of the study. This makes it difficult to obtain meaningful answers on the basis of existing work for two main reasons. Firstly, it means that most studies were not specifically designed to answer such questions and hence different methodologies might be required in order to do so. Secondly, as this issue has not been the primary aim of the study, it precludes initial or preliminary theoretical exploration of the structure of insight and consequent possible theoretical predictions concerning outcome. Any significant results could only be examined in a post-hoc fashion and explanations limited by the inherent biases of such methods. Bearing in mind these caveats, empirical studies reporting on these associations can be divided into those showing no correlations between insight and socio-demographic variables (Table 3.1), and those studies

Table 3.1 Studies reporting NO association between insight and socio-demographic variables

Study	Patients*	Insight assessment	Result
Heinrichs *et al.* (1985)	$n = 38$	Patients dichotomised according to case-note descriptions	No differences between patients with and without insight in relation to age, gender or socio-economic status
Greenfeld *et al.* (1989)	$n = 21$	Interview structured along defined dimensions	No correlation with demographic variables
David *et al.* (1992)	$n = 91$	SAI PSE: insight item	No correlation with age or gender
Takai *et al.* (1992)	$n = 57$	PSE: insight item	No correlations with socio-demographic variables
McEvoy *et al.* (1993b)	$n = 26$	ITAQ Clinical vignettes	No correlation with age of onset, chronicity or illness activity
Young *et al.* (1993)	$n = 31$	SUMD: abridged	No correlation with age, education and chronicity
Amador *et al.* (1994)	$n = 348$	SUMD: abridged	No correlation with age, gender and education
Cuesta and Peralta (1994)	$n = 40$	AMDP: three items (LII)	No correlation with age, gender and education
Lysaker and Bell (1994)	$n = 92$	PANSS: item G12	No correlation with age, gender, race, education, age at first hospitalisation, length of longest full-time job
Peralta and Cuesta (1994)	$n = 115$	SAI AMDP: three items (LII)	No correlation with age, gender and education
Vaz *et al.* (1994)	$n = 64$	ITAQ	No correlation with age of onset, education
Ghaemi *et al.* (1995)	$n = 28$	ITAQ	No correlation with socio-demographic variables
Lysaker and Bell (1995)	$n = 44$	PANSS: item G12	No correlation with age, years of education
Almeida *et al.* (1996)	$n = 40$	SAI PSE: insight item	No correlation with age, age of onset, duration of illness
Collins *et al.* (1997)	$n = 58$	SAI	No correlation with gender
Dickerson *et al.* (1997)	$n = 87$	PANSS: item G12	No correlation with age, gender, age of onset, duration of illness, years of education

Table 3.1 (*cont.*)

Study	Patients*	Insight assessment	Result
Lysaker *et al.* (1998b)	*n* = 101	SUMD: abridged	No differences between patients with and without insight in terms of their backgrounds
Peralta and Cuesta (1998)	*n* = 54	AMDP: three items (LII)	No correlation between socio-demographic variables and insight at admission, discharge or change in insight
Schwartz (1998a)	*n* = 64	PANSS: item G12	No correlation with age, total years of treatment
Larøi *et al.* (2000)	*n* = 21	SUMD	No correlation with age, gender, education and age at onset
Chen *et al.* (2001)	*n* = 80	SUMD: abridged	No correlation with age, education, illness duration
Schwartz (2001)	*n* = 223	SUMD	No correlation with age, gender, substance abuse
McCabe *et al.* (2002)	*n* = 89	SAI	No correlation with socio-demographic variables
Arduini *et al.* (2003)	*n* = 64	SUMD: abridged	No correlation with age, gender, years of education, duration of illness

* Diagnoses not specified here, since detailed in text and subsequent tables, but majority of patients diagnosed with psychotic disorder, mainly schizophrenia, also schizoaffective, bipolar, affective and mixed psychoses.

Abbreviations: AMDP-LII: Lack of Insight Index from three items of the *Manual for the Assessment and Documentation of Psychopathology*; ITAQ: Insight and Treatment Attitude Questionnaire; PANSS: Positive and Negative Syndrome Scale; PSE: Present State Examination; SAI: Schedule for Assessing Insight; SUMD: Scale to Assess Unawareness of Mental Disorder.

showing at least some correlation between insight and socio-demographic variables (Table 3.2).

As can be seen from the tables, the studies are fairly balanced in terms of their sizes and the types of insight assessments used. Overall, many more studies report no association between insight and socio-demographic variables though they range on the numbers and types of socio-demographic variables included in the correlations analysis.

In terms of the associations reported, there seems to be little consistency in the results. Neither gender nor age appear to be significantly relevant factors, while the

Table 3.2 Studies reporting some correlation between insight and socio-demographic variables

Study	Patients*	Insight assessment	Results
Linn (1965)	n = 593	Answers to questions about what patients believed was wrong with them	Increased duration of illness associated with reduced insight
Soskis and Bowers (1969)	n = 32	Standardised questionnaire on attitudes to psychosis	Women have more positive attitude to psychosis than men
Appelbaum et al. (1981)	n = 50	Standardised questionnaire: seven conceptual categories	Men have greater insight than women. Younger age is associated with better insight
Wciórka (1988)	n = 100	Structured questionnaire on attitudes to illness	Patients with negative, isolating attitudes had lower levels of education
Caracci et al. (1990)	n = 20	Awareness of psychiatric disorder dichotomised (present/absent). Awareness of involuntary movements (0–3 rating)	Increased duration of illness associated with reduced awareness of psychiatric disorder and reduced awareness of involuntary movements
Taylor and Perkins (1991)	n = 30	1. Question whether they have mental health problem 2. Discrepancy between patients and staff on Awareness of Disabilities Scale	Poor insight associated with more previous hospital admissions, female patients, older age
Amador et al. (1993)	n = 43	SUMD	Age at first psychiatric evaluation associated with insight (greater retrospective awareness of achieved effects of medication associated with earlier age of psychiatric contact)
David et al. (1995)	n = 150	PSE item 104	Patients with better insight had parents from socio-economic classes I and II
Kemp and Lambert (1995)	n = 29	SUMD: abbreviated	Women showed increased insight (attribution of past illness) over course of hospital admission
Cuffel et al. (1996)	n = 89	Awareness of illness interview (recognition of mental illness and need for psychiatric treatment)	Women showed reduced awareness. Use of illicit drugs associated with increased awareness

Table 3.2 (*cont.*)

Study	Patients*	Insight assessment	Results
Fennig *et al.* (1996)	n = 189	Insight item from Hamilton Depression Rating Scale	Being married was associated with better insight. (No correlation with age, gender, ethnicity, etc.)
Johnson and Orrell (1996)	n = 318	Assessments based on case-note descriptions	Caucasian British patients rated as having more insight than other ethnic groups
MacPherson *et al.* (1996)	n = 64	SAI	Insight correlated with educational attainment
Kim *et al.* (1997)	n = 63	SAI	Impaired insight associated with later age of onset of illness
Lysaker *et al.* (1998a)	n = 81	PANSS: item G12	Increased insight associated with earlier age of first hospitalisation
Sanz *et al.* (1998)	n = 33	ITAQ SAI (and SAI-E) IPQ (preliminary) PANSS: item G12	Non-illicit drug use associated with higher levels of insight. Years of education correlated with insight (IPQ only)
Lysaker *et al.* (1999)	n = 74	PANSS: item G12	Patients with impaired insight were significantly older
Marks *et al.* (2000)	n = 59	SAIQ	Increased duration of illness associated with impaired insight
Weiler *et al.* (2000)	n = 187	ITAQ	No correlation with demographics except for bipolar patients in whom age at first admission associated with insight
White *et al.* (2000)	n = 150	SAI	Ethnicity not associated with insight but being born outside the UK associated with reduced insight. Insight not associated with education, strength of religious beliefs, social class, illicit drug use
Goldberg *et al.* (2001)	n = 211	PANSS: item G12	Association between insight and race: white patients rated greater insight than black patients. Association between current substance abuse and insight

Table 3.2 (*cont.*)

Study	Patients*	Insight assessment	Results
Pyne *et al.* (2001)	*n* – 177	Dichotomised according to answer whether patients believed they had a mental illness.	Duration of illness and younger age correlated with reduced insight in outpatients.

* Diagnoses not specified here, since detailed in text and subsequent tables, but majority of patients diagnosed with psychotic disorder, mainly schizophrenia, also schizoaffective, bipolar, affective and mixed psychoses.

Abbreviations: IPQ: Insight in Psychosis Questionnaire; ITAQ: Insight and Treatment Attitude Questionnaire; PANSS: Positive and Negative Syndrome Scale; PSE: Present State Examination; SAI: Schedule for Assessing Insight; SAI-E: Schedule for Assessing Insight – Expanded version; SAIQ: Self-Appraisal of Illness Questionnaire; SUMD: Scale to Assess Unawareness of Mental Disorder.

few studies that find associations, yield conflicting results (Table 3.2). Age at first admission to hospital was found in four studies to be related to insight (Kim *et al.*, 1997; Lysaker *et al.*, 1998a; Weiler *et al.*, 2000) or an aspect of insight (Amador *et al.*, 1993) with increased insight being associated with earlier age of hospital admission. Interestingly, in a larger study using the abbreviated version of the SUMD (which did not include ratings of retrospective awareness), this latter finding was not replicated (Amador *et al.*, 1994). Duration of illness was also found to be associated with insight in three studies with increasing length of illness correlating with poorer insight (Linn, 1965; Caracci *et al.*, 1990; Marks *et al.*, 2000). Pyne *et al.* (2001), on the other hand, only found an association between duration of illness and insight in their outpatients as opposed to their inpatients. Furthermore, their reported association was in the opposite direction from the previous studies in that patients with shorter duration of illness seemed to show poorer insight. Owing to the methodological issues raised earlier, it is difficult to draw very much from these results and there may be effects from various confounding factors, e.g. as severity of illness itself. A few studies reported a significant correlation between insight and education (MacPherson *et al.*, 1996; Rossell *et al.*, 2003) whilst Sanz *et al.* (1998), in their study comparing the use of several insight measures, found that insight was related to education only when insight was assessed with the IPQ instrument. The study by David *et al.* (1995), appears to be the sole to report a positive association between insight and higher social class.

Of interest are the studies that have started to explore the relationship between insight and ethnicity. Conducting a case-note study with the specific aim of examining the relationship between ethnicity and patients' insight, Johnson and Orrell (1996) found that white British patients were rated as having significantly more insight than other ethnic groups. Though, as the authors point out, the design of the study did not permit administration of standardised or detailed assessments of insight, nor could consideration be taken of interacting variables such as severity of psychopathology. Two further prospective studies found similar results: the study by White *et al.* (2000) did not find a specific relationship between insight and ethnicity but showed that being born outside the UK was associated with reduced insight. Goldberg *et al.* (2001) found that white patients were rated as having greater insight than black patients. On the other hand, Fennig *et al.* (1996) found no association between insight in patients presenting with first admission for psychosis and ethnicity. The question thus remains as to the nature of such differences between insight in different cultures, and to what extent they might reflect true differences in insight and to what extent socio-cultural biases are contributing. Whilst not directly assessing insight, Townsend (1975), in a study designed to explore cultural differences in concepts of mental illness, examined the attitudes of German psychiatric inpatients ($n = 112$) and American psychiatric inpatients ($n = 110$). He found significant differences in the way that mental disorders were conceived. The German patient group had a more biological/organic view of mental disorders on which they had little individual control. On the other hand, the American patient group had a more behavioural perspective towards mental illness in regards to which they felt they were able to exert some control. Differences in the ways in which mental disorders are conceived in general are likely to contribute to the views and understanding individuals will develop when affected.

3.2.2 Insight and past psychiatric illness

Does insight increase with experience of more episodes of illness? Do patients who have had more hospital admissions develop more insight into their illness and how this affects them? Or, are frequent hospital admissions an indicator of more severe illness and have little direct relationship with patients' insight? Once again, most studies have not been designed to answer those questions although many report on the correlation between insight and numbers of past hospital admissions (Table 3.3).

It is evident that most studies report no relationship between levels of insight and the numbers of previous hospital admissions. In the studies that do report some association, then it is generally in the direction of increased insight being associated with increased hospital admissions (Takai *et al.*, 1992; Amador *et al.*, 1993; Peralta & Cuesta, 1994; Ghaemi *et al.*, 1996). However, some authors also report the opposite finding with poor insight associated with more hospital admissions (Taylor & Perkins, 1991; Moore *et al.*, 1999). A more complicated relationship is described by Lysaker *et al.* (2003) who found that poor insight was associated with more hospital admissions only in patients with poor cognition (on the Wisconsin Card Sorting Test (WCST)) but not in patients with average cognitive function. Given the methodological issues involved, it is not really possible to interpret such results at this stage though various questions may be raised in the light of these findings. For example,

Table 3.3 Studies reporting on associations between insight and previous hospital admissions

Study	Patients*	Insight assessment	Result
Appelbaum et al. (1981)	n = 50	Standardised questionnaire: seven conceptual categories	No correlation with numbers of past admissions
Heinrichs et al. (1985)	n = 38	Patients dichotomised according to case-note descriptions	No correlation with numbers of past admissions
Greenfeld et al. (1989)	n = 21	Interview structured along defined dimensions	More previous hospital admissions associated with less insight (along one dimension)
McEvoy et al. (1989b)	n = 52	ITAQ	No correlation with numbers of past admissions
Taylor and Perkins (1991)	n = 30	1. Question whether have mental health problem 2. Discrepancy between patients and staff on Awareness of Disabilities Scale	More previous hospital admissions associated with less insight
David et al. (1992)	n = 91	SAI PSE: insight item	No correlation with numbers of past admissions
Takai et al. (1992)	n = 57	PSE: insight item	More previous hospital admissions associated with increased insight
Amador et al. (1993)	n = 43	SUMD	Moderate correlation between numbers of past hospital admissions and aspects of insight
McEvoy et al. (1993b)	n = 26	ITAQ Clinical vignettes	No correlation with numbers of past admissions
Young et al. (1993)	n = 31	SUMD: abridged	No correlation with numbers of past admissions
Amador et al. (1994)	n = 348	SUMD: abridged	No correlation with numbers of past admissions
Lysaker and Bell (1994)	n = 92	PANSS: item G12	No correlation with numbers of past admissions
Peralta and Cuesta (1994)	n = 115	SAI AMDP: three items (LII)	More past hospital admissions associated with increased insight

Table 3.3 (*cont.*)

Study	Patients*	Insight assessment	Result
Ghaemi *et al.* (1995)	$n = 28$	ITAQ	No correlation with numbers of past admissions
Lysaker and Bell (1995)	$n = 44$	PANSS: item G12	No correlation between numbers of past admissions and changes in insight
Ghaemi *et al.* (1996)	$n = 16$	ITAQ	More past hospital admissions associated with increased insight
Dickerson *et al.* (1997)	$n = 87$	PANSS: item G12	No correlation with numbers of past admissions
Lysaker *et al.* (1998a)	$n = 81$	PANSS: item G12	No correlation with numbers of past admissions
Lysaker *et al.* (1998b)	$n = 101$	SUMD: abridged	No correlation with numbers of past admissions
Sanz *et al.* (1998)	$n = 33$	ITAQ SAI (and SAI-E) IPQ (preliminary) PANSS: item G12	Correlation between numbers of past admissions and insight only significant with IPQ
Moore *et al.* (1999)	$n = 46$	SUMD	Poor insight correlated with more past admissions
Larøi *et al.* (2000)	$n = 21$	SUMD	No correlation with numbers of past admissions
White *et al.* (2000)	$n = 150$	SAI	Weak association between increasing insight and increased numbers of past admissions
Goldberg *et al.* (2001)	$n = 211$	PANSS: item G12	No correlation with numbers of past admissions
Pyne *et al.* (2001)	$n = 177$	Dichotomised according to answer whether patients believed they had a mental illness	Inpatients: reduced insight associated with increased numbers of past admissions. Outpatients: reduced insight associated with reduced numbers of past admissions

* Diagnoses not specified here, since detailed in text and subsequent tables, but majority of patients diagnosed with psychotic disorder, mainly schizophrenia, also schizoaffective, bipolar, affective and mixed psychoses.

Abbreviations: IPQ: Insight in Psychosis Questionnaire; ITAQ: Insight and Treatment Attitude Questionnaire; PANSS: Positive and Negative Syndrome Scale; PSE: Present State Examination; SAI: Schedule for Assessing Insight; SAI-E: Schedule for Assessing Insight – Expanded version; SUMD: Scale to Assess Unawareness of Mental Disorder.

do patients who show greater insight perhaps seek medical help more frequently and are more willing to accept hospital admissions? Some indirect support could be given to this view by the results of studies showing that informal patients show greater insight than patients admitted involuntarily (McEvoy *et al.*, 1989c; David *et al.*, 1992; Ghaemi *et al.*, 1995; Upthegrove *et al.*, 2002). On the other hand, the study by Pyne *et al.* (2001) suggests a more complicated association between patients' insight and hospital admissions showing that a significant relationship was only evident in outpatients whereas inpatients at the time of the study showed the opposite association. Results also point to the possibility that perhaps some aspects of insight might be more relevant in the association between hospital admissions than others (Greenfeld *et al.*, 1989; Amador *et al.*, 1993; Sanz *et al.*, 1998). An interesting recent study explored the question in a different way by comparing insight (SUMD) in first episode psychosis patients ($n = 144$) with insight in multiple episode psychosis patients ($n = 312$) (Thompson *et al.*, 2001). They found that a significantly greater proportion of multiple episode psychotic patients were aware of having a mental disorder and were aware of the effects of medication than first episode psychosis patients. The researchers thus suggested that over time patients might show increased insight into their illness as they learn from their experiences, become less defensive and become adept at using medical terms. They did caution, however, that using medical terms may not necessarily reflect true insight. The question of the contribution made by past experience towards the attainment of insight therefore remains to be answered. Empirical work in this field is additionally difficult because of the problems involved in trying to control for the multitude of variables likely to be important in the development of insight.

3.2.3 Insight and prognosis

Is it important for patients to have good insight? Does having good insight into one's illness relate to a better or worse prognosis? Or, is insight perhaps independent of the condition itself and related more to individual and/or socio-cultural factors? Again these are the sorts of questions that need to be asked in order to determine more clearly the nature of insight as a clinical phenomenon, and its significance and relationship with clinical and other factors. There have been few studies specifically reporting on the association between insight and prognosis and, in particular, fewer prospective studies. One of the additional difficulties in exploring insight in regards to this area relates to the assessment of prognosis itself, i.e., how can this be best evaluated? For example, some studies use the number of subsequent re-hospitalisations over a time period as an indicator whilst others use duration of an index admission or response to medication, etc. Clearly, however, these variables are assessing quite different things in relation to the patient's prognosis (e.g. short term versus long term, hospitalisation versus response to management, etc.), which complicates things further when it comes to making comparisons between studies (Table 3.4).

Table 3.4 Studies reporting on association between insight and clinical outcome

Study	Patients*	Insight assessment	Clinical outcome	Results
Eskey (1958)	$n = 300$	Categorised on basis of mental state examination (insight, partial insight, no insight)	Duration of hospital admission	No correlation between insight and length of admission
Kahn and Fink (1959)	$n = 63$	Denial Personality Score dichotomised to high- and low-denial groupings	Response to ECT	Explicit verbal denial associated with better response to ECT
Hankoff et al. (1960a)	$n = 169$	Denial of illness questionnaire (rating 1–4)	Response to medication. Hospitalisation rate over 6 months	Denial associated with better response to medication but more hospitalisation
Hankoff et al. (1960b)	$n = 103$	Denial of illness questionnaire (rating 1–4)	Psychiatric progress notes	Denial associated with better prognosis when treated with placebo
Linn (1965)	$n = 593$	Answers to questions about what patients believed was wrong with them	Duration of hospital admission	No evidence that insight predicted better prognosis
Small et al. (1965)	$n = 68$	Structured questionnaire on attitudes about treatment and hospitalisation	Numbers of re-hospitalisation and/or transfers to chronic care institutions over 16–20 months	Positive change in attitudes associated with better prognosis
Soskis and Bowers (1969)	$n = 32$	Standardised questionnaire on attitudes to psychosis (3–7 years post-discharge)	Numbers of re-hospitalisation. Post hospital adjustment scales (KAS 1 and 2), BFR	No correlation between attitudes and re-hospitalisation rates. Positive attitudes correlated with higher levels of post hospital adjustment
Exner and Murillo (1975)	$n = 148$	Discrepancy between patients and relatives ratings on Katz Adjustment Scale	Relapse: needing re-hospitalisation within 12-month post-discharge	Greater discrepancy (poorer insight) predicted relapse

Table 3.4 (*cont.*)

Study	Patients*	Insight assessment	Clinical outcome	Results
Roback and Abramowitz (1979)	n = 24	Tolor–Reznikoff Test (clinical vignettes)	Hospital Adjustment Scale Symptom checklist	Increased insight associated with better hospital adjustment but more distress
McGlashan and Carpenter (1981)	n = 30	Soskis and Bowers attitude scales	Quantity and quality of work and social relations, absence of symptoms, fullness of life	Less negative attitudes associated with better outcome
Heinrichs et al. (1985)	n = 38	Patients dichotomised (insight versus no insight) according to case-note descriptions	Resolution of psychotic relapse. Retrospective study	Increased insight predicted successful resolution of relapse on outpatient basis. Reduced insight associated with more hospitalisation
Lelliott et al. (1988)	n = 49 OCD	Structured interview on attitudes to symptoms	Medication and behaviour therapy	No difference in outcome between patients with poor and good insight
McEvoy et al. (1989a)	n = 52	ITAQ	Rates of re-hospitalisation over 30–40 months since discharge	Good insight associated with less re-hospitalisation
Greenfeld et al. (1991)	n = 30 Anorexia nervosa (DSM-IIIR)	Schedule for assessment of insight into illness	Body mass index changes during hospitalisation	Good insight associated with positive outcome measures
Taylor and Perkins (1991)	n = 30	1. Question whether have mental health problem 2. Discrepancy between patients and staff on Awareness of Disabilities Scale	Functioning level. Subjective well-being Compliance with services	Denial associated with longer contact with services but less distress

Table 3.4 (*cont.*)

Study	Patients*	Insight assessment	Clinical outcome	Results
Amador *et al.* (1993)	n = 43	SUMD	Duration of hospital admission	Modest correlation between insight and length of admission
Foa *et al.* (1999)	n = 20 OCD	Structured interview on fixity of beliefs	Response to behaviour therapy	Poor insight associated with worse outcome (see text, section 3.2.9)
Eisen *et al.* (2001)	n = 71 OCD (DSM-IV)	BABS	Response to sertraline treatment (open label study)	Degree of insight did not predict response to sertraline

*Diagnoses not specified here, since detailed in text and subsequent tables, but majority of patients diagnosed with psychotic disorder, mainly schizophrenia, also schizoaffective, bipolar, affective and mixed psychoses. Exceptions are indicated.

Abbreviations: BABS: Brown Assessment of Beliefs Scale; BFR: Brief Follow-up Rating; ITAQ: Insight and Treatment Attitude Questionnaire; KAS: Katz Adjustment Scale; OCD: Obsessive-Compulsive Disorder; SUMD: Scale to Assess Unawareness of Mental Disorder.

It can be seen that results of studies are varied. Slightly more studies appear to suggest that better insight is associated with improved clinical outcome (Small *et al.*, 1965; Exner & Murillo, 1975; McGlashan & Carpenter, 1981; Heinrichs *et al.*, 1985; McEvoy *et al.*, 1989a; Greenfeld *et al.*, 1991; Amador *et al.*, 1993). A few studies report no association with prognosis (Eskey, 1958; Linn, 1965; Eisen *et al.*, 2001) and some suggest that insight is associated with worse clinical outcome (Kahn & Fink, 1959; Hankoff *et al.*, 1960b). Yet others indicate more mixed results with insight relating to some aspects of good but also to some aspects of worse outcome (Hankoff *et al.*, 1960a; Roback & Abramowitz, 1979; Taylor & Perkins, 1991). However, given the particular variability between the studies not only in how insight is assessed but also in the different clinical outcome indicators and different patient groups, the relationship between insight and prognosis cannot yet be determined.

3.2.4 Insight and severity of psychopathology

Perhaps most empirical studies exploring insight have focused on the relationship between patients' insight into their illness and the severity of their mental disorder. Does insight deteriorate with increasing severity of illness? Immediately, however, this raises further complications in terms of addressing the meaning of severity of mental illness, for, how is that best assessed? Will insight relate more to the degree of psychopathology in terms of numbers of concomitant symptoms, or perhaps to the types or patterns of symptoms/syndromes experienced? Or, is severity better determined by levels of functional ability? Studies in this area again yield very variable results (Table 3.5).

The variability in the results is of different types. Firstly, a number of studies show no association at all between the degree of patients' insight into mental disorder and the severity of their mental disorder (e.g. McGlashan & Carpenter, 1981; McEvoy et al., 1993a, b; Cuesta & Peralta, 1994; Lysaker & Bell, 1994; David et al., 1995; Lysaker & Bell, 1995; McEvoy et al., 1996; Flashman et al., 2000; Eisen et al., 2001). Secondly, a number of studies report a direct relationship between poor insight and global severity of mental disorder, i.e. the poorer the patient's insight, the more severe his/her mental illness (e.g. David et al., 1992; Takai et al., 1992; Young et al., 1993; Kemp & Lambert, 1995; Fennig et al. 1996; Young et al., 1998; Rossell et al., 2003; Eisen et al., 2004). Thirdly, another group of studies find that whilst there is no (or little) direct association between insight and global severity of illness, there is an association between 'positive' symptoms/syndromes (Almeida et al., 1996; Collins et al., 1997; Kim et al., 1997; Lysaker et al., 1998; Schwartz 1998a, b; Carroll et al., 1999). On the other hand, other studies disagree with the association with positive syndromes and instead report on an association between poor insight and more severe 'negative' symptoms/syndromes (McPherson et al., 1996; Cuesta et al., 2000; Larøi et al., 2000; McCabe et al., 2002). Other studies report an association between poor insight and severity of both positive and negative symptoms (Keshavan et al., 2004; Mintz et al., 2004). Fourth, some studies find rather that poor insight is associated with specific symptoms or groups of symptoms (Heinrichs et al., 1985; Lysaker et al., 1994; Vaz et al., 1994; Dickerson et al., 1997; Debowska et al., 1998; Baier et al., 2000). And in these latter studies, the symptoms, that elicit the association, themselves differ, e.g. 'severity of grandiosity' correlated with poor insight in the study by Heinrichs et al. (1985) and 'formal thought disorder' correlated with poor insight in the Baier et al. (2000) investigation. Then there are studies, which report association between only some dimensions of insight with different aspects of illness severity (Amador et al., 1993; Amador et al., 1994; Vaz et al., 1994; Buckley et al., 2001; Yen et al., 2003; Sevy et al., 2004). For example, the study by Sevy et al. (2004) in 96 patients with schizophrenia reported an association between poor awareness of current symptoms and all factors of severity derived from the PANSS. However, the lack of awareness of having a mental illness and its social consequences was correlated only with the positive factor from PANSS. Similarly, the lack of awareness of achieved effects of medication correlated only with the autistic preoccupation factor from the PANSS and no correlations at all were obtained between misattribution of symptoms and any of the PANSS factors. The authors conclude that different components of insight are related in different ways to the various

Table 3.5 Studies reporting on association between insight and severity of psychopathology

Study	Patients (diagnostic classification)	Insight assessment	Psychopathology assessment	Results
McGlashan and Carpenter (1981)	$n = 30$ Schiz. (DSM-II) inpatients and follow-up	Soskis and Bowers attitude scales	Global psychopathology ratings	No correlation between attitudes to psychosis and severity
Heinrichs et al. (1985)	$n = 38$ Chronic schiz. Retrospective case-note study	Patients dichotomised: with and without insight	BPRS	No relationship between insight and severity. Poor I associated with more severe grandiosity score
McEvoy et al. (1989b)	$n = 52$ Schizophrenia (DSM-III) inpatients	ITAQ	BPRS CGI	No consistent relationship between insight and severity
David et al. (1992)	$n = 91$ Mixed psychotic (PSE) Mainly inpatients	SAI PSE: insight item	PSE total score	Less I associated with more severe psychopathology (SAI measure only)
Marková and Berrios (1992b)	$n = 43$ Schizophrenia, depression. (DSM-IIIR), inpatients, admission and discharge	IPQ (preliminary). Semi-structured interview	BPRS HDRS	Poor I associated with greater severity at admission (BPRS) and more depression at d/s
Takai et al. (1992)	$n = 57$ Schizophrenia (DSM-IIIR).	PSE: insight item.Subjective ratings (FBS). Ratios of FBS and BPRS.	BPRS 4-positive symptoms (SADS). 5-negative symptoms (SANS).	Less I associated with greater BPRS scores. Less I associated with increased scores on both positive and negative symptom scores (SADS, SANS)
Amador et al. (1993)	$n = 43$ Schiz./schizaff. (DSM-IIIR), inpatients	SUMD Insight item from HDRS.	SAPS SANS HDRS	No relationship between I and severity, except: – current awareness and reduced total SAPS

Table 3.5 (*cont.*)

Study	Patients (diagnostic classification)	Insight assessment	Psychopathology assessment	Results
				− retrospective awareness and reduced depression
McEvoy et al. (1993a)	n = 25 Schiz./schizaff. (DSM-III), outpatients	ITAQ: modified	BPRS CGI	No correlation between I and severity
McEvoy et al. (1993b)	n = 26 Schiz./schizaff. (DSM-III), inpatients	ITAQ Clinical vignettes	Global Assessment Scale	No correlation between I and severity
Young et al. (1993)	n = 31 Chronic schiz. (DSM-IIIR), in and outpatients	SUMD	Likert scales of severity for each symptom	Poor I associated with increased severity of symptoms
Amador et al. (1994)	n = 348 Mixed psychotic, affective (DSM-IIIR), inpatients	SUMD: abridged	SAPS SANS	Some correlation between low I and higher SAPS. General level of awareness unrelated to symptom severity except delusions, thought disorder, social isolation
Cuesta and Peralta (1994)	n = 40 Schiz. (DSM-IIIR) inpatients	AMDP: three items (LII)	SAPS SANS	No correlation between I and severity
Lysaker and Bell (1994)	n = 92 Schiz./schizaff. (DSM-IIIR)	PANSS: item G12	PANSS	No correlation between I and severity (global, positive and negative)
Lysaker et al. (1994)	n = 85 Schiz./schizaff. (DSM-IIIR)	PANSS: item G12	PANSS	No correlation between I and severity (global, positive and negative). Poor I associated with some items: poor rapport, conceptual

Table 3.5 (*cont.*)

Study	Patients (diagnostic classification)	Insight assessment	Psychopathology assessment	Results
				disorganisation, stereotyped thinking, suspiciousness, etc
Michalakeas *et al.* (1994)	*n* = 77 females Schiz., mania, depression (DSM-IIIR), inpatients, admission and discharge	ITAQ	BPRS	Schiz. patients – no correlation between I and BPRS. More I correlated with less severity at discharge. Manic patients: poor insight correlated with severity at admission and discharge
				Depression Patients: no correlation between I and severity at any time
Peralta and Cuesta (1994)	*n* = 115 Schiz. (DSM-IIIR) inpatients	AMDP: three items. SAI	SAPS SANS	Poor I associated with fewer depressive symptoms
Vaz *et al.* (1994)	*n* = 64, males Acute Schiz. (DSM-IIIR) Inpatients	ITAQ: 2 factors: F1: awareness of illness. F2: awareness of need for Rx	PANSS	No correlation between total I or F1 and global severity Correlation between F2 and global severity. Correlation between F1: somatic preoccupation, poor rapport; F2: hostility, poor rapport
David *et al.* (1995)	*n* = 150 Mixed psychoses (DSM-IIIR), inpatients, follow-up	PSE: item 104	PSE total score	No correlation between I and global severity
Ghaemi *et al.* (1995)	*n* = 28 Acute mania (DSM-IIIR) inpatients	ITAQ	BPRS CGI	No correlation between I and global severity

Table 3.5 (*cont.*)

Study	Patients (diagnostic classification)	Insight assessment	Psychopathology assessment	Results
Lysaker and Bell (1995)	$n = 44$ Schiz./schizaff. (DSM-IIIR), rehabilitation	PANSS: item G12	PANSS	No correlation between I and severity (global positive and negative)
Kemp and Lambert (1995)	$n = 29$ Schiz. (DSM-IIIR) Inpatients (T1 and T2)	SUMD: modified	PANSS	Poor I associated with greater severity (positive, and negative and total) and grandiosity and less depression
Almeida et al. (1996)	$n = 40$ Late paraphrenia (ICD-9) In- and out and day patients	SAI PSE: item 104	PSE BPRS SAPS HEN	No correlation with negative symptoms. Poor I associated with worse BPRS and more positive symptoms
Fennig et al. (1996)	$n = 189$ Schiz., Bipolar, psychotic depression, other psychoses	Insight item from Hamilton Depression Rating Scale	SAPS SANS	Poor I associated with severity at baseline. Severity not predictive of I at 6-month follow-up
MacPherson et al. (1996)	$n = 64$ Schiz. (DSM-IIIR)	SAI	PANSS	No correlation between I and positive syndrome score but correlation between poor I and more severe negative syndrome score
McEvoy et al. (1996)	$n = 32$ Schiz. (DSM-IIIR)	ITAQ	BPRS	No correlation between I and severity
Collins et al. (1997)	$n = 58$ Schiz. (DSM-IIIR) outpatients	SAI	PANSS Calgary Depression Scale	Strongest association between poor I and positive symptoms score Small correlation between poor I and negative symptoms score Poor I associated with worse depression

Table 3.5 (*cont.*)

Study	Patients (diagnostic classification)	Insight assessment	Psychopathology assessment	Results
Dickerson *et al.* (1997)	*n* = 87 Schiz./schizaff. (DSM-IIIR), outpatients	PANSS: item G12	PANSS	Poor I associated with severity of symptoms, particularly delusions, paranoia, different abstract thinking, poor rapport, etc More I related to more severe anxiety
Ghaemi *et al.* (1997)	*n* = 30 Seasonal affective disorders (DSM-IIIR)	SUMD modified for mood	HDRS CGI	Better I associated with more severe depression
Kim *et al.* (1997)	*n* = 63 Schiz. (ICD-10) Inpatients and outpatients	SAI	BPRS SANS HDRS	Poor I associated with more severe positive symptoms No correlation with negative symptoms
Cuesta *et al.* (1998)	*n* = 100 Acute schiz. (DSM-IIIR), inpatients	PANSS: item G12, AMDP: three items	PANSS	Poor I associated with more severe symptoms in disorganised and excited dimensions and with more severe negative symptoms
Debowska *et al.* (1998)	*n* = 61 Paranoid schiz. (DSM-IIIR), inpatients	PANSS: item G12 four items re Rx attitude	PANSS Inventory of delusion contents	Poor I associated with more severe delusions and hostility (positive scale) and with more severe negative symptoms
Lysaker *et al.* (1998a)	*n* = 81 Schiz./schizaff. (DSM-IIIR)	PANSS: item G12	PANSS	Poor I associated with more severe positive symptoms No correlation with negative symptoms
Lysaker *et al.* (1998b)	*n* = 101 Schiz./schizaff. (DSM-IIIR)	SUMD: abridged	PANSS Schedule for deficit syndrome	Poor I associated with more severe positive symptoms No correlation with negative symptoms

Table 3.5 (*cont.*)

Study	Patients (diagnostic classification)	Insight assessment	Psychopathology assessment	Results
Sanz et al. (1998)	n = 33 Mixed psychotic disorders (DSM-IV), mainly inpatients	ITAQ SAI (and SAI-E) IPQ (preliminary) PANSS: item G12	PANSS BPRS: expanded BDI CGI	Correlations varied according to I rating used. SAI and PANSS correlated with total severity. All measures correlated with grandiosity item. SAI, ITAQ, PANSS ratings of I correlated with depression severity
Schwartz (1998a)	n = 64 Schiz. (DSM-IV)	PANSS: item G12	PANSS	Poor I associated with more severe positive symptoms No correlation with negative or general symptoms
Schwartz (1998b)	n = 66 Schiz. (DSM-IV) outpatients	SUMD	PANSS	Poor I associated with more severe positive symptoms No correlation with negative or general symptoms
Smith et al. (1998)	n = 33 Schiz./schizaff. (DSM-IV), in and outpatients	SUMD	BPRS SAPS SANS	No correlation with severity except: good I associated with more depression and less disorganised symptoms
Young et al. (1998)	n = 129 Schiz., bipolar (DSM-IIIR), in and outpatients	SUMD	BPRS	Poor I associated with greater global severity
Carroll et al. (1999)	n = 100 Schiz. (DSM-IIIR) Inpatients prior to discharge	ITAQ	PANSS MADRS	Poor I associated with more severe positive symptoms and less depressed mood. Improvement in I

Table 3.5 (*cont.*)

Study	Patients (diagnostic classification)	Insight assessment	Psychopathology assessment	Results
				related to worsening mood but not to improvement in positive symptoms
Lysaker et al. (1999)	n = 74 Schiz./schizaff. (DSM-IIIR), inpatients and following rehabilitation	PANSS: item G12	PANSS	Poor I associated with more severe positive symptoms at admission and after 5 months. No correlation between I and symptoms after 1 year
Baier et al. (2000)	n = 37 Schiz./schizaff. Inpatients and outpatients	IS Davidhizar et al. (self-rating insight scale)	SAPS SANS	No correlation with severity except: poor I associated with more formal thought disorder
Caracci et al. (1990)	n = 78 Chronic schiz. (DSM-IIIR), outpatients	Questions on awareness of mental disorder (insight present or absent)	Rockland Tardive Dyskinesia Scale	Poor I associated with more severe orofacio-lingual dyskinesia
Cuesta et al. (2000)	n = 75 Schiz., affective and schizaff. disorders (DSM-IV), index, follow-up	SUMD ITAQ AMDP: three items	CASH: positive and negative syndrome scores	Poor I-SUMD/AMDP associated with worse negative symptoms. No correlation with affective dimension
Flashman et al. (2000)	n = 30 Schiz., schizaff., (DSM-IV)	SUMD	BPRS SAPS SANS	No correlation between I and severity
Larøi et al. (2000)	n = 21 Schiz. (DSM-IV)	SUMD	BPRS	No correlation between I and severity except for association between poor I and anergia category

Table 3.5 (*cont.*)

Study	Patients (diagnostic classification)	Insight assessment	Psychopathology assessment	Results
Smith T.E. *et al.* (2000)	*n* = 46 Schiz./schizaff. (DSM-IV), outpatients	SUMD: abridged	SANS SAPS BPRS	Poor I associated with more formal thought disorder and worse depression and better positive symptoms. *No correlation with negative symptoms
Weiler *et al.* (2000)	*n* = 187 Mixed psychoses, affective disorders (DSM-IIIR), inpatients, admission, d/s	ITAQ	BPRS	Improvement in I associated with improvement in severity of symptoms
White *et al.* (2000)	*n* = 150 Schiz. (DSM-IV, ICD-10), in and outpatients	SAI	PANSS Calgary Depression Scale	Poor I associated with greater severity of psychotic symptoms. No correlation with depression but poor I associated with more depression when psychotic symptoms partialled out
Buckley *et al.* (2001)	*n* = 50 Schiz./schizaff. (DSM-IV) inpatients	SUMD	BPRS	No correlation between severity and awareness of illness/effects of Rx. Some correlations between I and positive and negative syndromes. Poor I associated with more depression
Cassidy *et al.* (2001)	*n* = 53 Bipolar (mania and mixed) (DSM-IV)	ITAQ	SMS PANSS: G items	Poor I weakly related to greater severity. Strong correlation with delusions and disorganisation. Better I associated with more depression

Table 3.5 (*cont.*)

Study	Patients (diagnostic classification)	Insight assessment	Psychopathology assessment	Results
Chen *et al.* (2001)	*n* = 80 Mixed psychoses and affective disorders (DSM-IV), inpatients, admission and d/s	SUMD: abridged	BPRS	No correlation with total severity. Improvement in I scores related to positive symptoms scores
Eisen *et al.* (2001)	*n* = 71 OCD (DSM-IIIR)	BABS	Y-BOCS	No correlation between I and severity of OCD
Francis and Penn (2001)	*n* = 29 Schiz., bipolar and schizaff. disorders (DSM-IV), outpatients	ITAQ PANSS: item G12 IS	BPRS	Poor I associated with total severity, anergia and thought disorder. No correlation with affective/disorganised syndromes
Goldberg *et al.* (2001)	*n* = 211 Schiz., bipolar, other psychotic and affective (DSM-IV), in/outpatients	PANSS: item G12	PANSS	Poor I associated with more positive and negative symptoms. No correlation with general (G items)
Pyne *et al.* (2001)	*n* = 177 Schiz. Inpatients and outpatients	Insight: present or absent on response to question if think that mentally ill	Modified Symptom Checklist-90	Good insight associated with worse depression
Schwartz (2001)	*n* = 223 Schiz. (DSM-IV) Outpatients	SUMD	SCI-FARS	Poor I associated with more severe depressive symptoms
McCabe *et al.* (2002)	*n* = 89 Chronic schiz. (DSM-IIIR), outpatients	SAI	SANS SAPS	Poor I associated with more avolition-apathy (SANS). Subscales of I correlated with some symptoms but majority of I variance not

Table 3.5 (*cont.*)

Study	Patients (diagnostic classification)	Insight assessment	Psychopathology assessment	Results
				explained by symptom severity
Vaz *et al.* (2002)	*n* = 82 Schiz. (DSM-IV) Outpatients	SAI	PANSS	Poor I associated with more severe psychopathology
Rossell *et al.* (2003)	*n* = 78 males Schizophrenia (DSM-IV)	SAI-E	SANS SAPS	Poor I associated with more severe psychopathology, particularly: delusions, formal thought disorder and inappropriate affect
Yen *et al.* (2003)	*n* = 33 Bipolar: currently manic (DSM-IV)	SAI SAI-E	Young's Mania Rating Scale (YMRS)	No association between I (SAI) and severity of mania Poor I on SAI-E associated with more severe mania
Drake *et al.* (2004)	*n* = 257 1st episode psychoses (Schizophrenia spectrum, DSM-IV) f/u 72% at 18 months	IS (Birchwood) PANSS: item G12	PANSS: delusions Delusion Scale: PSYRATS PANSS: anxiety, depression, guilty and avolition items	Insight not strongly associated with paranoia Insight at admission strongly associated with (predicted) depression but only weak at follow-up
Keshavan *et al.* (2004)	*n* = 535 1st episode psychoses (Schizophrenia spectrum, DSM-IV)	PANSS: item G12	PANSS: CGI	Poor I associated with positive, negative and general psychopathology (especially thought disorder)
Eisen *et al.* (2004)	*n* = 64 OCD (DSM-IV) *n* = 85 BDD (DSM-IV)	BABS	Y-BOCS BDD-YBOCS	Poor I associated with more severe symptoms only in BDD (not OCD)

Table 3.5 (*cont.*)

Study	Patients (diagnostic classification)	Insight assessment	Psychopathology assessment	Results
Mintz *et al.* (2004)	*n* = 253 1st episode psychoses (Schizophrenia spectrum, DSM-IV). f/u: 180 at 12 months	PANSS: item G12. Patients high insight or low insight	PANSS Calgary Depression Scale	Poor I associated with higher levels of positive and negative symptoms at baseline and f/u assessments
Sevy *et al.* (2004)	*n* = 96 Schizophrenia (DSM-IV)	SUMD: revised	PANSS: analysed in relation to five factors	Different components of I correlated with different PANSS factors (see text)

Abbreviations: AMDP-LII: Lack of Insight Index from three items of the Manual for the Assessment and Documentation of Psychopathology; BABS: Brown Assessment of Belief Scale; BDD: Body Dysmorphic Disorder; BDD-Y-BOCS: Yale-Brown Obsessive Compulsive Scale modified for Body Dysmorphic Disorder; BDI: Beck Depression Inventory; BPRS: Brief Psychiatric Rating Scale; CASH: Comprehensive Assessment Schedule History; CGI: Clinical Global Impressions global severity item; HDRS: Hamilton Depression Rating Scale; HEN: High Royds Evaluation of Negativity Scale; I: Insight; IPQ: Insight in Psychosis Questionnaire; IS: Insight Scale; ITAQ: Insight and Treatment Attitude Questionnaire; MADRS: Montgomery and Asberg Depression Rating Scale; OCD: Obsessive Compulsive Disorder; PANSS: Positive and Negative Syndrome Scale; PSE: Present State Examination; PSYRATS: Psychotic Symptom Rating Scales; Rx: Treatment; SADS: Schedule for Affective Disorders; SAI: Schedule for Assessing Insight; SAI-E: Schedule for Assessing Insight – Expanded version; SANS: Scale for the Assessment of Negative Symptoms; SAPS: Scale for the Assessment of Positive Symptoms; Schiz.: Schizophrenia; Schizaff.: Schizoaffective disorder; SCI-FARS: Structured Clinical Interview for the Functional Assessment Rating Scale; SMS: Scale for Manic States; SUMD: Scale to Assess Unawareness of Mental Disorder; Y-BOCS: Yale-Brown Obsessive Compulsive Scale; YMRS: Young's Mania Rating Scale.

aspects of the patient's illness (Sevy *et al.*, 2004). Reporting on an opposite direction of association between insight and severity of illness, one study examining insight in patients with anorexia nervosa found that good insight related to more severe illness as assessed by duration of hospitalisation and degree of emaciation (Greenfeld *et al.*, 1991). Finally, some studies using several insight assessment measures at the same time report on different associations between insight and severity of illness with the different measures used (Sanz *et al.*, 1998; Cuesta *et al.*, 2000).

In the light of the variable outcomes of these empirical studies, it is clear that the relationship between insight and severity of illness is not yet possible to define definitively. The finding that some studies have reported improvements in patients' insight over time, which seem to be independent of improvements in psychopathology over the same time (McEvoy *et al.*, 1989b; Jørgensen, 1995; Fennig *et al.*, 1996; Cuesta *et al.*, 2000), further complicates the overall picture. In addition, the studies summarised in Table 3.5 vary considerably in methodological design which creates problems in making comparisons and obtaining consistent results. Thus, studies range in size ($n = 21$–348), diagnostic heterogeneity (some studies include only patients with schizophrenia, others have a range of psychotic disorders, some include patients with affective disorders with or without psychosis, some are acute, others chronic, some are inpatients and others outpatients, etc.), methods of insight assessment and measures of outcome. At the most, all that can be said at present concerning the relationship between patients' insight and severity of mental illness is that it is likely to be complicated. Many factors will play a part in the complications, not just the difficulties around defining and assessing insight, but also the problems of defining severity of mental illness and the need to consider a great many different factors that are likely to be contributing to an individual mental state.

3.2.5 Insight and cognitive function

Over the last decade particular interest has focused on examining the relationship between insight and cognitive function or impairment. Much of this interest has arisen as a result of, firstly, the findings that various cognitive deficits occur commonly in patients with severe mental illness, particularly schizophrenia (David & Cutting, 1994; McKenna, 1994). And secondly, analogies have been made between loss of awareness or anosognosia in patients with neurological conditions (see Chapter 4) with loss of insight in patients with mental disorders (Amador et al., 1991; Young et al., 1993; Mullen et al., 1996; Amador & Kronengold, 1998). The underlying questions behind the empirical studies in this area thus relate to whether impaired insight can be linked aetiologically with impaired neurocognitive function, particularly executive function, that can be found in patients with severe mental illness. Studies exploring this relationship are summarised in Tables 3.6 and 3.7.

It is evident that studies claiming a significant relationship between insight and cognitive function (Table 3.7) are roughly equal in numbers to those finding no such relationship (Table 3.6). The two groups of studies are generally comparable in terms of their sizes, in the range of insight assessments used, and in the range and specificity of neuropsychology measures employed to evaluate cognitive function. Amongst the studies suggesting an association between poor insight and impaired cognitive function, a few find that insight relates to general cognitive function, i.e. measures of IQ (e.g. Lysaker & Bell, 1994; Young et al., 1993; Lysaker et al., 1994; Fennig et al., 1996), but, in general, this has not been replicated by other studies (e.g. Takai et al., 1992; MacPherson et al., 1996; Larøi et al., 2000; Marks et al., 2000; Drake & Lewis, 2003). The most consistent finding amongst the positive cognitive function associations has been a correlation between some (general or selective) impairment on performance in tests of 'executive' or frontal lobe function and poor insight (Young et al., 1993; Lysaker & Bell, 1994; Lysaker et al., 1994; Voruganti et al.,

Table 3.6 Studies reporting NO association between insight and cognitive function

Study	Patients	Insight assessment	Neuropsychology assessment	Results
Caracci et al. (1990)	n = 20 Chronic schiz. (DSM-III)	Rated absent or present on enquiry re-awareness of mental illness	Full scale IQ	No correlation with IQ
Takai et al. (1992)	n = 57 Schiz. (DSM-IIIR)	PSE: item 104 FBS, ratio of FBS/BPRS	WAIS (total, verbal and performance IQ)	No correlation with IQ (total, verbal performance)
McEvoy et al. (1993a)	n = 43 Schiz./schizaff. (DSM-IIIR)	ITAQ	WMS (I, II) Peabody Picture Vocabulary Test Bender Gestalt Test Benton's Controlled Word Association Test	No correlation between insight and performance on any tests
Cuesta and Peralta (1994)	n = 40 Schiz. (DSM-IIIR)	AMDP: three items	MMSE, WAIS (seven subtests), Rey., Trail (A, B) Making Test, Bender's Visual-Motor Test, subtests from Spanish Neuropsychological Battery	No correlation between I and performance (Poor I associated with better performance on verbal memory and delayed visual memory.)
Cuesta et al. (1995)	n = 49 Schiz, schizaff., bipolar manic (DSM-IIIR)	AMDP: three items	WCST	No correlation between I and performance on WCST
David et al. (1995)	n = 150 Mixed psychoses (DSM-IIIR)	SAI PSE: item 104	NART or WAIS-R (vocab), Iager scale, Trail (A, B) Making Test, tests of frontal lobe function (Reitan, 1958)	No correlation between I (SAI) and IQ (but PSE item associated with IQ) No correlation with any other tests
Almeida et al. (1996)	n = 40 Late paraphrenia (ICD-9)	SAI PSE: item 104	NART, CAMCOG, Digit and Spatial Span, Verbal Fluency Test, RMTW/F, Computerised tests*	No correlation between I and any cognitive test

Table 3.6 (*cont.*)

Study	Patients	Insight assessment	Neuropsychology assessment	Results
Ghaemi *et al.* (1996)	*n* = 16 Acute mania (DSM-IIIR)	ITAQ	WAIS-R, WMS, COWAT, Finger Tapping Test, Luria tests on visual perception, language, construction	No correlation between I and cognitive impairment
Kemp and David (1996)	*n* = 74 Mixed psychoses (DSM-IIIR)	SAI	NART, Verbal Fluency Test, Cognitive Estimates Test, Trail (A, B) Making Test, MMSE	No correlation with performance on any test (Only hypothetical contradiction associated with frontal tests scores.)
MacPherson *et al.* (1996)	*n* = 64 Schiz. (DSM-IIIR)	SAI	NART and MMSE	No correlation with IQ (but poor I associated with worse MMSE)
Collins *et al.* (1997)	*n* = 58 Schiz. (DSM-IIIR)	SAI	WCST	No correlation with WCST score
Dickerson *et al.* (1997)	*n* = 87 Schiz./schiza ff. (DSM-IIIR)	PANSS: G12	WAIS-R, WMS, Rey., WCST, Trail (A, B) Making Test, HWAST, Chicago Fluency Test	No correlation between I and any tests
Sanz *et al.* (1998)	*n* = 33 Mixed psychotic (DSM-IV)	ITAQ SAI IPQ prelim PANSS: G12	MMSE, NART, WCST, Star Cancellation Test, Trail Making Test	No correlation between I on any measure and any tests
Carroll *et al.* (1999)	*n* = 100 Schiz. (DSM-IIIR)	ITAQ	NART, Quick Test, RBMT	No correlation with any test
Goldberg *et al.* (2001)	*n* = 211 Schiz., bipolar, other (DSM-IV)	PANSS: G12	RBANS, WCST, WRAT-R, WAIS-R	No correlation with IQ or any test
Schwartz (2001)	*n* = 223 Schiz. (DSM-IV)	SUMD	Cognitive deficits from the FARS	No correlation with cognitive impairment
McCabe *et al.* (2002)	*n* = 89 Chronic schiz. (DSM-IIIR)	SAI	Luria Nebraska Neuropsychology Battery	No association between global cognitive impairment and any I dimension

Table 3.6 (*cont.*)

Study	Patients	Insight assessment	Neuropsychology assessment	Results
				(Re-labelling dimension on SAI correlated with motor and arithmetic functions). Cognitive deficit failed to predict poor insight
Arduini *et al.* (2003)	*n* = 64 Schiz., bipolar (DSM-IV)	SUMD: abridged	WCST	No correlation with WCST in either or both patient groups
Freudenreich *et al.* (2004)	*n* = 122 Schiz. (DSM-IV)	SUMD: modified	WCST, WAIS-III – IQ, CVLT, Stroop, Benton's Controlled Word Association Test	No association between symptom awareness and cognitive variables
Mintz *et al.* (2004)	*n* = 253 Schiz. spectrum, DSM-IV F/u: *n* = 180 at 1 year	PANSS: item G12	Cognitive Battery: COWAT, category fluency, verbal, auditory, visual memory, WCST, visuo-constructive skills, attention, Trails A,B, etc	No association between insight and cognition at baseline or at follow up assessments

* Computerised tests: Simultaneous and Delayed-Matching-to-Sample Task, Extra-Dimensional and Intra-Dimensional Attention Shift Task, Spatial Working Memory Task, Tower of London Task.

Abbreviations: AMDP-LII: Lack of Insight Index from three items of the Manual for the Assessment and Documentation of Psychopathology; BPRS: Brief Psychiatric Rating Scale; FARS: Functional Assessment Rating Scale; FBS: Frankfurter Befindlichketsskala; I: Insight; IPQ: Insight in Psychosis Questionnaire; ITAQ: Insight and Treatment Attitude Questionnaire; PANSS: Positive and Negative Syndrome Scale; PSE: Present State Examination; SAI: Schedule for Assessing Insight; Schiz.: Schizophrenia; Schizaff.: Schizoaffective Disorder; SUMD: Scale to Assess Unawareness of Mental Disorder.

Neuropsychology abbreviations: CAMCOG: Cognitive section of the Cambridge Examination for Mental Disorders of the Elderly; COWAT: Controlled Word Association Test; HWAST: Halstead-Wepman Aphasia Screening Test; MMSE: Mini-Mental State Examination; NART: National Adult Reading Test; RBANS: Repeatable Battery for the Assessment of Neuropsychological Status; RBMT: Rivermead Behavioural Memory Test; Rey.: Rey's Complex Figure Test; RMTW/F: Recognition Memory Test for Words and Faces; WAIS (-R): Wechsler Adult Intelligence Scale (Revised); WCST: Wisconsin Card Sorting Test; WMS: Wechsler Memory Scale; WRAT-R: Wide Range Achievement Test-Reading.

Table 3.7 Studies reporting SOME association between insight and cognitive function

Study	Patients	Insight assessment	Neuropsychology assessment	Results
David et al. (1992)	n = 91 Psychotic (PSE)	SAI PSE: item 104	NART	Better I (on SAI but not PSE) associated with higher IQ
Young et al. (1993)	n = 31 Chronic schiz. (DSM-IIIR)	SUMD	WCST, verbal fluency test, trails A and B, WAIS-R IQ	Poor I associated with worse performance on WCST and worse IQ. No correlation with verbal fluency or trails
Lysaker and Bell (1994)	n = 92 Schiz./schizaff. (DSM-IIIR)	PANSS: item G12	WCST, Slosson Intelligence Test	Poor I associated with lower IQ, poorer performance on WCST
Lysaker et al. (1994)	n = 85 Schiz./schizaff. (DSM-IIIR)	PANSS: item G12	WCST, Slosson Intelligence Test, Gorham Proverbs Test (GPT)	Poor I associated with lower IQ, poor performance on WCST, bizarre/ idiosyncratic thought on GPT
Lysaker and Bell (1995)	n = 44 Schiz./schizaff. (DSM-IIIR)	PANSS: item G12	WCST, Slosson Intelligence Test, Digit Symbol Subtest (WAIS-R), Gorham Proverbs	Greater levels of cognitive impairment predicted less improvement in I
Cuffel et al. (1996)	n = 89 Schiz. (DSM-IIIR)	Interview rating awareness of illness	Neurobehavioural Cognitive Status Examination	Poor I associated with cognitive impairment
McEvoy et al. (1996)	n = 32 Schiz. (DSM-IIIR)	ITAQ	WAIS-R (block, vocab), Judgement of Line Orientation, Rey., Finger localisation test, R-L orientation, COWAT, FFT, WCST	Poor total I associated with poor R-L orient Subscale from ITAQ (poor awareness of mental illness) associated with impaired WCST, block, R-L orientation
Voruganti et al. (1997)	n = 52 Schiz. (DSM-IIIR)	PANSS: item G12	COGLAB (includes WCST, vigilance, span of apprehension, illusion task, reaction time, etc.)	Poor I associated with poor performance on span of apprehension, backward masking task and WCST
Lysaker et al. (1998a)	n = 81 Schiz./schizaff. (DSM-IIIR)	PANSS: item G12	WAIS-R, WCST, subtests of WMSR, HVLT, CPT	Poor I associated with impaired WCST scores No correlation with other tests

Table 3.7 (*cont.*)

Study	Patients	Insight assessment	Neuropsychology assessment	Results
Young *et al.* (1998)	*n* = 129 Schiz., bipolar (DSM-IIIR)	SUMD	WAIS-R, WCST	In schiz. poorer I associated with poor performance on WCST and poor IQ. No correlation in bipolar. Weaker in acute mania
Mohamed *et al.* (1999)	*n* = 46 Schiz. (DSM-IIIR)	SUMD, subscales relating to negative and positive symptoms	WAIS-R, Verbal Fluency Test, Design Fluency Test, Trail (B) Making Test	Poorer awareness and misattribution of negative symptoms associated with poorer performance on some fluency and WCST tasks
Larøi *et al.* (2000)	*n* = 21 Schiz. (DSM-IV)	SUMD	WAIS (Block, vocab), Finger Tapping Test, Kimura Figures, WCST, Trail (A, B) Making Test	Poor I associated with worse performance on WCST and block design. No correlation with IQ or any other test
Marks *et al.* (2000)	*n* = 59 Schiz./schizaff. (DSM-IV)	SAIQ PANSS: item G12 SUMD	WCST, WAIS-III subtests, Stroop Test, HVLT, Logical memory of WMS, AMNART	Two factors from SAIQ correlated with WCST, letter-number sequencing and similarities No correlation with IQ or other tests
Smith *et al.* (2000)	*n* = 46 Schiz./schizaff. (DSM-IV)	SUMD: abridged	WAIS-R, SPAN, DSDT, CVLT, Verbal Fluency Test, WCST, BFRT	Worse symptom attribution associated with poor performance on WCST
Buckley *et al.* (2001)	*n* = 50 Schiz./schizaff. (DSM-IV)	SUMD	Trail (A, B) Making Test	Only poor past awareness of mental disorder associated with poor TMT performance
Chen *et al.* (2001)	*n* = 80 Psychoses and affective (DSM-IV)	SUMD: abridged	WCST	Improvement in I correlated with improvement in WCST performance
Upthegrove *et al.* (2002)	*n* = 30 Schiz. (ICD-10)	SAI-E	Serial 7s, digit span backwards, working memory span	Poor I associated with poor digit span performance. No other correlation

Table 3.7 (*cont.*)

Study	Patients	Insight assessment	Neuropsychology assessment	Results
Lysaker *et al.* (2002)	*n* = 132 Schiz./schizaff. (DSM-IV)	SUMD: abridged	WCST Letter Number Sequencing of WAIS III	Poor I associated with poorer executive function. Mixed results for partial insight
Drake and Lewis (2003)	*n* = 33 Schiz./schizaff. Schiz. form, delusional dis. (DSM-IV)	SUMD, IS, SAI-E, ITAQ Davidhizar (three I factors derived)	Trail (A, B) Making Test Frontal Lobe Score, Brixton test, Hayling test, Abstraction, theory of mind visual jokes test	Better I (especially relabelling factor) associated with less perseveration and better set shifting. No correlation with abstraction
Rossell *et al.* (2003)	*n* = 78 Schiz. (DSM-IV)	SAI-E	WAIS-R (shortened) CPT, COWAT, visual span (WMS), NART	Poor I associated with worse NART IQ and poorer performance on WCST-categories. No other correlations
Keshavan *et al.* (2004)	*n* = 535 Schizophrenia spectrum (DSM-IV)	PANSS: item G12	WAIS-R, WCST, verbal fluency WMSR, RVLT, CPT	Poor I associated with poor performance on RVLT and frontal lobe tasks

Abbreviations: I: Insight; IS: Insight Scale; ITAQ: Insight and Treatment Attitude Questionnaire; PANSS: Positive and Negative Syndrome Scale; PSE: Present State Examination; SAI: Schedule for Assessing Insight; SAI-E: Schedule for Assessing Insight – Extended version; SAIQ: Self-Appraisal of Illness Questionnaire; Schiz.: Schizophrenia; Schizaff.: Schizoaffective Disorder; SUMD: Scale to Assess Unawareness of Mental Disorder.

Neuropsychology abbreviations: AMNART: American version of the NART; BFRT: Benton Facial Recognition Test; COGLAB: Cognitive Laboratory computerised test battery; COWAT: Controlled Word Association Test; CPT: Continuous Performance Test; CVLT: California Verbal Learning Test; DSDT: Digit Span Distractibility Test; FFT: Figural Fluency Test; HVLT: Hopkins Verbal Learning Test; NART: National Adult Reading Test; Rey.: Rey's Complex Figure Test; RMTW/F: Recognition Memory Test for Words and Faces; RVLT: Rey Auditory Verbal Learning Test; SPAN: Span of Apprehension Test; WAIS (-R): Wechsler Adult Intelligence Scale (Revised); WCST: Wisconsin Card Sorting Test; WMS(R): Wechsler Memory Scale (Revised).

1997; Lysaker *et al.*, 1998; Young *et al.*, 1998; Larøi *et al.*, 2000; Drake & Lewis, 2003; Rossell *et al.*, 2003; Keshavan *et al.*, 2004). However, the studies often differ in the specific frontal lobe impairments found (Table 3.7) or some aspects/dimensions of poor insight (McEvoy *et al.*, 1996; Mohamed *et al.*, 1999; Marks *et al.*, 2000; Smith

et al., 2000; Buckley *et al.*, 2001; Lysaker *et al.*, 2002). Nevertheless, many other studies specifically exploring this relationship have failed to find an association between
poor insight and impairment on tests of frontal lobe function (Cuesta & Peralta,
1994, Cuesta *et al.*, 1995; David *et al.*, 1995; Almeida *et al.*, 1996; Kemp & David, 1996;
Collins *et al.*, 1997; Dickerson *et al.*, 1997; Sanz *et al.*, 1998; Goldberg *et al.*, 2001;
Schwartz, 2001; Arduini *et al.*, 2003; Freudenreich, *et al.* 2004; Mintz *et al.*, 2004).
Curiously, one study reports a stronger association between poor insight and
impaired temporal lobe function (Keshavan *et al.*, 2004).

An interesting hypothesis, attempting to explain such inconsistency of results in
studies exploring the relationship between insight and cognitive deficits, is suggested by Startup (1996). He proposes that the relationship between insight and
cognitive deficits might more usefully be conceived as curvilinear on account of
the contribution of psychological or motivational factors in the manifestation of
insight. In other words, existing neurological and psychological theories put forward to explain impairments of insight are not mutually exclusive and might contribute proportionately according to the level of cognitive impairment suffered by
the individual. In a study involving 26 patients with schizophrenia (DSM-IIIR),
Startup administered a number of tests sensitive to frontal lobe dysfunction
(Cognitive Estimates, Verbal Fluency, Trail (B) Making Test, Stroop Test and Stylus
Maze Test), and used the ITAQ to assess insight. He was able to demonstrate that a
quadratic, rather than a linear, model could help explain the relationship between
insight and cognitive deficits, accounting for 56% of the variance. Following on
from this, Lysaker *et al.* (2003) carried out a cluster analysis on 64 patients
with schizophrenia spectrum disorder and, using the PANSS insight item, they
divided patients into those with good insight and those with poor insight. On
administering tests of frontal lobe function (WCST), they obtained three groups of
patients, namely, patients with good insight and average performance on WCST;
patients with poor insight and average performance on the WCST, and patients
with poor insight and poor performance on the WCST. They thus concurred with
Startup (1996) that perhaps there are subgroups of patients who may show poor
insight for different reasons: poor cognition on the one hand might underlie
problems in understanding reality in one group and a tendency to ignore or
deny unpleasant things might contribute more to impairment of insight in
another group.

Overall, however, it is evident from these studies that the relationship between
insight into mental illness and cognitive function also continues to be unclear.

3.2.7 Insight and brain structure

On the basis of similar neuro-cognitive arguments, namely, that insightlessness in
severe mental illness may be the result of cognitive deficits or even akin to anosognosia

in neurological disorders, a few studies have attempted to explore the relationship between poor insight and structural brain abnormalities. Takai *et al.* (1992) found that poor insight in schizophrenic patients was associated with ventricular enlargement on MRI. Similarly, Flashman *et al.* (2000) found that poor insight in patients with schizophrenia or schizoaffective disorders was associated with smaller brain size and intracranial volumes on MRI scanning. Patients were dichotomised into those with and without awareness of symptoms on the basis of SUMD scores. On this occasion, no correlations were found with global frontal lobe volumes. On the other hand, David *et al.* (1995) found no association between levels of insight and ventricular enlargement on CT scanning in 128 patients with mixed psychotic disorders. Likewise, Rossell *et al.* (2003) in a large MRI study found no correlation between insight in 71 patients with schizophrenia and their grey, white, cerebro spinal fluid (CSF) or total brain volume. A recent study by Larøi *et al.* (2000) examining insight in 20 patients with chronic schizophrenia found that there was a significant association between frontal cortical atrophy and poorer insight (SUMD). A similar finding was reported by Flashman *et al.* (2001) who found that poor insight (SUMD) in 15 patients with schizophrenia correlated with reduced volumes in frontal lobe regions. They specified further correlations between individual aspects of insight as assessed by the SUMD and reported that unawareness of symptoms was associated with smaller middle frontal gyrus volumes whereas misattribution of symptoms was correlated with smaller superior frontal gyrus volumes.

3.2.8 Insight in relation to psychosocial functioning and quality of life

Questions have also been asked about the relationship between patients' insight into their mental illness and their level of psychosocial functioning, pre-morbid adjustment and, more recently, various quality of life variables. Few studies, however, have addressed these questions directly and most have reported on associations with insight as secondary aims. Again, as can be seen from the summaries of studies (Table 3.8), results are variable and inconclusive. In part at least, this is likely to be on account of the studies examining quite different areas of functioning or quality of life and only few studies examining such aspects in detail.

Results of these studies can be roughly divided into three groups. A number of studies seem to show no relation between insight and levels of psychosocial functioning (Cuesta & Peralta, 1994; Ghaemi *et al.*, 1995; Schwartz, 1998a, b; Baier *et al.*, 2000; Schwartz, 2001; Marková *et al.*, 2003) or pre-morbid adjustment (David *et al.*, 1995). In most of these studies, the level of psychosocial functioning was assessed by the Global Assessment Scale (Endicott *et al.*, 1976) or its modification in the form of Global Assessment of Functioning (APA, 1987/1994). Other studies, on the other hand, and using a more varied range of measures of function and quality of life (Table 3.8), suggest a relationship between poor insight and

Table 3.8 Studies reporting on association between insight and level of functioning/quality of life

Study	Patients	Insight assessment	Measure of function/quality	Results
O'Connor and Herrman (1993)	n = 41 Residual Schiz. (DSM-IIIR)	SAI	LSP	Poor insight associated with worse social functioning
Amador et al. (1994)	n = 348 Psychotic, affective (DSM-IIIR)	SUMD: abridged	GAS: current, past year, past 5 years	Poor awareness associated with poorer function on current and past year. No correlation with past 5 years
Cuesta and Peralta (1994)	n = 40 Schiz. (DSM-IIIR)	AMDP: three items	GAF: current, past year; Strauss-Carpenter Scale	No correlation between I and functioning
Lysaker et al. (1994)	n = 85 Schiz./schizaff. (DSM-IIIR)	PANSS: item G12	Work Personality Profile	Poor I associated with fewer weeks participation (work, rehab), poorer social skills and personal presentation
Peralta and Cuesta (1994)	n = 115 Schiz. (DSM-IIIR)	AMDP: three items SAI	GAF current, past year; Strauss-Carpenter Scale	Poor I associated with lower functioning in past year
David et al. (1995)	n = 150 Mixed psychoses (DSM-IIIR)	PSE: item 104	Maternal interviews, pre-morbid adjustment (PS)	No correlation with pre-morbid social adjustment
Ghaemi et al. (1995)	n = 28 Acute mania (DSM-IIIR)	ITAQ	GAS	No correlation with functioning
Dickerson et al. (1997)	n = 87 Schiz./schizaff. (DSM-IIIR)	PANSS: item G12	SFS	Poor I associated with poorer frequency of social activities
Lam and Wong (1997)	n = 40 Bipolar 1 (DSM-IV)	SAI	SPS	Poor insight weakly associated with lower level of social functioning
Debowska et al. (1998)	n = 61 Paranoid schiz. (DSM-IIIR)	PANSS: item G12	CSPAS	Poor I associated with pre-morbid adjustment disorders in early adulthood

Table 3.8 (*cont.*)

Study	Patients	Insight assessment	Measure of function/quality	Results
Lysaker et al. (1998b)	n = 101 Schiz./schizaff. (DSM-IIIR)	SUMD: abridged	QOL	Poor I (particularly awareness of social consequence of illness) associated with poorer social function (independent of deficit symptoms)
Schwartz (1998a)	n = 64 Schiz. (DSM-IV)	PANSS: item G12	GAF	No correlation with psychosocial functioning
Schwartz (1998b)	n = 66 Schiz. (DSM-IV)	SUMD	GAF	No correlation with psychosocial functioning
Doyle et al. (1999)	n = 40 Acute schiz. (DSM-IIIR)	IS: median score divided patients into high I (n = 20) and low I (n = 20)	SOL-I LQOLP	No correlation between I and quality of life scores But patients with high insight had positive correlation with objective/ subjective indicators of quality of life
Smith et al. (1999)	n = 46 Schiz./schizaff (DSM-IV)	SUMD	SBS QOLI	Poor I associated with social behavioural deficits Subjective quality of life not correlate with I
Baier et al. (2000)	n = 37 Schiz./schizaff.	IS DSS	GAF	No correlation with psychosocial functioning
Larøi et al. (2000)	n = 21 Schiz. (DSM-IV)	SUMD	GAF	Poor I associated with worse psychosocial functioning
White et al. (2000)	n = 150 Schiz. (DSM-IV)	SAI	QOLI Items from IMSR GAF, GARF	Higher I associated with more close friends and family but with less satisfaction with relationships
Francis and Penn (2001)	n = 29 Schiz./schizaff.	ITAQ PANSS: item	Social skills and interactions in two	Better I associated with better social skill, less

Table 3.8 (*cont.*)

Study	Patients	Insight assessment	Measure of function/quality	Results
	and bipolar (DSM-IV)	G12 IS	contexts taped and rated; CES	strangeness, greater self-disclosure of mental illness. No correlation with specific social skills (eye contact, fluency, fidgeting, etc.)
Goldberg *et al.* (2001)	*n* = 211 Psychoses and affective (DSM-IV)	PANSS: item G12	BQOLI Overall social and non-verbal skills	Better I associated with better overall social skills. No correlation with non-verbal skills or quality of life
Pini *et al.* (2001)	*n* = 236 Psychoses and affective (DSM-IIIR)	SUMD	GAF	Some dimensions of I associated with GAF: poor awareness of anhedonia and a sociality associated with worse psychosocial function
Schwartz (2001)	*n* = 223 Schiz. (DSM-IV)	SUMD	FARS	No association with self-care deficits, inter-personal problems or family relationship problems
Marková *et al.* (2003)	*n* = 64 Schiz. (DSM-IV)	IPQ PSE: item 104	GAS	No correlation with functioning

Abbreviations: AMDP-LII: Lack of Insight Index from three items of the Manual for the Assessment and Documentation of Psychopathology; BQOLI: Brief Quality of Life Interview; CES: Customer Experience of Stigma; CSPAS: Cannon-Spoor Premorbid Adjustment Scale; DSS: Davidhizar *et al.* – Self-Rating Scale for Insight; FARS: Functional Assessment Rating Scale; GAF: Global Assessment of Functioning; GARF: Global Assessment of Relational Functioning; GAS: Global Assessment Scale; I: Insight; IMSR: Interview Measure of Social Relationships; IPQ: Insight in Psychosis Questionnaire; IS: Insight Scale; ITAQ: Insight and Treatment Attitude Questionnaire; LQOLP: Lancashire Quality of Life Profile; LSP: Life Skills Profile; PANSS: Positive and Negative Syndrome Scale; PSE: Present State Examination; QOL: Quality of Life Scale (Heinrichs *et al.*, 1984); QOLI: Quality of Life Interview (Lehman, 1988); SAI: Schedule for Assessing Insight; SBS: Social Behaviour Scale; Schiz.: Schizophrenia; Schizaff.: Schizoaffective Disorder; SFS: Social Functioning Scale; SOL-I: Standard of Living Questionnaire; SPS: Social Performance Schedule; SUMD: Scale to Assess Unawareness of Mental Disorder.

poorer psychosocial function and quality of life (O'Connor & Herrman, 1993; Lysaker *et al.*, 1994; Peralta & Cuesta, 1994; Dickerson *et al.*, 1997; Lysaker, *et al.*, 1998b; Larøi *et al.*, 2000; Pini *et al.*, 2001). One study reports that poor insight is associated with some pre-morbid adjustment disorders in late adolescence and in early adulthood (Debowska *et al.*, 1998). Finally, there are studies, which yield mixed results and generally these employ more detailed measures of different aspects of psychosocial functioning and/or quality of life. For example, using the Quality of Life Interview together with a Social Behaviour Scale, Smith *et al.* (1999) found that whilst poor insight in schizophrenic/schizoaffective patients was related to social behavioural deficits, their subjective quality of life assessments were not related to insight. In contrast, White *et al.* (2000) found that better insight in patients with schizophrenia was related not only to having more close friends and family but also to less satisfaction with their relationships. And other studies, also using more detailed social skills and quality of life measures, have suggested that poor insight relates to impairment in some social skills but not in others (Francis & Penn, 2001; Goldberg *et al.*, 2001).

3.2.9 Insight and psychiatric diagnosis

Do patients with schizophrenia have worse or a different sort of insight into their illness than patients with other mental disorders? Does insight depend to some extent on the type of mental disorder affecting an individual? Perhaps surprisingly such questions have not been addressed to any great extent. Overwhelmingly, empirical studies exploring insight into mental disorders have tended to focus predominantly on patients with schizophrenia and schizoaffective disorders. Of the studies that have included patients with various psychoses and affective disorders, only some have reported on any differences in insight held between different patient groups (Table 3.9).

Little can be said conclusively on the basis of the results summarised. Some studies suggest no significant differences in insight between different patients groups (David *et al.*, 1992; David *et al.*, 1995; Arduini *et al.*, 2003). Other studies point to differences between diagnostic groups but the differences themselves are variable. Most of these studies indicate that patients with schizophrenia seem to show less insight than patients in other diagnostic groups (Amador *et al.*, 1994; Michalakeas *et al.*, 1994; Fennig *et al.*, 1996). Nevertheless, some investigations claim that patients with schizophrenia have similar levels of insight to patients with bipolar and other psychotic disorders but poorer insight than that of patients with schizoaffective or other affective disorders (Weiler *et al.*, 2000; Pini *et al.*, 2001). On the other hand, other studies suggest that insight in schizophrenic patients is similar to that of schizoaffective patients (Cuesta *et al.*, 2000; Smith *et al.*, 2000) or even better than that of schizoaffective patients and manic patients

Table 3.9 Studies reporting on differences in insight between diagnostic groups

Study	Patients	Insight assessment	Results
Greenfeld *et al.* (1989)	*n* = 21 (SZ-9, BP-5, Unip.-4, atypical psychology: three) DSM-III	Interview along defined dimensions	Patients with depression more likely to attribute psychosis to physical illness
David *et al.* (1992)	*n* = 91 (SZ-52, paranoid psychosis −12, depressive psychosis −7, manic psychosis −4, mixed aff. and neurotic − 11, uncertain − 5) PSE CATEGO	SAI PSE: item 104	No difference in degree of I between patients with SZ and those with other diagnoses
Amador *et al.* (1994)	*n* = 348 (SZ-221, SA-49, BP-40, PMDD-24, non-psychotic MDD-14) DSM-IIIR	SUMD: abridged	Patients with SZ showed greater deficits in awareness than any other diagnostic group. Patients with BP (mania) showed similar levels of unawareness except had more awareness into delusions
Michalakeas *et al.* (1994)	*n* = 77 (women) (SZ-42, Mania-13, MDD-22) DSM-IIIR	ITAQ	Patients with SZ had poorest I, followed by patients with mania, and patients with MDD had highest I
David *et al.* (1995)	*n* = 150 (SZ-69, SA-12, AP-38, OP-31) DSM-IIIR	PSE: item 104	No difference in I between diagnostic groups
Swanson *et al.* (1995)	*n* = 41 (SZ-21, Mania-20) DSM-IIIR	Clinical vignettes	Patients with SZ less I than patients with Mania
Fennig *et al.* (1996)	*n* = 189 (SZ-86, BPp-52, PD-35, OP-16)	Insight item from HDRS	I highest in PD. Majority of BP gained I at f/u. SZ – poor I and less change over time
Kemp and David (1996)	*n* = 74 (SZ-43, SZF-7, BPm-17, BPd-3, SA-4) DSM-IIIR	SAI	Insight higher in non-SZ diagnostic groups

Table 3.9 (*cont.*)

Study	Patients	Insight assessment	Results
Sanz *et al.* (1998)	n = 33 (SZ-18, SA-6, BPm-6, PD-3) DSM-IV	ITAQ, SAI IPQ prelim PANSS: item G12	Patients with BPm and SA had lowest I, followed by SZ, whilst patients with PD had highest I (only with SAI)
Young *et al.* (1998)	n = 129 (SZ-108, BP-21 [12 manic]) DSM-IIIR	SUMD	No difference in I between SZ and BP (but when mania excluded, then poorer I in SZ) I in SZ was global correlating with other aspects of self-awareness (not the case for I in BP)
Weiler *et al.* (2000)	n = 187 (SZ-81, BP-40, MDD-33, SA-14, other-19) DSM-IIIR	ITAQ	Patients with SZ, BP and other psychoses had poorer I than SA and MDD. At d/s, patients with 'other' psychosis had lowest I
Cuesta *et al.* (2000)	n = 75 (SZ-37, SA-11, AP-27) DSM-IV	SUMD, ITAQ, AMDP: three items	Patients with SZ and SA had similar I but worse than patients with AP
Goldberg *et al.* (2001)	n = 211 (Psychotic: mostly SZ/SZF-158, Mood: mostly BP-52) DSM-IV	PANSS: item G12	Patients with mood disorders (including BP) had better I than patients with psychotic disorders
Pini *et al.* (2001)	n = 236 (SZ-29, SA-24, BP-153, UD-30) DSM-IIIR	SUMD	Patients with SZ had poorer I than SA and Unip. but same level of I as BP
Arduini *et al.* (2003)	n = 64 (SZ-42, BP-22) DSM-IV	SUMD: abridged	No difference in degree of I between patients with SZ and BP
Eisen *et al.* (2004)	n = 149 (OCD-64, BDD-85) DSM-IV	BABS	Patients with BDD had poorer I than patients with OCD

Abbreviations: AMDP-LII: Lack of Insight Index from three items of the Manual for the Assessment and Documentation of Psychopathology; AP: Affective Psychosis; BABS: Brown Assessment of Belief Scale; BDD: Body Dysmorphic Disorder; BP: Bipolar Affective Disorder; BPd: Bipolar Depression; BPm: Bipolar Manic; BPp: Bipolar Psychotic Disorder; HDRS: Hamilton Depression Rating Scale; I: Insight; IPQ: Insight in Psychosis Questionnaire; ITAQ: Insight and Treatment Attitude Questionnaire; MDD: Major Depressive Disorder without psychosis; OCD: Obsessive Compulsive Disorder; OP: Other Psychosis; PANSS: Positive and Negative Syndrome Scale; PD: Psychotic Depression; PMDD: Major Depressive Disorder with Psychosis; PSE: Present State Examination; SA: Schizoaffective Disorder; SAI: Schedule for Assessing Insight; SUMD: Scale to Assess Unawareness of Mental Disorder; SZ: Schizophrenia; SZF: Schizophreniform Disorder; UD: Unipolar Depression.

(Sanz *et al.*, 1998). Factors likely to contribute to the inconsistencies in this area include not just the differences in insight assessments but also the specific diagnostic criteria used. In addition, the proportions of patient numbers in the different diagnostic categories vary considerably across the studies described.

There have been few systematic empirical studies exploring insight in conditions other than the various psychoses. Why the exploration of insight empirically should be limited to the psychoses is not so clear, except presumably that since loss of insight has long been intrinsic to the definitional criteria of certain psychotic symptoms such as delusions (Berrios, 1994b), examination of insight has been promoted by the conditions where its loss is so dramatically apparent. Indeed, as far as the so-called anxiety, dissociative disorders, milder depressive disorders, etc. (i.e., those conditions traditionally conceived in the 'neurotic' sphere where, conventionally, insight is assumed to be present), are concerned, much of the empirical work has taken place predominantly in the psychodynamic field (Chapter 2). However, it is of interest, that some of the traditional views concerning the notion that the presence of insight can be used as a criterion to differentiate between the psychoses and the so-called neuroses have begun to be challenged in practical as well as in theoretical ways. For example, in recognition of the increasingly common observations that patients with obsessive-compulsive disorders (OCD) show a wide range of insight, particularly as far as regarding their obsessions/compulsions as senseless is concerned (e.g. Insel & Akiskal, 1986; Lelliott *et al.*, 1988), then the DSM-IV Field Trial, using a structured scale, specifically explored insight in 431 patients with OCD (Foa & Kozak, 1995). Their conclusions, confirming that patients with OCD do show a range of insight resulted in a change made to the previous definitional criteria of DSM-IIIR, and a new specifier of 'OCD with poor insight' was introduced into DSM-IV (American Psychiatric Association, 1994). Nevertheless, there has not yet been much work exploring the relationship between insight in patients with OCD and other clinical correlates. Some small earlier studies yield mixed results. For example, one study suggested that patients with poor insight into their obsessions/compulsions showed worse clinical outcome after exposure treatment (Foa, 1979). On the other hand, a larger study by Lelliott *et al.* (1988) found no difference in outcome following behaviour therapy between those patients with and without insight. Another more recent study found that patients with poorer insight in OCD (i.e. patients who had strong beliefs in the feared consequences of not carrying out their compulsions) had worse outcome following behaviour therapy than those who expressed less strong beliefs in the consequences of not carrying out their compulsions (Foa *et al.*, 1999) (Table 3.4). However, the same study also found that patients who showed less insight into their OCD (in terms of articulating fears concerning consequences of obsessional beliefs) seemed to benefit more from the behaviour treatment than those who showed better insight. In other words, the researchers found different types of outcome according to level or severity of poor insight expressed by the patients. Using a semi-structured rating scale assessing insight in 71 patients with OCD, Eisen *et al.* (2001) found that insight improved as symptoms of OCD improved though insight itself was not found to be a predictor of clinical response to pharmacotherapy. The semi-structured rating scale used in the study, the Brown Assessment of Beliefs Scale (BABS), was originally devised to assess delusional beliefs in terms of components of insight, such as conviction, fixity of belief, response to different explanations, perceptions of others' views, etc. (Eisen *et al.*, 1998). Again, this arose in recognition of the observation that patients with delusions showed a range or continuum of insight and hence delusional beliefs should not, simply by definition, be associated with insightlessness. Using the same semi-structured rating scale assessing insight into beliefs, Eisen *et al.* (2004) compared insight in patients with obsessive-compulsive disorder and those with body dysmorphic disorder (BDD). The authors found that patients with BDD had significantly worse insight than patients with OCD even though severity of illness was comparable in the two groups. The authors suggested that it was the type of beliefs held by the BDD group that was significant, particularly beliefs around others' perception of patients' views, as well as more delusional ideation that contributed to the poorer insight held.

Greenfeld *et al.* (1991) carried out a longitudinal study exploring insight in 30 patients with Anorexia Nervosa. Using their structured schedule for assessment of insight, they found that the presence of insight predicted clinical outcome (Table 3.4). In contrast to the results reported in relation to changes in insight over time (e.g. McEvoy *et al.*, 1989b), patients with anorexia nervosa were found to maintain a relatively consistent level of insight between their acute illness (hospitalisation) and follow-up (after discharge from hospital). The other interesting and contrasting finding (compared with much of the work on insight in psychoses), was that the researchers reported a correlation between high levels of global insight and more severe illness (in terms of degree of emaciation and longer hospital admissions) (Table 3.5). The authors speculated that perhaps the longer duration of hospital admission as well as the more severe emaciation promoted patients to confront their illness and to learn about the reality of their problems. These are interesting issues raised by the studies, both in OCD/BDD and in anorexia nervosa, but there needs to be much more research in these areas and in other non-psychoses disorders in order to develop further understanding about the nature of insight in these conditions.

Only some studies have explored insight empirically solely in affective disorders (Ghaemi *et al.*, 1995; 1996; Ghaemi *et al.*, 1997; Peralta & Cuesta, 1998; Pallanti *et al.*, 1999; Cassidy *et al.*, 2001; Yen *et al.*, 2003) and these vary in their aims. Thus, the studies by Ghaemi *et al.* (1995; 1996) examined insight in patients with acute mania and found that patients tended to show poor insight and that this did not improve over the course of hospital admission. In contrast, Yen *et al.* (2003) reported an overall improvement in insight in patients with mania as their manic symptoms resolved though they found also that in some cases patients' insight remained either unchanged or worsened. Pallanti *et al.* (1999), on the other hand, focusing on clinical differences between patients with bipolar I and II disorders, found that patients with bipolar II disorders seemed to show poorer insight than bipolar I patients. A different study, reported by Peralta and Cuesta (1998), explored differences in insight (using the AMDP: 3 items) between patients with mania ($n = 21$) and patients with depression ($n = 33$) and looked at the effects of psychotic symptoms in relation to insight. They found that manic patients tended to show less insight than depressed patients, that patients with depression and psychotic symptoms had less insight than those with depression and without psychotic symptoms (this same association with psychotic symptoms did not hold for patients with mania), and that mood-congruent and mood-incongruent psychotic symptoms did not differ in relation to contributing to insight. In another approach, Ghaemi *et al.* (1997) examined insight change in patients with seasonal affective disorder before and after light therapy, and found higher levels of insight associated with more severe depressive ratings but no significant change in insight following treatment. Lastly, and in yet a different vein, the study by Cassidy *et al.* (2001) explored differences in insight between patients with pure manic disorders ($n = 42$) and those with mixed manic disorders ($n = 11$). Using the ITAQ, they found that patients with the mixed manic episodes showed greater insight than those with pure manic episodes and linked this with more depressive symptoms experienced by the former. Again, as with other variables, no definitive statements can be made concerning the nature of insight in relation to affective disorders. However, the studies do raise the issue of the relationship between depression and insight.

3.2.10 Insight and depression

Questions around the relationship between insight and depression have tended to be embedded, generally speaking, within the psychological and motivational conceptions of the nature of insight. In other words, within these frameworks, impairment of insight in relation to mental disorders is viewed as a form of denial, a strategy employed to protect the self from the psychological consequences of having knowledge about a particular disorder and its effects. It would follow, therefore, that patients with greater insight, or less denial, by understanding more fully the implications of having a particular disorder, would naturally be likely to become distressed or depressed. In general, empirical studies exploring associations between insight and depression have sought to either support or disprove this broad premise. More recently, related cognitive models couching the possible relationship between insight and depression in terms of self-esteem factors, have also been proposed though empirical results have not been conclusive (Iqbal *et al.*, 2000; Drake *et al.*, 2004).

As already seen in the previous section (Table 3.9), there is some suggestion that patients with depressive disorders show better insight into their illness than patients with schizophrenic/schizoaffective/other psychotic disorders. Cassidy *et al.* (2001) study indicated, in addition, that patients with mixed manic states (i.e. with increased depressive symptoms) had more insight than patients with pure manic states (without depressive symptoms). However, as was discussed, numbers of studies are small and results are variable.

Clearly, by far the most empirical studies on insight have been carried out in patients with schizophrenia and other psychotic disorders. In these studies, therefore, depression tends to be rated on the basis of presence of depressive symptoms or patterns of depressive symptoms usually by adding cumulative scores on depressive items from general psychopathology instruments or occasionally using depressive rating scales such as the Hamilton Depression Rating Scale or the Calgary Depression Rating Scale. Thus, several studies have reported on the association between insight and degree of depression. Results here, as in other areas, are variable. However, most of the studies do seem to find an association between better insight and worse depression (Smith *et al.*, 1998; 2000; Carroll *et al.*, 1999; Moore *et al.*, 1999; Iqbal *et al.*, 2000; White *et al.*, 2000; Pyne *et al.*, 2001; Schwartz, 2001) though some studies have qualified this association on longitudinal follow-up finding that better insight is associated with worse depression at baseline but not at 6 weeks (Kemp & Lambert, 1995), 12 months (Mintz *et al.*, 2004) or 18 months follow-up (Drake *et al.*, 2004). Some studies find this association only with some aspects of insight, e.g. the Amador *et al.* (1994) study found that schizophrenic patients with depressive symptoms showed better awareness of specific symptoms (current thought disorder, blunt affect, anhedonia) than schizophrenic patients without depressive symptoms. Similarly, the study by Carsky *et al.* (1992) showed that patients with greater acknowledgement of symptoms and poor functioning had more depressive symptoms but that this association did not hold in relation to acknowledgement of the need for treatment. Some studies find no relationship between insight and depression in mixed psychotic patients (Amador *et al.*, 1993; Kim *et al.*, 1997; Cuesta *et al.*, 2000), and a few studies apparently find an association in the opposite direction, i.e., poor insight (or aspects of insight) associated with worse depression (O'Connor & Herrman, 1993; Collins *et al.*, 1997; Buckley *et al.*, 2001; Sevy *et al.*, 2004). An interesting study, explicitly testing a hypothesis of psychological mechanisms underlying insight (specifically invoking mechanisms of self-deception), was reported by Dixon *et al.* (1998). Using a discrepancy method of assessing insight (i.e. differences between patients' and relatives' evaluations) in 41 schizophrenic patients, they found that subjective ratings (i.e. those made by patients) of worse depression were associated with increased insight. In contrast, objective ratings (i.e. those made by relatives) of worse depression were associated with poorer insight. Subjective increased depression was also associated with greater insight into psychotic illness in the study by Sanz *et al.* (1998).

Related to the ideas about insight and depression, some investigations have also examined the association between insight and suicidal thoughts/behaviour in schizophrenic patients. In Amador *et al.* (1996) study, patients were categorised into those with and without recurrent suicidal thoughts/behaviours. An association was found between only some aspects of insight and suicidal thoughts. Thus, patients with greater awareness of specific symptoms (delusions, asociality, blunted affect, anhedonia) showed more suicidal thoughts and behaviours. Similarly, Schwartz and Petersen (1999) found a specific association between suicidality ratings (on the FARS) and only some aspects of insight. They found that only increased insight into the need for treatment was associated with increased suicidality ratings, whereas there was no such association with insight into mental disorder or into its social consequences. This finding contrasts (if depressive symptoms and suicidal thoughts are taken as reflecting similar distress) with Carsky *et al.* (1992) study where no relationship was found between depression and insight into need for treatment but it was found between depression and insight into mental illness. Recent longitudinal studies of patients with schizophrenia spectrum disorders found that patients with good insight had experienced more suicidal attempts than those with poor insight (Bourgeois *et al.*, 2004; Mintz *et al.*, 2004). Bourgeois *et al.* (2004) suggested that depression and hopelessness were factors mediating this. They also reported that changes in insight associated with treatment over 2 years helped reduce risk of suicide attempts. The association between insight and depression was found at baseline measurements but not at 1-year follow-up in the study by Mintz *et al.* (2004).

3.2.11 Insight and compliance with treatment

Poor compliance with treatment is a source of major problems in the management of patients with severe mental illness as it carries important implications for patients' well-being and prognoses (McEvoy, 1998). Increasingly, research has focused on determining possible factors which influence compliance and which could be used to find new ways of improving adherence to treatments (Buchanan, 1992; Kemp & David, 1996). The role that insight into mental illness might have in relation to compliance with treatments has been examined in several studies. Most such studies suggest that poorer insight into illness is associated with poorer compliance with treatments (Lin *et al.*, 1979; Marder *et al.*, 1983; Bartkó *et al.*, 1988;

McEvoy *et al.*, 1989b; Amador *et al.*, 1993; MacPherson *et al.*, 1996; Mutsatsa *et al.*, 2003) though some suggest only a weak correlation (Van Putten *et al.*, 1976) or no correlation (Taylor & Perkins, 1991) and even a negative relationship (Whitman & Duffey, 1961). McEvoy *et al.* (1989a, b) found that schizophrenic patients with better insight on hospital admission (ITAQ) were more compliant with treatments at initial and early assessments but that good insight at this stage did not associate with compliance at long-term (2–3 year) follow-up. Similar results were reported by Cuffel *et al.* (1996) in their study of 89 schizophrenic patients in that better insight (based on semi-structured interview addressing patients' recognition of illness and need for psychiatric treatment) was associated with recent adherence to outpatient treatment and medication but not with later use of services and adherence to medication.

Studies examining the relationship between insight into mental illness and compliance with offered treatments are, however, particularly difficult to interpret. Some of the problems relate to the difficulty in evaluating treatment adherence itself (McEvoy, 1998) but the main problem concerns the assessments of insight in these circumstances and the consequent meaningfulness of results. Specifically, the problem consists of the circularity that results when insight is defined, in part at least, by acceptance of treatment (e.g. Lin *et al.*, 1979; McEvoy *et al.*, 1989a; David, 1990; Buchanan, 1992; Amador *et al.*, 1993; Cuffel *et al.*, 1996). Rating insight then becomes tantamount to rating verbal compliance and difficulties arise in determining the individual aspects of the putative explored relationship. It is not that it is invalid to address the question of a relationship between verbal compliance with treatment and actual adherence to treatment for that will necessarily provide important information in terms of understanding views and concerns of patients, and help to plan future management. Indeed, studies have shown that there is not a direct relationship between articulated attitudes towards treatment and actual behavioural adherence (McEvoy *et al.*, 1989b). The issues here, however, are twofold. First is the question of whether there are any theoretical grounds to consider verbal compliance with treatment as a component of insight (Marková & Berrios, 1995a; McCabe *et al.*, 2000). Second is the question whether it is meaningful to treat verbal compliance *qua* insight as a variable against which actual treatment adherence is assessed (David, 1990; Lambert & Baldwin, 1990). Interestingly, there is some suggestion from the few studies where insight assessment does not, to any great extent, incorporate attitudes to treatment, that the relationship between insight and adherence to treatment is more complicated. For example, in the study by Goldberg *et al.* (2001), better insight (assessed by the PANSS: item G12) was associated with more positive attitudes towards medication but was not correlated with self-reported ratings of medication compliance. And, similarly, the study by Sanz *et al.* (1998) which compared insight evaluated by different scales found that better insight, as assessed by ITAQ, SAI and PANSS, showed significant association with adherence to medication, as well as compliance with attendance at mental health centres. However, insight assessed by the IPQ (preliminary version) did not correlate with medication adherence although it did relate to continued contact with mental health centres.

3.2.12 Insight and other clinical variables

Lastly, there are a few studies examining the relationship between insight and other clinical features which are interesting but which, because of the lack of sufficient work in these areas, can do little more than suggest further avenues of exploration. Taylor and Perkins (1991), e.g. explored the relationship between 'insight' (denial/exaggeration of problems) and patients' feelings of identity, i.e., in regards to whether patients related more to feeling as 'community members' or as 'patients'. Contrary to their expectations, they found no association between patients' perceived identities and denial of illness. On the other hand, McEvoy *et al.* (1996) examined the relationship between schizophrenic patients' insight and their social understanding or common sense. Using the *Social Knowledge Questionnaire*, to determine patients' understanding of social behaviours, and the ITAQ to assess insight, they found that higher insight was related to better social knowledge in 32 patients with schizophrenia. Interestingly, using the SAI to assess insight, Upthegrove *et al.* (2002), also examining the association between insight and social knowledge in schizophrenic patients ($n = 30$), found no association between levels of insight and social knowledge, and argued for independence of these concepts. From a slightly different perspective, Vaz *et al.* (2002) examined social interaction (using the Social Cognitions and Object Relations Scale (SCORS)) as a form of social knowledge about the environment in patients with schizophrenia, and found a correlation between good insight (SAI) and understanding of social causality dimension on the SCORS. They posited the importance of conceiving insight as a multidimensional structure that needs to take account of a wider context of social knowledge and interpersonal relationships.

Another viewpoint in relation to insight was examined by Lysaker *et al.* (1999) in their investigation of likely personality factors that could be important in contributing to insight and changes in insight in patients with schizophrenic disorders. Their study suggested that some personality factors, such as extraversion and psychoticism, might be predictive of fewer fluctuations in insight over time. In a later study, Lysaker *et al.* (2002) examined the relationship between patients' insight and coping style (using avoidance and positive reappraisal scales of the Ways of Coping Scale). They reported that, in their sample of 132 patients with schizophrenia or schizoaffective disorders, patients unaware of their symptoms showed a greater preference for positive reappraisal than partially aware or unaware patients (SUMD). In addition, they found that patients unaware of the consequences of their illness endorsed a greater preference for escape-avoidance as a coping style. Within the acknowledged limitations of the study design, the researchers suggest that, perhaps, different types of coping strategies might be differentially related to deficits in different aspects of insight and raise the importance of exploring this further particularly in terms of developing and enhancing rehabilitation strategies. Indeed, in another study, Lysaker *et al.* (2003) found that a subgroup of patients (schizophrenia spectrum disorders) with poor insight and average executive function (WCST) scored significantly more on the distancing (passive dismissal) coping strategy than patients with poor insight and impaired executive function. Discussion in these areas can only be speculative at this point but the issue is highlighted that insight in its multidimensional sense may be underpinned by a variety of different mechanisms.

In a novel approach seeking to modify patients' insight into their psychoses by allowing self-observation into their acute psychotic state by means of videotapes, Davidoff *et al.* (1998) found that patients' insight into their illness improved compared with those patients not exposed to such videos despite comparable levels of psychopathology. The researchers thus suggested that self-observation in recovered patients of their acute illness may be a useful means of developing patients' insight.

Moore *et al.* (1999) explored levels of self-deception or denial in schizophrenic patients using the Balanced Inventory of Desirable Responding. They found that patients with poorer insight had fewer depressive symptoms and had higher scores on the self-deception measure, and suggested that the mechanism of impaired insight in these patients might relate to the psychological process of denial.

A few studies have looked at the relationship between patients' insight into mental illness and their insight into abnormal movements (dyskinesia), and generally found that poor insight into mental disorder is associated with poor insight into involuntary movements (Caracci *et al.*, 1990; Cuesta & Peralta, 1994; Arango *et al.*, 1999). Using the SUMD, Arango *et al.* (1999) found that unawareness of dyskinesia correlated only with some aspects of poor insight into mental illness. They also reported that schizophrenic patients with the deficit syndrome had less awareness of abnormal movements than those without a deficit syndrome and that unawareness of dyskinesia was not related to the severity of the dyskinesia itself. The latter finding was likewise reported by Macpherson and Collis (1992) who also suggested that patients with manic-depressive psychoses (ICD-9) were significantly more likely to be aware of their tardive dyskinesia than patients with schizophrenia. However, the nature of the relationship between insight into such drug-induced abnormal motor movements and into mental illness itself has not been the focus of much conceptual or theoretical work. It is therefore difficult to infer very much in terms of understanding insight or its relationships on the bases of these empirical studies alone. However, they do raise important issues that need to be considered particularly as far as insight as a relational concept is concerned (Chapter 7).

Other occasional correlations have been sought between insight into mental disorder and different clinical variables. For example, Cuesta and Peralta (1994) found no association between insight into mental disorder and the presence of neurological soft signs. The rationale in examining this relationship was to look for an association between neurological/cognitive dysfunction (using the soft neurological signs as proxy 'organic' variables) as a mechanism to 'explain' poor insight.

3.3 Conclusion

Over the last 15 years considerable interest has been taken in the empirical exploration of insight in patients with mental illness and predominantly those with psychotic disorders. Whilst clinical interest in the notion of insight has been apparent since insight was conceptualised as a clinical phenomenon, this specific research interest seems to have been generated following the relatively recent attempts at the operationalisation of the concept of insight. In turn, this has resulted in the development of a number of structured measures of insight thus facilitating its quantitative assessment and hence encouraging the surge of correlational studies.

In different ways, the underlying purpose of empirical studies, whether explicitly stated or implicitly understood, has been to elucidate the nature of insight as a clinical phenomenon. The primary questions have focused on three main issues. First has been the question concerning the extent to which impairment of insight could be considered intrinsic to the mental illness process itself. Thus, studies have examined the relationship between patients' insight and clinical variables related to the mental disorder, such as severity of illness, specific symptomatology, cognitive impairment, brain dysfunction, etc. Second has been the question concerning the extent to which impaired insight could be considered as an individual reaction to the mental illness. In order to try to answer this, studies have examined the association between patients' insight and various mood disorders or reactions or specific personality variables. Third has been the question concerning the extent to which patients' insight might be shaped by individual and external or environmental factors. Studies have attempted to explore this by examining the relationship between patients' insight and socio-demographic variables, cultural factors, past experiences, educational/social knowledge, etc. Secondary questions explored by empirical studies have related mainly to the clinical implication of having impairment of insight, i.e., whether insight can be considered a prognostic factor and consequently whether efforts should be made to help change patients' insight.

It is evident, however, that clear or definitive answers to the above questions are difficult to obtain. As this chapter has shown, the outcomes of empirical studies in these areas yield, to varying extents, mixed and inconclusive results. Whilst differences in study methodologies, e.g. patient samples (diagnostic categories, acute/chronic, numbers, outpatients/inpatients, etc.) and outcome measures, are likely to contribute to this variability in results, a significant factor must be to do with the difficulties involved in 'capturing' insight empirically. As is apparent, such difficulties reside in a number of areas. Firstly, the conceptualisation of insight theoretically has proved complex and work in this area has demonstrated this in the wide range of definitions proposed. Such definitions vary in specificity, breadth, focus and their detail or components. The numbers and range of definitions put forward are reflective of the inherent complexity of the concept of insight itself and, indeed, the view of insight as a multidimensional structure has become the dominant conceptualisation amongst researchers. Secondly, and as a result of different definitions of insight, various assessment instruments have been devised, differing in contents (types and specificity of judgements, details, etc.), in the way in which insight is elicited (clinician versus self-ratings), the ratings employed (categorical/continuous scores), etc. Thirdly, additional difficulties are posed by the problems of the translation process itself, i.e., the conversion from a theoretical concept of insight to an empirical measure designed to capture the identified components of the theoretical construct. The various measures that have been detailed in this chapter reflect to different extents the researchers' original conceptualisation. For all these reasons, it is perhaps not surprising that empirical studies exploring the relationship between patients' insight and clinical variables yield such mixed results.

The fact that so far empirical work has been unable to produce conclusive results should not, however, detract from the importance of the research carried out in this area. What is raised and highlighted by these studies is the complexity of the concept of insight, its relational nature (Chapter 7) and the issue that *different* aspects of insight are elicited in *different* studies and by *different* methods and are likely to be important in different ways and for *different* reasons. Consequently, future work needs to look again at firstly exploring the structure of insight at a conceptual or theoretical level, which would enable the clearer delineation of specific aspects of insight. Secondly, work needs to address the problems and limitations of the translation process so that the clinical phenomena of aspects of insight can be more clearly demarcated. Only then, decisions can be made concerning which aspects of insight might be usefully examined in relation to particular variables. These issues are explored in more detail in Part II.

Insight in organic brain syndromes: insight into neurological states

4.1 Introduction

Over the past 10–15 years, and paralleling the interest in the empirical examination of insight in 'functional' psychiatric disorders, there has likewise been a proliferation of studies focusing on exploring patients' insight into organic brain syndromes, particularly, dementias (Marková & Berrios, 2000; Clare, 2004). Studies in this area have concentrated predominantly on examining the relationship between patients' insight and clinical variables, e.g. the severity or type of brain lesion/dementia, the presence of affective disorder, etc. There has been, in addition, more emphasis on developing specific measures to assess insight as well as on exploring possible neurological and neuropsychological mechanisms underlying impaired insight. As with studies on insight in functional psychiatric disorders, outcomes have yielded variable and inconsistent results (Marková & Berrios, 2000). Many of the problems encountered in the empirical study of insight in functional psychiatric disorders, such as, differences in the definitions of insight and underlying concepts, differences in methods of assessing insight and different outcome measures employed, are likewise evident in the studies of insight in patients with dementia and are likely to be contributing to the variability in results. However, there are, in addition, issues more specific to the exploration of insight in dementia and these also need to be considered.

Firstly, the clinical status of the dementias themselves is of particular significance. Dementias, or chronic organic brain syndromes, are conditions which, in contemporary times, cross different clinical disciplines, occupying neurological, neuropsychological, psychiatric, etc., domains in clinically relevant ways. Consequently, studies exploring insight in patients with dementias are subject to the additional influences of the specific conceptual frameworks of insight held by these different clinical disciplines. Secondly, and relating to this first issue, the clinical features themselves of the dementias are also likely important contributors to the mixed results obtained in studies exploring insight. Dementias are characterised by a range of diverse symptoms and signs as a result of organic, psychiatric, psychological and functional changes. Problems therefore can include various specific cognitive impairments (including memory), neurological deficits, affective changes, psychotic symptoms, personality and/or behavioural disturbances, functional disabilities, and can also relate to the experience of having the condition as a whole. These problems are different in kind from each other and demand different ways of assessing insight. Studies exploring insight into dementias therefore will be influenced by the problems that are chosen as the 'objects' of insight assessment and, in turn, the latter will influence the particular concept of insight used by researchers. This theoretical point will be explored more fully in Chapter 7. However, the issue here is that the different types of symptoms and signs characterising the dementias have resulted in a much wider range of instruments assessing insight. Such instruments assess different aspects of insight and will therefore contribute to the variability in study outcomes more than has been the case with studies assessing insight in functional psychiatric disorders.

Particularly influential in studies exploring insight in dementia has been the work on insight or awareness into neurological states. This chapter therefore provides an introduction to Chapter 5 and briefly examines such work concentrating on the neurological and neuropsychological conceptualisations of insight. Chapter 5 follows on to review the empirical studies on insight in dementia and focuses particularly on the differences between various approaches to insight assessment and their consequences on the aspect of insight elicited. Both chapters also review the results of studies exploring insight in relation to different clinical variables.

4.2 Insight into neurological states

In contrast to the way in which interest in insight developed in general psychiatry where attention was drawn to the phenomenon when patients were observed to *show some insight* into their madness, interest in insight in relation to neurological states developed from the opposite perspective. Namely, patients with marked neurological abnormalities were, surprisingly, observed to *show no insight* or awareness into their problems. Thus, since the late nineteenth century, the literature provides descriptions of patients, seemingly oblivious to prominent and major neurological deficits, who maintained their 'unawareness' and/or explicitly denied any disability in the face of confrontative evidence to the contrary (e.g. Anton, 1899). Babinski (1914) coined the term 'anosognosia' to refer to the unawareness or denial of hemiplegia seen in patients following a stroke. The term has, since then, also been used to refer to the unawareness displayed in patients with other neurological or neuropsychological syndromes. These include cortical blindness (Anton's syndrome), aphasia (Rubens & Garrett, 1991), hemiballismus (Roth, 1944), amnesic syndromes (McGlynn & Schacter, 1989), dementia (Reed *et al.*, 1993; Smith *et al.*, 2000, see below), tardive dyskinesia (Myslobodsky, 1986) and deficits seen following head injury (Prigatano, 1991) and others.

Irrespective of the particular neurological/neuropsychological impairment involved, the concept of anosognosia has, in contrast to the concept of insight in general psychiatry, been consistent in generally referring to the more specific and fairly narrow meaning of unawareness of a particular impairment. In a similar fashion, a variety of different terms have been employed (and used interchangeably) in the neurological/neuropsychological literature to refer to the concept, including, e.g. loss of insight, unawareness, impaired awareness, impaired self-awareness or impaired self-consciousness and denial. Nonetheless, the underlying concept has been that of unawareness in its narrow sense, i.e. without any reference to more wider judgements made by the subject. The one exception is in the use of the term 'denial' which has been used, in addition (though not consistently), in a psychodynamic sense to refer to a concept where the subject is understood to have awareness at some level (conscious or otherwise) but, for various reasons is unable or unwilling to acknowledge this (Weinstein & Kahn, 1955). This distinction between unawareness, as an inability to be aware of a deficit on neurological/neuropsychological grounds, and denial, as an inability to be aware of a deficit on psychodynamic or motivational grounds, is significant. It marks the division between two broad lines of conceptualisation of loss of insight in neurological states that has been evident in various forms since the late nineteenth century (McGlynn & Schacter, 1989; Prigatano & Schacter, 1991). And, both conceptualisations of unawareness have been important in the empirical work on loss of insight in relation to dementia (see below). In addition, the neurological or neuropsychological concept of unawareness/anosognosia has been particularly influential in the more recent empirical work on insight in psychoses seeking to associate poor insight with neuropsychological deficits and neuroanatomical substrates (see Chapter 3).

One question needs to be addressed before moving on to briefly look at some of the models of unawareness in neurological states and related empirical work in this area. This is the question concerning any difference between conceptualisation of unawareness in the neurological/neuropsychological sense (excluding 'denial' in the motivational sense) and unawareness or loss of insight in the general psychiatric sense of the concept. This is important for two reasons. First, research work often extends ideas and results between different clinical areas, e.g. in studies making analogies between anosognosia in neurology and loss of insight in psychiatry. Second, it draws attention to the confusion that is often generated by the interchangeable use of various terms and will thus help to clarify the meaning of the underlying concept.

Although literally meaning a lack of knowledge of disease, anosognosia or unawareness in the neuropsychological sense refers to a much narrower notion of knowledge than is usually understood by lack of insight or unawareness in the general psychiatric sense. In the former, and likely as a result of its direct link to a specific obvious impairment, the concept is much closer to the notion of a lack of conscious-ness of a problem. In other words, it is lack of knowledge at the most basic level, a loss of *perception*, which is invoked; that is, the ability to interpret apparent changes in experienced sensory stimulation. The patient with anosognosia for blindness cannot *perceive* he is blind. He is not making a correct interpretation of his apparently disturbed sensory input. Similarly, the patient with anosognosia for hemiplegia cannot *perceive* his disability, again he is not making a correct interpret-ation of a neurologically apparent impairment of ability to move his limbs. The concept is one of loss of perception, i.e. perception in the sense of the most primary of knowledge involving direct interpretations of sensations. Clearly, as the concept is extended to relate to a wider range of disabilities/neuropsychological impair-ments, then these sensations become more complex structures incorporating internal perceptions as well as sensations, e.g. in anosognosia for memory impairment. But the core concept remains one of an impairment of perception or consciousness of something. Within this framework, i.e. the inherent loss or impairment of basic knowledge, there is not the scope for including other forms of judgements in the way these are incorporated into the wider notion of lack of insight in relation to psychiatric disorders.

It is important at this point to clarify another issue. Referring to the neurological or neuropsychological conceptualisation of unawareness/loss of insight might give the impression that there is only the one definition, only the one way of conceiving loss of awareness in this field. In fact, that is far from the case. Here too, as in other clinical areas, there are a multitude of definitions and models put forward in attempts to describe and define a concept that remains complex and irreducible except in very simplistic terms. The literature on consciousness or awareness is extremely vast both in trying to explain normal mental and brain states as well as pathological states. It encompasses perspectives from neurology, philosophy, psych-ology, particularly cognitive neuropsychology, etc. and is a testament to the com-plexity of the problem and the difficulties in trying to bring together phenomenal, subjective qualities and neurological function/dysfunction into a common language (Picton & Stuss, 1994). It is well beyond the scope of this chapter to review such work and detailed and comprehensive texts can be found elsewhere (e.g. Brain, 1958; Marcel & Bisiach, 1988; Milner & Rugg, 1992; Hameroff *et al.*, 1996; Velmans, 1996; Edelman, 2003). The essential point for the purposes of this chapter is that, accept-ing the qualifications above, within the broad neurological/neuropsychological framework, the core conception of impaired insight is that of impaired awareness or consciousness. As such, it does not entail the secondary elaborations or judgements that are intrinsic to the concept of insight in general psychiatry.

This narrower concept is reflected in the clinical phenomena of unawareness that are elicited in neurological states and, as is described below, in the instruments designed to assess these. Once again, it is necessary to provide some qualifications. Unawareness in this narrower sense is generally conceived and elicited clinically as a unitary phenomenon, i.e. patients are viewed as having or not having awareness of their disability or aspects of their disability. (Some researchers argue that unawareness, as applied in neurological states, is not a unitary phenomenon. However, it is the term 'unitary' that is the source of confusion here rather than the way in which unawareness is conceived and elicited.) Nevertheless, there have also been some attempts to widen the notion and incorporate additional judgements to capture more of the type of 'knowledge' patients have concerning their disabilities. For example, Critchley (1953) refers to other forms of anosognosia and includes judgements concerning ascribed ownership of paralysed limbs, their location in space, their detachment from the body, names given to them, etc. Weinstein and Kahn (1955) include similar judgements and, in addition, extend the concept by including clinicians' judgements of patients' behaviours and incorporating clinical phenomena, such as withdrawal, mood changes and inattention. Likewise, Cutting (1978) brings together so-called 'anosognosic phenomena' with anosognosia in his study examining clinical correlations with unawareness of hemiplegia. There, he includes not just unawareness of the disability but also a range of attitudes towards the disability (e.g. anosodiaphoria, misoplegia, personification, somatoparaphrenia). Nevertheless, these sorts of elaborations on the part of the patient are intrinsic to the abnormal awareness state itself, representing the primary pathological interpretations of the abnormal perception. This can be likened to the way that some psychotic patients might interpret delusionally what is happening to them. In this sense, Weinstein and Kahn (1955) likewise refer to the 'anosognosic delusion'. However, this is not the same as the more involved judgements demanded of psychiatric patients with respect to insight into their illness where such judgements extend into relating abnormal experiences to the self and to their consequences to the self. In other words, although further judgements are being assessed in these patients with unawareness of hemiplegia, these judgements remain, in a sense, primary. They cannot extend beyond the basic description of the specific experience. In part, this is directly due to the perspective from which insight in neurological states is sought and this will be discussed in detail in Chapters 7 and 8. In brief, however, by definition, it is not possible to demand judgements concerning the detailed consequences of a problem if a problem is not actually experienced or perceived. Thus, the phenomenon of awareness in neurological states remains focused on its narrow sense.

The recognition that unawareness/anosognosia is specific and selective, i.e. patients could show awareness of some deficits (frequently mild ones) and yet be unaware of others in the face of more extensive pathology (McGlynn & Schacter, 1989; Bisiach & Geminiani, 1991; Jehkonen et al., 2000), or, show dissociation between verbal denial and behavioural concomitants (Berti et al., 1998), has, however, helped to broaden the notion and the instruments used to assess unawareness. For example, in brain injury, attention has been paid to the different resulting deficits or disabilities, e.g. behavioural problems, affective disorders, personality changes, etc. and 'awareness' has been examined in relation to these (Prigatano, 1991; Sherer, *et al.*, 1998; 2003b). Similarly, Blonder and Ranseen (1994) focused on examining unawareness for cognitive and affective deficits rather than unawareness for hemiplegia in patients who had suffered strokes. Conceptualisation and evaluation of unawareness in neurological states has therefore broadened in a number of ways but, as is seen below, the core concept of unawareness remains narrow and relatively circumscribed.

It is useful, for two main reasons, to briefly review some of the approaches assessing impaired insight or unawareness in neurological states. Firstly, this helps to illustrate more clearly the differences in conceptualisation of awareness/unawareness between neurology/neuropsychology and general psychiatry. Secondly, the approaches in this clinical area have been particularly influential in the methods developed for exploring insight in patients with dementia.

4.2.1 Assessments of impaired insight/anosognosia in neurological states

Since the early case reports (e.g. Anton, 1899; Babinski, 1914; Roth, 1944; Redlich & Dorsey, 1945; Stengel & Steele, 1946), studies in anosognosia have in recent years become more systematic. Larger numbers of patients have been examined and attempts have been made to evaluate the degree of anosognosia in structured ways (Cutting, 1978; Bisiach *et al.*, 1986; Prigatano *et al.*, 1986; Starkstein *et al.*, 1992; 1993a; Sherer *et al.*, 1998a; 2003a). As with the various insight measures in general psychiatry, a variety of assessment methods have been developed to study unawareness in neurological states. Ratings range from simple dichotomous divisions, i.e. anosognosia is described as 'present' or 'absent' (Cutting, 1978; Hier *et al.*, 1983a, b; Levine *et al.*, 1991), to multiple categorisations based on several point scales (Bisiach *et al.*, 1986; Cappa *et al.*, 1987; Blonder & Ranseen, 1994). Such instruments also vary from clinician-rated scales with set criteria in hemiplegia (Cutting, 1978; Bisiach *et al.*, 1986; Starkstein *et al.*, 1992) to patient-rated deficits using questionnaires (Levine *et al.*, 1991). More detailed and structured methods to assess unawareness have been devised in relation to the multiple deficits sustained following head injury. In this area in particular, discrepancy measures have been used to assess awareness. In other words, patients' awareness of their disabilities is defined, empirically, as a function of the difference between theirs and their relatives' perception of deficits as rated on structured questionnaires given to them both (Sunderland *et al.*, 1984; Oddy *et al.*, 1985; Prigatano *et al.*, 1986; Sherer *et al.*, 1998). Discrepancy measures have likewise been adopted in relation to amnesic syndromes (Schacter, 1991; 1992) and, more recently, in dementia research (see Chapter 5).

The assumption underlying such methods is that relatives/carers or clinicians are providing a 'correct' appraisal of the patients' deficits against which patients' perceptions are judged. However, it would seem plausible, as others have suggested (McGlynn & Schacter, 1989), that relatives' assessments of patient function are also likely to be influenced by a number of factors which could lead them to overestimate and/or to underestimate levels of impairment in patients. Such judgements demanded of carers/relatives must depend on a variety of factors, not only on the nature of the function in question, but also including type and frequency of contact, the quality of relationship with the patient, individual observational capacity, the effects of stress and affective disorders and psychological reactions such as denial. In fact, with respect to unawareness of memory deficits, most work in this area suggests that carers' assessments of patients' memory deficits correlate reasonably well with 'objective' tests of patients' memory function (McGlone et al., 1990; Feher et al., 1991; Koss et al., 1993). Nonetheless, some studies have indicated that discrepancies are greater (and hence patients' insight is poorer) when the burden of care is perceived as greater by the carers (De Bettignies et al., 1990).

Much of the detailed and structured work in assessing impaired insight or anosognosia in neurological states has been carried out in amnesic syndromes and in traumatic brain injury. Foremost amongst the studies examining anosognosia in amnesic syndromes has been the work by Schacter and colleagues (e.g. McGlynn & Schacter, 1989; Schacter, 1991; 1992). To illustrate the type of assessment of awareness developed in these areas it is useful to look at the comprehensive measure described by Schacter (1991). Comprising of three main components, the first part consists of a 'General Self-Assessment Questionnaire' in which patients rate on a 7-point scale the degree to which they experience difficulty with various aspects of memory compared to before their illness. Relatives also complete this scale. The second part consists of an 'Everyday Memory Questionnaire' in which a number of hypothetical situations are described and patients are asked to rate the probability that they would remember information in these situations (both currently and before their illness) after delays of a minute, an hour, a day and a week. In addition, they are asked to make similar ratings of their relatives' abilities to remember in these situations. Likewise, the relatives also complete this for themselves and the patients. The last part consists of an 'Item Recall Questionnaire' in which patients have to predict how many items they would remember (currently and prior to illness) if they were shown lists of 10 items (further subdivided into 'easy' and 'difficult' items), and are subsequently tested at each of the delays.

In the area of traumatic brain injury there have likewise been a number of comprehensive measures developed to assess impaired awareness of various deficits using comparisons between patients' ratings of deficits and ratings made by relatives or clinicians or performance on specific tests (Prigatano et al., 1986; Anderson & Tranel,

1989; Allen & Ruff, 1990; Gasquoine & Gibbons, 1994; Sherer *et al.*, 1998a). The '*Patient Competency Rating Scale*' (Prigatano *et al.*, 1986) evaluates patients' awareness of deficits on the basis of discrepancies between patients' judgements of how difficult they find tasks in certain areas (activities of daily living, cognitive functioning, interpersonal functioning and emotional regulation) and the same judgements made by relatives/clinicians. Ratings are scored on a Likert scale ranging from 1 (can't do) to 5 (can do with ease). Comparisons between patients' judgements and relatives or clinicians' judgements determine the degree of unawareness in patients by means of subtracting relatives/clinician scores from those derived from patients. Similarly, Gasquoine and Gibbons (1994) report the use of Gasquoine's '*Self-awareness Questionnaire*' for patients with more severe head injury which also compares patients and staff ratings in areas including awareness of: head injury, physical impairment, communication difficulties, functional impairment and sensory/cognitive impairment. The '*Awareness Questionnaire*' developed by Sherer *et al.* (1998a) likewise evaluates patients' awareness of deficits on the basis of discrepancies between patients' judgements and relatives and/or clinician judgements. However, the content of this questionnaire focuses on ratings made comparing current and pre-injury functional abilities (cognitive area, behavioural/affective area and motor/sensory area). Ratings are scored on a Likert scale ranging from 1 (much worse) to 5 (much better). Again, impaired awareness is evaluated by subtracting scores of relatives' or clinicians' ratings from the patients' self-ratings.

Similar approaches to evaluating insight have been taken in relation to patients with dementia and will be reviewed in Chapter 5. However, what is evident from the sorts of measures described above, is that the phenomenon of awareness or unawareness elicited is, compared with the phenomenon elicited in general psychiatry, much sharper in definition and narrower in content. Patients are assumed to either 'know' or 'not know' that they have a memory problem, or behavioural difficulty, or emotional changes, etc. Awareness is rated variously according to either the perceived severity of the problem, or the frequency with which it is bothersome, or the change from a previous state, or predicted ability on specific tests. Irrespective of such ratings, the phenomenon is still focused on a unitary concept of awareness in its narrow sense. This does not mean to say that the concept of awareness is regarded as an all-or-none phenomenon and Schacter (1992) explicitly argues against such a point of view. Rather, it means that the qualitative differences in awareness are related directly and specifically to the tasks demanded of the patients whether this is a *judgement of severity*, a *comparison* with previous function or with others, or *prediction* (and subsequent check) of performance on specific tests. In comparison, the conceptualisation of insight in general psychiatry has necessitated different types of judgements on the part of the patient which have determined a much wider, albeit less clearly defined phenomenon whose qualitative aspects relate to a broader recognition of pathology and its consequences for the individual.

4.2.2 Models underlying impaired insight/anosognosia in neurological states

One of the aims behind the refinement of instruments assessing awareness and carrying out larger studies has been to explore possible mechanisms that might explain unawareness or anosognosia in neurological states. Numerous theories have been proposed and are comprehensively reviewed by McGlynn and Schacter (1989). However, it is worthwhile to highlight some of the models developed as not only have they contributed to the proposed explanations of insightlessness in relation to dementia but they have also guided much of the recent empirical work on impaired insight in relation to general psychiatry. Such theories can be roughly divided into two broad groups, namely: (i) the *neuroanatomical and the neuropsychological* theories, linked to the conceptualisation of awareness in its narrow sense of consciousness as detailed above and (ii) the *motivational*, linked with the psychoanalytic conceptualisations of awareness/insight.

4.2.2.1 Neuroanatomical and neuropsychological theories

Although arising from different perspectives, these two groups of theories/models seeking to explain awareness and impaired awareness in neurological states may, for the purposes here, be usefully reviewed together. This is because, firstly, they share the common core conceptualisation of unawareness and, secondly, because of increasing convergence between the postulated neuropsychological processes and specific neuroanatomical structures (e.g. Stuss & Benson, 1986; Schacter, 1990; 1991).

A variety of neuroanatomical theories have been put forward as possible aetiological bases to anosognosia. Diffuse generalised brain disease (Stengel & Steele, 1946) has generally been deemed insufficient to cause anosognosia, particularly, since patients can be well orientated and have little evidence of general intellectual impairment (Babinski, 1914; Roth, 1949; Cutting, 1978). Some specific support for this view is also provided by Schacter (1991) from a neuropsychological perspective. Using his detailed measure of awareness of memory deficits (see above), he described a different pattern of results obtained from two densely amnesic patients. One patient, whose amnesia was secondary to a ruptured aneurysm of the anterior communicating artery (ACAA rupture), showed poor awareness of memory deficits and overestimated his ability to recall items on the questionnaire as compared with his wife who made more accurate predictions. In contrast, the other patient, whose amnesia was secondary to herpes simplex encephalitis, showed much greater awareness of her memory problems with ratings on the questionnaires consistent with her spouse's ratings and with her performance on testing. Both patients had equivalent severity of memory deficits as measured by the tests and the intelligence quotient (IQ) of the second patient was actually much lower than that of the first, suggesting that the difference in awareness of deficits was unlikely to be due to generalised intellectual impairment. In addition, the specificity of anosognosia for a particular deficit or deficits, in the face of awareness of other impairments, also goes against the view that generalised brain disease might underlie anosognosia.

More interest has thus focused on focal brain lesions as possibly underlying anosognosia, e.g. thalamic (Roth, 1944; Redlich & Dorsey, 1945; Watson & Heilman, 1979) or striatal damage (Healton *et al.*, 1982). Most focus, however, has been directed at the right hemisphere, and particularly the parietal region has been implicated (Hier *et al.*, 1983a; Price & Mesulam, 1985; Bisiach *et al.*, 1986; Goldberg & Barr, 1991; Rubens & Garrett, 1991; Bisiach & Geminiani, 1991; Starkstein *et al.*, 1992; Heilman *et al.*, 1993). In general, though, findings have been inconclusive and although anosognosia does seem to be more prevalent in patients with right hemispheric lesions, it is also associated with left hemispheric damage (Cutting, 1978). Experimental studies examining individual hemispheric function by inducing temporary hemianaesthesia with intracarotid barbiturate injections have likewise yielded mixed results. Some studies find anosognosia restricted to patients receiving right sided injections (and hence left hemiplegia) (Buchtel *et al.*, 1992; Gilmore *et al.*, 1992) and others find no difference in the frequency of unawareness following right and left sided injections (Kaplan *et al.*, 1993; Dywan *et al.*, 1995). Anosognosia/ unawareness in these experimental studies was elicited as a memory of the event rather than elicited at the time of the hemiplegia developing which, as the researchers pointed out, might influence the validity of the findings.

Numerous mechanisms subserving right hemisphere damage as the basis for anosognosia have been suggested, including, e.g. disturbance of the body scheme (Roth, 1944; Roth, 1949), 'disconnection' from the speech areas (Geschwind, 1965), and personality disorder (Horton, 1976). However, there is little empirical evidence provided for such mechanisms and, as others have argued, a body scheme disturbance would not explain the unawareness manifest in relation to cognitive or behavioural deficits or indeed to traumatic experiences (Weinstein & Kahn, 1955). Nor is there evidence that patients are aware of deficits but are unable to express this awareness (McGlynn & Schacter, 1989). The notion that unawareness develops as a result of impaired position sense and sensory loss has also been refuted since researchers found that neither somatosensory loss nor spatial neglect were sufficient to account for anosognosia of hemiplegia in patients with right hemispheric strokes (Bisiach *et al.*, 1986; Levine *et al.*, 1991; Berti *et al.*, 1998).

Probably one of the most consistent findings has been the association between anosognosia and frontal lobe dysfunction (McGlynn & Schacter, 1989; Goldberg & Barr, 1991). And, much of cognitive neuropsychological work has likewise focused on the frontal lobes as the central structures for self-monitoring and so-called executive functioning (Stuss & Benson, 1986; Baddeley, 1987). An interesting model attempting to account for the different types of awareness in neurological deficits, primarily related to memory, was proposed by Schacter (1990). This model, termed DICE (dissociable interactions and conscious experience), postulated the existence of a 'conscious awareness system' (CAS) which has direct links to individual 'knowledge modules' such as lexical, conceptual, spatial, etc., as well as to an episodic memory information system. Schacter suggested that whilst such modules/systems are in constant or ongoing operation during normal mental and behavioural states, it is only when the CAS is activated and when it interacts with such systems, that a conscious experience of the particular information is obtained. Concentrating on memory deficits, Schacter went on to discuss how damage at different levels in such a system could explain both global and specific impairments of awareness. He then put forward different levels of explanation within this model to account for the various types of unawareness in both deficits and function (implicit memory, see below). A *first-order* level of explanation, he said, would involve damage or impairment within the CAS or with its individual connections. However, he favoured a *second-order* level of explanation which would involve dysfunction at the level of the knowledge modules themselves. Schacter then went on to postulate that the CAS was a posterior system involving the inferio-parietal lobes, with connections to the 'executive system' situated in the frontal lobes (McGlynn & Schacter, 1989; Schacter, 1990; 1991). The model thus is an attempt to provide both a structural and functional explanation of impairment in awareness and the dissociations in awareness found in relation to different 'modules' or functions. In line with cognitive theory, it assumes modularity of mental processes and hence the level of explanation is directed at postulated individual cognitive systems and particularly at the proposed connections between them. Models sharing similarity of approaches in terms of integrating postulated cognitive processes and neuroanatomical structures can be found also in Stuss and Benson (1986), Bisiach *et al.* (1986), Mesulam (1986), Heilman (1991), and Prigatano (1991) amongst others. More recently, such models have been further elaborated and refined in attempts to capture the full heterogeneity found amongst anosognosic phenomena (e.g. Agnew & Morris, 1998).

Stuss and Benson (1986) make a conceptual distinction between *self-awareness* and *awareness of deficits* in behavioural disorders such as neglect and aphasia. The former is viewed as the highest psychological attribute of the frontal lobes, interacting closely with organised function systems subserving various psychological processes, e.g. attention, language and memory. Thus, damage to the frontal lobes would result in a general disturbance of self-awareness, which, because of the varied nature of the 'self', in turn would lead to fractionation of disordered self-awareness (Stuss, 1991). Awareness of deficits, on the other hand, is viewed as relating to the specific functional systems themselves, such as language. Hence, impaired awareness of deficit would involve impaired knowledge associated with the specific system and would be related to dysfunction in posterior or basal brain regions. This view is reiterated by others (Bisiach *et al.*, 1986; Mesulam, 1986; Prigatano, 1991). Indeed, Bisiach *et al.* (1986) emphasise this point, stating that anosognosia for a specific deficit 'betrays a disorder at the highest levels of organisation of *that function*. This implies that monitoring of the internal working is not secured in the nervous system by a general superordinate organ, but is decentralised and apportioned to the different functional blocks to which it refers' (p. 480, my emphasis). Thus, whilst sharing some similarities with Schacter's (1990) model in terms of endowing individual cognitive or psychological process with intrinsic 'monitoring' functions, we find here, in addition, a conceptual and an anatomical separation between impaired awareness for a specific deficit and impaired awareness of the self. Stuss's hierarchical model of awareness develops this further and proposes four levels of awareness linked to different anatomical substrates: (i) arousal, (ii) perceptual analysis of incoming stimuli and engagement in complex motor activity, (iii) initiation and self-monitoring of goal-directed behaviour and, (iv) self-awareness (Picton & Stuss, 1994; Clare, 2004). Thus, the conceptualisation of awareness at the highest level, in *theoretical* terms becomes, in this neurological/neuropsychological frame, a much broader concept, distinct from anosognosia, and, closer perhaps to the theoretical notion of insight in general psychiatry.

Empirical evidence pointing to the contribution of frontal lobe dysfunction in the development of anosognosia has come from a variety of sources. For example, it has been observed that patients with the amnesic syndrome as a result of frontal lobe impairment tend to be unaware of their memory deficit whereas patients with amnesic syndromes as a result of temporal lobe damage tend to show some awareness of their memory difficulties (McGlynn & Schacter, 1989; Schacter, 1991). Nevertheless, there have also been reports of patients with amnesic syndrome and frontal lobe dysfunction who had preserved awareness of memory deficits (Luria, 1976; Vilkki, 1985; Schacter, 1991). The prevalence of frontal lobe damage in patients with unawareness of deficits following head injury (Prigatano, 1991) has, on the other hand, supported a putative aetiological role for the frontal lobes in awareness of dysfunction. With respect to cerebrovascular accidents, Starkstein *et al.* (1993b) found that patients with anosognosia for hemiplegia ($n = 8$) were significantly poorer on neuropsychological tasks of frontal lobe function compared with patients without anosognosia ($n = 8$), though there were no differences on computerised tomographical (CT) scan lesions. On the other hand, neuropsychological tests did not discriminate between patients with and without awareness of deficits following head injury (Prigatano, 1991). However, in this instance, patients with reduced awareness of deficits had greater incidence of frontal and parietal lesions on magnetic resonance imaging (MRI) or CT scans. Similar work correlating unawareness with neuroimaging changes and frontal lobe neuropsychological tests has been carried out in general psychiatry (and Chapter 3) and in dementia research (and Chapter 5) and likewise yields mixed results.

4.2.2.2 Motivational theories

In contrast to the preceding neurological/neuropsychological approaches, others have argued that the pathogenesis of anosognosia can be explained in terms of psychological processes or motivational factors within the patient. The main proponents of these theories were Weinstein and Kahn (1955) who argued that anosognosia, or denial of illness, was an adaptive response to avoid distress or a catastrophic reaction to the recognition of disability. The authors were less concerned with the actual mechanism of this process and referred, instead, to the dynamic approaches of Schilder, Goldstein and Sandifer. They concentrated on providing a descriptive account of patients' behaviours which, they argued, could be interpreted as symbolic representations of their 'adaptation' to disability. Weinstein and Kahn (1955) did stress the point that such interpretations of behaviours (particularly in relation to implicit denial) were very much dependent on the perspective of the observer and his/her theoretical preconceptions. Basing their ideas on comprehensive observations of 104 patients with various forms of brain damage and anosognosia, they distinguished between two kinds of behaviour indicative of denial. First, they referred to *explicit verbal denial* which involved complete denial of illness, denial of major disability, minimisation or attribution to some benign cause, projection of disability outside of the self and temporal displacement of the disability. Second, they described *implicit denial* which was suggested by behaviour such as withdrawal, inattention, pain asymbolia, alteration in sexual behaviour, hallucinations and mood changes. In both categories of denial, the authors contended, that it was the symbolism behind either the words (explicit) or the behaviours (implicit) that signified the adaptational nature of the behaviours and made 'simple unawareness' of the disability less likely. Thus, for example, a patient complained about the 'hammering and the sawing on his head [but] still denied that he had had a craniotomy' (Weinstein & Kahn, 1955, p. 69) or patients might misname objects related to their illness and yet at the same time show they understood their use. One patient, expressing her denial through reduplication of her left arm, claimed that the extra paralysed hand belonged to a close friend. Weinstein and Kahn (1955) suggested that this expression of denial symbolised the close relationship between the two women. Similarly, whilst patients were denying their illness, they nevertheless behaved like other patients on the ward and accepted medication and medical management normally. Thus, argued Weinstein and Kahn (1955, p. 70), 'it cannot be said that the patient "forgets" or is "unaware" that he is ill but rather that he expresses his feelings about it in a particular language'.

Whilst proposing psychological mechanisms, Weinstein and Kahn stressed, nonetheless, the necessity for the presence of brain dysfunction itself in contributing to the presence and expression of the multiple forms of denial or anosognosia. They did not claim that the brain dysfunction caused the denial but argued that the level of brain function determined the 'integration of the pattern in which the denial is expressed'. In other words, it was the alteration in the brain function that provided the environment or 'milieu' in which the denial could be expressed but the latter itself was determined by individual psychological factors. Consequently, they proposed, it was not the localisation of the lesion or the type of disability itself that were specifically related to the presence or type of denial shown by the patient although they did stipulate that deeper brain structures had to be affected. Rather, it was the individual's personality and previous experience that determined the type of denial manifested, i.e. 'the symbolic modalities in which he habitually expressed his motivations' (p. 97). The non-specificity of the brain lesion in this regard also helped to explain why such a range of disabilities or dysfunctions might be denied, not just hemiplegia or blindness but the fact of having an operation or some distressing family or social event. Anosognosia or denial using this model is thus conceived as developing within a dynamic interplay of brain and personality motivational factors though the specific mechanisms remain unclear. Weinstein (1991) later stated, '... The existence and form of denial/anosognosia are determined by the location and rate of development of the brain lesion, the situation in which the denial is elicited, the type of disability, and the way the patient perceives its meaning on the basis of his past experience' (p. 254).

On the basis of questionnaires and interviews exploring individual/personality factors with relatives of patients showing denial, Weinstein and Kahn (1955) suggested that a particular personality type predisposed to the development of denial. Such patients, they claimed, premorbidly considered illness as a weakness or failure and were strongly concerned about the opinions of others and had strong drives to do well and to succeed. Subsequently, Weinstein et al. (1994) attempted to capture such personality traits empirically by means of their Denial Personality Ratings in their research on denial or anosognosia in dementia. On the other hand, personality factors, as assessed by the Eysenck Personality Questionnaire (scales for measuring extroversion, neuroticism, psychoticism and a lie scale), were not found to distinguish between patients who denied ($n = 20$) and those who did not deny ($n = 10$) their hemiplegia following acute stroke in the study by Small and Ellis (1996). The same study did suggest, however, that whilst relatives did not class patients with denial as being perfectionists, nevertheless, the patients with denial rated themselves as having difficulty in admitting to illness in general compared with patients who did not show denial.

As McGlynn and Schacter (1989) point out, there are a number of problems with viewing anosognosia or unawareness of deficits predominantly in terms of motivational or psychological processes. For example, it is difficult to account for the specificity of anosognosia seen frequently in neurological states. Nor, if unconscious psychological mechanisms are postulated, should the site of the lesion make much difference. Likewise, the time course of anosognosia is often inconsistent with the views on onset and course of motivated denial. Emphasising these difficulties, Lewis (1991) distinguished between *psychogenic* and *neurogenic* denial. However, she stressed the importance of interaction of both psychological and neurological factors in the overall production of denial.

4.2.3 Empirical studies of impaired insight in relation to neurological states

Much of the empirical work on impaired insight in neurological states has, in fact, been focused on looking for associations between anosognosia and specific brain lesions (as described above). However, there have also been other areas of interest. A few studies have examined the relationship between impaired insight/anosognosia and different neurological impairments (e.g. hemiplegia, hemianopia, amnesia) and clinical variables such as severity of impairment or lesion, presence of emotional problems or neuropsychological impairment. These have been comprehensively reviewed elsewhere (Vuilleumier, 2000). As in other clinical areas overall results are mixed and inconsistent. Importantly, however, there is some suggestion that anosognosia is a poor prognostic factor for functional recovery following stroke (Gialanella & Mattioli, 1992; Pedersen *et al.*, 1996; Appelros *et al.*, 2002).

Of particular clinical relevance has been the more recent work exploring the likely importance of awareness or degrees of insight in traumatic brain injury, particularly from the perspective of rehabilitation. Earlier studies had reported a high prevalence of impaired awareness of behavioural/cognitive problems amongst patients following traumatic brain injury (Sunderland *et al.*, 1984; Oddy *et al.*, 1985). This has been recognised as a significant factor complicating rehabilitation and influencing clinical outcome (Prigatano, 1991; Gasquoine & Gibbons, 1994; Sherer *et al.*, 1998b). Further studies have attempted to characterise such impaired awareness in order to determine its predictive value and also to enable rehabilitation strategies to be targeted appropriately. So far, the few studies that have been carried out in this regard have also yielded inconsistent results though they await replication (Sherer *et al.*, 1998b).

Studies examining the relationship between various clinical variables and the presence of impaired awareness yield mixed results. For example, some studies suggest that more severe head injury is associated with poorer awareness of disability (Levin *et al.*, 1987) while others find no such association (Anderson & Tranel, 1989; Gasquoine, 1992; Sherer *et al.*, 2003b). Similarly, some studies find an association between level of cognitive impairment and level of awareness of disability (Anderson & Tranel, 1989) and others find no such association (Prigatano & Altman,

1990; Prigatano *et al.*, 1997). Some studies suggest that patients with greater awareness of their disabilities have more emotional distress or depression (Gasquoine, 1992; Godfrey *et al.*, 1993; Wallace & Bogner, 2000). A more consistent finding reports patients, following traumatic brain injury, as being more aware of their physical deficits than of their non-physical, i.e. emotional and cognitive problems (Gasquoine, 1992; Gasquoine & Gibbons, 1994; Prigatano, 1996; Sherer *et al.*, 1998b; Hart *et al.*, 2004). Overall, however, there have been too few studies to conclude very much about the relationship between awareness of disability and characteristics of the traumatic head injury. Moreover, the studies are diverse methodologically, employing different measures of evaluating awareness, of severity of head injury, of emotional and cognitive states, etc.

In regard to patient awareness and rehabilitation following head injury, Sherer *et al.* (2003b) report that early self-awareness is associated with older age at admission to rehabilitation and with prediction of employability at discharge from inpatient rehabilitation (Sherer *et al.*, 2003b). Their study, examining 129 patients with traumatic brain injury, used the *Awareness Questionnaire* (Sherer *et al.*, 1998a). Whilst needing replication, it highlights the need for early assessment of patients' awareness in the prediction of various functional activities and stresses the need for further research to determine if treatment programmes directed at impaired awareness might help functional outcomes.

A number of interesting approaches to characterising impaired awareness have been put forward with a view to devising treatment programmes directed at impaired awareness following traumatic brain injury. For example, based on different time frames, Crosson *et al.* (1989) proposed a nested conceptualisation of awareness differentiating between awareness of the problem generally (intellectual awareness), awareness of the problem when manifest (emergent awareness) and awareness of the problem in advance (anticipatory awareness). The type of deficit in awareness shown by the patient then determined the particular compensatory strategy that could be employed in rehabilitation work. On the other hand, Allen and Ruff (1990) suggested that patients' assessment of their cognitive abilities was guided by three processes, namely *awareness* (the ability to recognise problems), *appraisal* (the ability to compare the current state with previous functioning) and *disclosure* (the willingness to articulate or report their understanding of their state to others). For rehabilitation purposes it would thus be important for the clinician to assess the patient from the perspective of each of these processes.

A different approach, but sharing some similarities with the above, was taken by Langer and Padrone (1992) who described a tripartite model for conceptualising impaired awareness after brain injury attempting to integrate both the neurological/ neuropsychological and the motivational concepts of awareness. Thus, they identified three components of awareness, namely, *information* (actually having the right information in order to be able to be aware of it), *implication* (to be aware of implications of the information) and *integration* (having the information and knowing the implications of this and behaving accordingly). Patients could have impairments of any of these components which would then manifest as deficits in awareness. For example, if they did not have the right information, then they would appear to be unaware of the problem. If they had the information but could not see the implications then they would also show impaired awareness. And if they had the information and were potentially aware of its implications and yet behaved as if they did not have it, then they would be denying their problems. Again, depending on the level of impairment, treatment in terms of rehabilitation could be tailored accordingly. Such approaches await further empirical testing and may have important therapeutic implications. Moreover, they are indicative of a further broadening of the concept of awareness in this area as different sorts of judgements are being incorporated in the structure of awareness as a whole.

4.3 Impaired awareness of function in neurological states

Anosognosia has been defined as unawareness of deficit but, in relation to neurological states, much interest has been directed, in addition, at unawareness or impaired insight of *function* or knowledge. Thus, akin to the clinical accounts produced in the late nineteenth century on patients with anosognosia in neurological impairments, observations were recorded of other patients who appeared to show no overt awareness or insight into their abilities or preserved function. Korsakoff (1889), in his original descriptions of the amnestic syndrome, was particularly interested in this aspect of insight. Thus, whilst commenting on the lack of concern (rather than lack of awareness) shown by patients about their memory impairment, he was struck also by the level of their *unconscious knowledge*. In other words, patients did not seem to be aware that they knew certain things and, on questioning, would specifically deny that this was the case. Thus, Korsakoff noted that whilst such patients might not recognise him despite repeated daily contact, they nevertheless recognised that he was a doctor. Furthermore, months or even years after their illnesses, patients could recollect conversations or events occurring during their illness of which they had no awareness at the time. Consequently, he postulated, memory traces must be laid down at an unconscious level. In addition, Korsakoff observed that the unconscious knowledge was evident to differing extents in relation to different aspects of memory. For example, patients would show pleasant and sympathetic behaviour towards certain individuals and events but hostile or unsympathetic behaviour towards others. Therefore, he believed, this suggested that patients preserved unconsciously *affective* responses in the face of a lack of conscious recollection of the people/situations evoking such responses (Korsakoff, 1889).

The theoretical notion of unconscious knowledge or memory in the 'healthy' subject, i.e. knowledge or memory of which an individual is not consciously/overtly aware can be traced, in various forms, back to the seventeenth century to the writings of Descartes, Leibniz and others (for a historical review see Schacter, 1987). In the context of a general interest in unconscious mental processes in the nineteenth century, a number of physiologists highlighted the importance of the unconsciousness in the constitution of memory itself (Hering, 1870/1920; Butler, 1880/1920). For example, the Viennese physiologist Hering (1870/1920, p. 72), emphasised that memory, '... whose results, it is true, fall, as regards one part of them, into the domain of consciousness, while another part and not less essential part escapes unperceived as purely material processes'. Since such early theoretical observations in relation to normal function and anecdotal reports in various clinical states (e.g. Korsakoff, 1889; Janet, 1904), the concept of 'unconscious knowledge' in various guises has only developed as the focus of systematic research in cognitive (and to some extent behaviourist) psychology since the middle of the twentieth century (Reber, 1993; Schacter, 1995).

In general terms, two parallel research programmes appeared to develop independently, one focusing on 'unconscious learning' or implicit learning (Reber, 1993), and the other focusing on 'unconscious memory', later termed 'memory without awareness' (Jacoby & Witherspoon, 1982) or 'implicit memory' (Graf & Schacter, 1985). Some efforts have been made to bring together and integrate the cognitive models and approaches used in each of these areas (Reber, 1993). More recently, these approaches have also been applied to the area of metacognition (Metcalfe & Shimamura, 1994; Reder, 1996, see also Chapter 2). The common issues have revolved around the idea that much of normal mental processing, be it learning, perceiving, remembering, etc. seems to take place without the individual being consciously or explicitly aware of these. Cognitive psychological research has focused on developing different tests to explore the contribution or otherwise of consciousness to such mental processes. Indeed much of the terminology referring to unconscious or implicit mental processes in these contexts has to be viewed as reflecting subjects' responses to, and results from, specific neuropsychological tests rather than necessarily representing distinct mental phenomena. In other words, it is important when considering this research to bear in mind some of the crucial assumptions on which studies are based. Most importantly, there is firstly the assumption concerning the putative divisions of the mind or mental functions as conceived in neuropsychological models both in terms of the 'modules' of cognition and their interrelationships and their contents of 'cognition'. Secondly, there is the assumption that the specific tests are 'pure' in the sense that they can actually distinguish between conscious/explicit processing and unconscious/implicit mental processing, and, in fact, this has been challenged (e.g. Jacoby & Kelley, 1992; Rugg,

1995) with the consequence that there is continued refining of such tests and models. Thus, in regards to implicit memory in this particular neuropsychological context, the term has been defined in a specific technical sense: 'Implicit memory is revealed when performance on a task is facilitated in the absence of conscious recollection; explicit memory is revealed when performance on a task requires conscious recollection of previous experiences' (Graf & Schacter, 1985, p. 501).

The neuropsychological tasks used to elicit implicit memory have involved primarily repetition priming tests and skill-learning tasks (Schacter, 1987). Much work has been carried out in researching implicit memory in healthy subjects but, interestingly, implicit memory has also been demonstrated in patients with amnesic syndromes, who are thus able, for example, to show effects of priming on memory tests without recalling the priming itself (Warrington & Weiskrantz, 1968; 1974; 1982; Cermak *et al.*, 1985; Shimamura, 1986; McAndrews *et al.*, 1987; Schacter, 1991). In other words, dissociations between implicit and explicit memory can be demonstrated suggesting that these may represent different aspects of memory which may be disturbed independently. Furthermore, various impairments in implicit memory itself and further dissociations between different types of implicit memory tasks used (e.g. verbal/non-verbal material, words/non-words, patterns, perceptual, auditory, etc.) have been found in patients with amnesic syndromes indicating that dysfunction can occur at specific (task-determined) levels (Schacter, 1995). For example, it was found that while priming effects for common words and idioms in amnesic patients is comparable to control subjects, amnesic patients seem to fail to show priming effects for non-words (Cermak *et al.*, 1985). Other studies have found preserved implicit memory in amnesic patients using skill-learning tasks. Patients were taught to learn and retain new skills such as computer training and yet they remained 'unaware' of having such training or skills (Glisky *et al.*, 1986). Clearly, demonstration of the presence of implicit memory as well as of different types of impaired implicit memory in patients with amnesic syndromes (and patients with dementia) has been dependent on such very specific neuropsychological tasks.

The question that remains, however, concerns the structure of awareness and its relationship to other mental structures. And how can the impairments in different aspects of awareness be explained and understood? As far as neuropsychological approaches are concerned, implicit memory or knowledge has tended to be addressed predominantly from the perspective of the mental functions themselves rather than from the perspective of an awareness or consciousness system although the latter has been postulated in an abstract form in relation to the mental functions (e.g. Schacter, 1990). For example, explanations for implicit memory, rather than being directed at the awareness aspect of the concept, have focused on memory itself in terms of how it is retrieved, the contribution of context and the possibility of multiple as opposed to single memory systems. This has led to some researchers suggesting that the notion of implicit memory is redundant outside the specific constraints of neuropsychology testing (Willingham & Preuss, 1995).

Impaired insight/awareness of knowledge or function has been described also in other neurological syndromes. Most striking perhaps is the example of 'blindsight', where there is 'visual capacity in a field defect in the absence of acknowledged awareness' (Weiskrantz, 1990, p. 166). The patient described by Weiskrantz had a left hemianopia following excision of a malformation within the occipital lobe, yet, was able to perform visual tasks in his left field at a level that was significantly higher than chance. At the same time, he appeared unaware of his ability to perform at such a level, expressing surprise when informed he had 'guessed' correctly. Likewise, patients with visual neglect responded to priming tasks despite overt denial of the presence of stimuli in their neglected field, again indicating the presence of some form of unconscious or implicit appraisal (Berti & Rizzolatti, 1992). Similarly, in prosopagnosia, where patients are unable to recognise familiar faces overtly, implicit recognition has nevertheless been suggested by the fact that such patients show increased autonomic responses (skin conductance responses, respiration rate/depth) on testing with familiar faces (Bauer, 1984; Tranel & Damasio, 1988; Benton & Tranel, 1993).

A number of mechanisms have been proposed to explain such phenomena, including, e.g. damage to one of two postulated separate channels (holding different types of retinal information) involved in visual perception (Perenin & Jeannerod, 1975, 1978; Perenin et al., 1980). A different type of 'neural disconnection' has been put forward by Weiskrantz (1988; 1990) who suggested that there was a split between the capacity to perceive and an awareness or commentary on this, thus implying damage to a parallel 'monitoring' system. Another 'disconnection' hypothesis, at a more neuroanatomical level, based on damage to selective neural paths from the visual system to the limbic systems, was proposed by Bauer (1984, p. 466) in relation to prosopagnosia. He suggested that in prosopagnosia there is damage to the 'ventral' path which, following Bear (1983), is a 'modality-specific "foveal system that recognises objects [faces] by multiple attributes" and mediates modality-specific orienting and stimulus-response learning'. The 'dorsal' path, on the other hand, which carries emotional tone or 'relevance' for the face, is intact, and hence, there is the observed autonomic arousal on presentation of familiar faces (Bauer, 1984; 1993). As already mentioned, Schacter (1990) in relation to the amnesic syndromes, including implicit or unconscious awareness of memory, suggested a mechanism involving impairment to the memory system itself rather than invoking damage at the level of an awareness or monitoring system.

In these and other instances, e.g. in blindtouch (Paillard et al., 1983), the 'object' of awareness or insight relates to *function* or *knowledge*. Clearly, this contrasts with the previously discussed research on anosognosia or impaired insight, where the 'object' of awareness related to *deficits* or *impairment* in function. Likewise, insight in general psychiatric disorders and dementias has focused predominantly on pathology, on abnormalities or impairments as a result of illness rather than on functioning or abilities (though for recent studies on implicit memory in dementia, see Chapter 5). Whilst this distinction has been made at a definitional level and different mechanisms have been postulated, this remains a relatively unexplored area at a conceptual level. In other words, what is the relationship between these types of impaired awareness, and how do they relate within the notion of insight as a whole? If there is implicit awareness or knowledge with respect to capacity/function, is there also implicit awareness with respect to deficits?

Furthermore, closer examination of the implicit/covert awareness exhibited in the different clinical situations suggests that perhaps these phenomena may not necessarily be of the same type. For example, in patients with prosopagnosia, their covert recognition of familiar faces is demonstrated by their autonomic responses in the face of their overt inability to recognise these faces. Similarly, amnesic patients demonstrate implicit memory through their ability to use knowledge or skills they have learnt previously, without recognising that this is the case. With blindsight, however, it has been shown that awareness of the ability to discriminate visual objects varies according to the presented stimulus (location, distance, salience). In addition, even though the patients may say they are 'guessing', it appears that they are aware of a 'feeling' or different perception: 'wave-like impression' (Weiskrantz, 1990, p. 167). A similar phenomenon was described by Paillard *et al.* (1983) in their patient with deafferentiation in her right hand, who was able to discriminate tactile stimulation, though was unable to experience the stimulation as a 'touch' sensation. The question then has to be posed as to whether the observed phenomenon is really impaired awareness, or whether the patient is describing (or having difficulty describing) a qualitatively different perceptual experience which guides the discriminating capacity. In other words, it might be that in this case, 'awareness' is intact, but appears impaired because of the difficulties in linking a 'foreign' perceptual experience with tasks dependent on a 'normal' visual/tactile experience.

Some mention should also be made of some related research examining awareness that falls perhaps in a level between the above implicit type of awareness or knowledge and the previously considered conscious or explicit awareness/knowledge. The *'feeling of knowing'* phenomenon has been studied in the field of metacognition and used as a test of 'metamemory', i.e. 'knowledge about one's memory capability and knowledge about strategies that can aid memory' (Shimamura & Squire, 1986, p. 452). Patients are asked to judge, on the basis of a 'feeling of knowing', whether they would 'recognise' the correct answers to questions even if they did not know the answers spontaneously. Recognition of things on the basis of a 'feeling of knowing' has been conceived in cognitive neuropsychology as a form of awareness though viewed from a different perspective and couched in different terms. Indeed, 'metamemory' is conceptualised as an independent 'cognitive' system which can become impaired separately from memory itself (Shimamura & Squire, 1986; Shimamura, 1994). Interestingly, the 'feeling of knowing' is not considered as constituting an aspect of insight in Gestalt cognitive psychological terms (Metcalfe, 1986b, see Chapter 2) where again, the specialised perspectives of that discipline preclude a broader notion.

Finally, a brief reference has to be made to experimental situations where the notion of awareness, albeit in a somewhat different sense, has also been raised. Penfield (1975) described 'experiential' phenomena evoked upon stimulation of the temporal cortex in patients with epilepsy. Patients reported complex hallucinations, illusions, memory flashbacks, etc. accompanied by a sense of reality of the experience, though, at the same time, were aware of what was happening in the operating room. Penfield suggested that this double awareness was possible because of the independence of the 'mind' from brain mechanisms. In other words, 'although the content of consciousness depends in large measure on neuronal activity, awareness itself does not' (Penfield, 1975, p. 55). In similar studies, Gloor *et al.* (1982), found that it was necessary to stimulate the limbic structures in order to confer the sense of 'experiential immediacy' to the evoked phenomena. They thus suggested that 'limbic activity may be essential for bringing to a conscious level percepts elaborated by the temporal neocortex' (p. 140). They further postulated that this was achieved by the limbic structures through the attachment of affective/motivational significance to the percept. In other words, and sharing corollaries with the model proposed by Bauer to explain covert recognition of faces in prosopagnosia, in order for an object to be consciously perceived, there has to be an affective dimension to the perceiving.

4.4 Conclusion

The study of insight in neurological states has developed from two main perspectives. First, has been the focus on patients' apparent unawareness of major neurological disability (anosognosia). Second, has been the exploration of patients' apparent unawareness of preserved function (implicit knowledge). In both areas of study, unawareness has been conceptualised in a much narrower sense than lack of awareness or insight in general psychiatry. The narrower conception of awareness is reflected both in the types of empirical measures designed to assess awareness clinically and in the neuroanatomical and neuropsychological models devised to explain specific impairments in awareness.

The 'neurological' approach is essential to consider for several reasons. First, as was seen in Chapter 3, recent studies exploring insight in general psychiatry are based on analogies of impairment of insight with anosognosia. Second, clarification of the concept of 'neurological' unawareness helps to determine differences and commonalities in the meanings/models of 'insight' used in different studies, particularly where related terms are used interchangeably (see Part II). Third, the 'neurological' approach has been particularly influential in the exploration of insight in the dementias. This is now examined in Chapter 5.

5

Insight in organic brain syndromes: insight into dementia

Empirical studies exploring patients' insight or awareness into dementia have been notably prolific, particularly over the past 15 years. In contrast to the relatively consistent approach taken to the study of insight in relation to neurological states, studies examining insight in the dementias are striking in the range of different approaches taken (Kaszniak & Christenson, 1996). As was suggested in the preceding chapter, a likely explanation for the differences seen may be in part due to the particular clinical nature of dementias themselves as well as their position in occupying neurological, psychological and psychiatric professional domains. It is perhaps not surprising that, much in the same way as research on insight in functional psychiatric syndromes, outcomes from studies exploring patients' insight into dementia and clinical variables (e.g. stage of dementia, severity of dementia, level of cognitive impairment, etc.) have been particularly mixed and inconsistent (Marková & Berrios, 2000).

This chapter reviews the empirical studies exploring insight in dementia and focuses on the specific conceptual issues arising from research in this area. First, differences in definitions and underlying concepts are explored. Then, the varied approaches taken to assess insight empirically are examined and related to the likely clinical aspects of insight elicited. Lastly, the results of studies exploring the relationship between patients' insight, and various clinical and socio-demographic variables are reviewed.

5.1 The meaning of insight in relation to dementia

The first question relates to the meaning of insight in dementia. What is meant by 'insight' in dementia? Does it share similarities with the other notions of insight discussed so far, e.g. insight in psychosis or in neurological states? Reviewing the literature on insight in dementia, however, shows that there are some difficulties in answering this question. These difficulties can be identified at various levels. First of all, it is apparent that there are differences in both the terms used and concepts involved between the various empirical studies. Secondly, there are striking variations between studies in terms of which features of dementia are the focus of insight evaluation, highlighting the importance of the relational aspects of insight in determining its meaning. Thirdly, a wide range of different methods of assessing insight have been used by researchers, carrying implications for the meaning of insight elicited in empirical studies. Before considering the results of empirical work on insight in dementia, it is necessary to examine these particular areas in more detail.

5.1.1 Terms and concepts

A number of related terms are used in studies aiming to explore the degree of patients' understanding or recognition of problems in relation to dementia. Such terms include '*loss/lack of insight*' (De Bettignies *et al.*, 1990; Mangone *et al.*, 1991; McDaniel *et al.*, 1995), '*lack/impairment of awareness*' or '*unawareness*' (Anderson & Tranel, 1989; McGlynn & Kaszniak, 1991a, b; Green *et al.*, 1993; Vasterling *et al.*, 1997; Wagner *et al.*, 1997, Clare *et al.*, 2002), '*anosognosia*' (Feher *et al.*, 1991; Reed *et al.*, 1993; Michon *et al.*, 1994; Migliorelli *et al.*, 1995; Smith C.A. *et al.*, 2000), '*denial*' (Sevush & Leve, 1993; Weinstein *et al.*, 1994; Deckel & Morrison, 1996), '*impaired self-awareness*' (Loebel *et al.*, 1990; Kaszniak & Christenson, 1996), '*self-monitoring/metamemory problem/self-assessment*' (Correa *et al.*, 1996; Theml & Romero, 2001) and '*self-consciousness*' (Gil *et al.*, 2001). This immediately raises a number of questions. First of all, do these various terms refer to a common underlying concept or do they perhaps reflect quite different concepts? Secondly, are these terms and concepts used in a consistent way within the research in this area? Thirdly, if there are differences in meanings, are these important from a clinical and/or research point of view?

At a theoretical level, the various terms clearly do imply different concepts. They are different with respect to their origins, i.e. arising in various historical contexts and within the specific frameworks relating to different professional disciplines, and consequently, they determine structures that are different from one another. We have already seen how the concept of insight in relation to mental illness developed, in the context of changing views around individuality, subjectivity, etc., as well as around mental illness itself. Within general psychiatry, the meaning of *insight* has thus retained a relatively broad structure. This incorporates individuals' understanding of their pathological experiences not only in terms of the latter's manifestation but also including judgements concerning the effects of such experiences, psychologically, socially and functionally. Different has been the conceptualisation of *denial* in psychoanalytic terms where a broader structure still has developed in the context of a deeper view of self-knowledge and the interaction of conscious and unconscious mental processes. Different again has been the development of *anosognosia* as a concept, emerging almost independently as a phenomenon, in the face of an individual's dramatic lack of understanding or recognition of a significant neurological deficit. And, linked so inherently to the neurological or neuropsychological impairment, the meaning within the neurology and neuropsychology fields has consequently been much narrower in structure. Similarly, the newer concepts of self-monitoring, and metamemory or metacognitive processes are products of approaches taken in cognitive and Gestalt neuropsychology and framed in the specific technical language that has developed with the increasing specialisation of these disciplines. The meanings invoked by those terms thus relate to the concepts bound by different categories (e.g. information processing) and they therefore determine different structures. A further issue that complicates the meaning of concepts referred to by such technical terms concerns the additional inclusion of the lay usage of the terms. This is particularly relevant in relation to the use of the term 'denial'. In the psychological conceptualisation, as described above, it has a two-fold meaning in that it refers firstly to an unawareness albeit implying awareness at some (deeper or unconscious) level and secondly it incorporates a psychological mechanism underlying and explaining the unawareness. Whilst the term 'denial' has been used in a number of different ways (Beaumont, 1999), generally, in lay language, it is used descriptively to refer simply to the refusal made by an individual to admit to an overt dysfunction or experience. In this latter sense, the meaning is clearly quite different in structure from the technical concept.

In practice, however, such conceptual distinctions are generally not explicated. Most studies examining insight or awareness in dementia tend not to define specifically the particular concept involved and, moreover, the different terms are frequently used interchangeably (e.g. Feher *et al.*, 1991; Verhey *et al.*, 1993; McDaniel *et al.*, 1995; Starkstein *et al.*, 1996; Smith C.A. *et al.*, 2000). This makes it sometimes difficult to identify the particular sense of the underlying intended concept. McGlynn and Schacter (1989) in their review of this area, in general neuropsychological impairments, highlight such difficulties and explicitly use the terms 'anosognosia', 'unawareness of deficit' and 'loss of insight' interchangeably. However, they make it clear that they are using these terms to refer to the underlying concept of unawareness in the narrow sense, and they specifically distinguish this concept from 'motivated denial' which they view as a separate phenomenon. In other words, they apply the broad distinction, that had emerged from research in this area in neurological states (Chapter 4), between the neurological/neuropsychological concepts of unawareness/anosognosia on the one hand, and the psychological concept of denial on the other.

With respect to studies in dementia, where there are explicit distinctions between various terms (and concepts), a further problem arises because the grounds on which distinctions are made, and meanings attributed to the terms, are different amongst researchers. For example, some researchers make a similar conceptual distinction, as described above (McGlynn & Schacter, 1989), using 'unawareness' and 'anosognosia' interchangeably (and in the neuropsychological sense) but distinguishing this categorically from 'denial' (Reed et al., 1993; Kotler-Cope & Camp, 1995). Others use all the terms (unawareness, denial, loss of insight and anosognosia) interchangeably, generally referring to a fairly narrow definition, focusing on the non-recognition (or non-acknowledgement) by the patient of cognitive or other impairments (Feher et al., 1991; Sevush & Leve, 1993; Verhey et al., 1993). Other meanings are not as clear. Reisberg et al. (1985), in one of the earliest systematic studies of awareness in patients with dementia, using the term 'anosognosia' (or 'lack of recognition of disease'), seem to refer to a broader concept incorporating both denial and lack of insight. They suggest that anosognosia in patients with dementia may be 'a product of decreased insight, itself an invariable symptom of the illness process ... (or) the product of denial or other so-called "psychological mechanisms of defense"' (Reisberg et al., 1985, p. 39). In other words, within their conception, 'anosognosia' is a descriptive term for the phenomenon observed when patients do not recognise their dementia. In contrast, loss of insight and denial are viewed as the mechanisms responsible, the former in terms of an organic process intrinsic to the disease itself and the latter in terms of a psychological reaction. Interestingly, Deckel and Morrison (1996), in their study on anosognosia in patients with Huntington's disease, conceive the relationship between denial and anosognosia somewhat differently. They refer to aspects of denial as representing an anosognosia. In other words, they view anosognosia as the neurologically determined process of unawareness. Weinstein et al. (1994), on the other hand, use the terms 'anosognosia' and 'denial' interchangeably but differentiate these from 'loss of insight', considering the latter as a distinct and unitary phenomenon. However, although anosognosia (or denial) is conceived in psychological terms (as a symbolic adaptation to having the disease), albeit in the necessary context of organic dysfunction, it is not entirely clear on what particular grounds this is differentiated from loss of insight. A different conceptualisation of 'anosognosia' is adopted by Starkstein et al. (1995a, p. 415) who, following Prigatano and Schacter (1991), define it as an 'apparent unawareness, misinterpretation or explicit denial' thus accepting a wider and more general notion. Taking yet a different approach, Mangone et al. (1991) conceive impaired insight following frontal lobe dysfunction as equivalent to 'confabulation'. In contrast, they equate impaired insight following right hemisphere dysfunction with 'anosognosia'. In other words, the concepts in this sense are defined by putative underlying brain mechanisms. Vasterling et al. (1995), on the other hand, make a distinction between the concepts of insight and awareness, defining the former in terms of the global loss of awareness in dementia and the latter in terms of a domain-specific awareness of deficit. Thus, here the researchers view insight as the broad concept incorporating the different types of awareness held in relation to different impairments of dementia.

A much broader and multidimensional conceptualisation of self-awareness or self-consciousness is offered by Gil *et al.* (2001). They conceive this as encompassing a wide range of perceptions relating to self-identity and, in empirical terms, they include awareness of the body, of mental processes (memory, autobiography, thoughts, etc.) and moral judgements. Likewise, conceiving insight as a broad and multidimensional structure but approaching this from a 'person-centred' perspective are the views held by Phinney (2002), and Howorth and Saper (2003). In the former, awareness is seen as inherent to the self and viewed as 'a way of being in the world, as an expression of lived experience that may be articulated through narrative' (Phinney, 2002, p. 331). This takes the concept away from some of the narrower 'cognitive' definitions and widens the notion to incorporate more qualitative aspects relating to the self. Similarly, Howorth and Saper (2003), whilst stressing the multidimensional aspects of insight as a concept, emphasise the importance of emotional awareness in its constitution.

The important issue emerging from an examination of the terms and concepts used in the studies exploring insight in patients with dementia is that studies refer to a wide range of different concepts of insight. Meanings of insight vary from simple descriptions of patients not acknowledging problems to more complex concepts incorporating postulated organic and/or psychological underlying mechanisms and range from narrow to wide inclusions (see also below). Some researchers seem to view lack of insight (or anosognosia) as a 'symptom' inherent to dementia progression (Auchus *et al.*, 1994) and others conceptualise lack of insight more in terms of disruption of a 'process' of self-monitoring (Correa *et al.*, 1996; Kaszniak & Christenson, 1996). Still others conceive insight in this context as a complex structure or 'ability' constituted by the interplay of a number of cognitive systems such that dysfunction at different levels or systems can give rise to different forms of anosognosia (Agnew & Morris, 1998; Duke *et al.*, 2002). In addition, some conceptions focus less on the cognitive aspects of insight but emphasise instead the importance of including emotional and behavioural aspects to insight and link this intrinsically to the self (Phinney, 2002; Howorth & Saper, 2003). Moreover, it is clear that researchers use the terms relating to insight in different ways and that the distinctions between terms, and the concepts they reflect, vary considerably from study to study.

5.1.2 Relational aspects of insight

The second issue contributing to the difficulties in determining the meaning of insight in dementia concerns the focus of insight in empirical studies. Insight is a relational concept and this carries crucial implications for the meaning of insight in different situations (Marková & Berrios, 2001). In other words, insight (or awareness) can only be understood or expressed in terms of its relation to something, be that a pathological state or a non-morbid experience. One cannot have insight without there being something to have insight about. The term 'object of insight assessment' has been used to refer to the particular mental or physical state (e.g. mental symptoms, mental illness, neurological abnormality, neuropsychological deficit, etc.) in relation to which insight is being assessed (Marková & Berrios, 2001). The importance of this relationship lies in the consequence that follows, namely, that the 'object' itself will determine to a significant extent the phenomenon (i.e. clinical manifestation) of insight and this theoretical issue is explored in detail in Chapter 7. For the purposes here, however, it is clear that studies examining insight in dementia vary also in terms of the 'object' chosen for insight assessment. In other words, empirical studies evaluate insight or awareness in relation to different aspects of the dementing illness, ranging from considering the illness as a whole to its individual features and impairments. Many researchers refer to 'domains' of awareness in this regard (Kotler-Cope & Camp, 1995; Vasterling *et al.*, 1995; Neundorfer, 1997) but, for the sake of consistency and for reasons that are discussed in Chapter 7, the term 'object' will be retained here.

Interestingly, compared with studies on insight in mental illness or neurological states, studies exploring insight in dementia are particularly noticeable by the number of different 'objects' of insight assessment. It is likely that this is a reflection of the special features of dementia which, as mentioned already, fall into a number of clinical domains (e.g. neurological impairments, psychological reactions, functional disabilities and psychiatric problems). Some of the earlier studies do not directly specify the object of insight and the general implication is that the insight assessed relates to the disease as a whole (e.g. Schneck *et al.*, 1982; Danielczyk, 1983). Many studies define *memory* or *cognitive impairment* as the object of insight and do not assess insight into other aspects of the dementia (Feher *et al.*, 1991; Reed *et al.*, 1993; Lopez *et al.*, 1994; Verhey *et al.*, 1995; Derouesné *et al.*, 1999; Sevush, 1999). Others concentrate solely on assessing patients' insight into their *functional abilities* (De Bettignies *et al.*, 1990; Mangone *et al.*, 1991). Still others assess insight in relation to a number of different 'objects'. For example, a number of studies examine insight into both cognitive deficits and functional impairments (Green *et al.*, 1993; Weinstein *et al.*, 1994; Ott *et al.*, 1996a; Harwood & Sultzer, 2002). Others include further objects of insight evaluation, such as *general health* and *mood disturbance* (Vasterling *et al.*, 1995; 1997), or knowledge of *progression of dementia* (Ott & Fogel, 1992) or *behavioural problems/ personality changes* (Starkstein *et al.*, 1995a; 1996) or *social function* (Seltzer *et al.*, 1997). Anderson and Tranel (1989) specified eight 'objects' of insight assessment, namely: reasons for hospitalisation, motor impairments, general thinking and intellect, orientation, memory, speech and language, visual perception and abilities on tests, and future activities. And, somewhat different 'objects' of insight assessment were evaluated by Kotler-Cope and Camp (1995), namely, language disorder, agitation, need for routine, depression, higher cognitive deficits, memory disorder, dementia, apraxia and disorientation. Interestingly, in addition to assessing insight into cognitive function and activities of daily living (ADL), the study by Giovannetti *et al.* (2002) also used *naturalistic action errors* as their object of insight assessment. In other words, the researchers here focused on assessing patients' awareness of any errors they made during normal (specified) every day tasks. Using their broader conceptualisation of insight or self-consciousness, Gil *et al.* (2001) on the other hand explored different objects again, including identity, cognitive disturbance, affective state, representation of the body, prospective memory, capacities for introspection and moral judgements.

In addition, even when the object of insight assessment is specified as memory or cognitive impairment, differences between studies are still present in regards to the type or aspect of memory impairment that is being evaluated. For example, some studies focus on insight into a *general memory problem* (Loebel *et al.*, 1990; Feher *et al.*, 1991; Verhey *et al.*, 1993; McDaniel *et al.*, 1995), while others assess insight into *specific memory/cognitive deficits* or tasks. In relation to the latter, Green *et al.* (1993) examine insight into remote memory, recent memory and attention whilst Michon *et al.* (1994) assess insight into global memory, recall, retention, remote memory for personal events, attention and metamemory. Some researchers, in addition, focus on patients' awareness of the *effects of memory impairment* (Sevush & Leve, 1993) or on the perception of *change in memory functioning* (McGlynn & Kaszniak, 1991a, b; Vasterling *et al.*, 1995).

5.1.3 Methods of insight assessment in dementia

In order to further clarify the various meanings of insight in relation to dementia, it is necessary to discuss some of the methods used to assess insight in empirical studies. Here again, a range of different measures have been developed to assess insight in patients with dementia. Indeed, the approaches in this clinical area, particularly as far as systematic measures are concerned, have been more numerous and more varied in scope than the measures developed to assess insight in general psychiatry (Chapter 3). Similarly, however, the problem arises as to whether the different insight measures are eliciting and assessing the *same* clinical phenomenon of insight or whether in fact they elicit different phenomena, with ensuing consequences for the comparison of study outcomes.

A detailed review of the various measures developed to assess awareness in dementia has been covered elsewhere (Clare *et al.*, 2005), but it is useful to examine some of the main differences between insight assessments. The earlier studies tend not to define their assessment criteria and patients are generally categorised into those having and those not having insight or awareness into their dementia on the basis of clinical judgement (Aminoff *et al.*, 1975; Gustafson & Nilsson, 1982; Neary *et al.*, 1986). More recently, however, attempts have focused on developing systematic methods of assessing insight in terms of both categorical and continuous ratings. Broadly, such insight measures can be divided into: (i) clinician-rated assessments, (ii) discrepancy measures and (iii) composite assessments which include a number of different measures.

5.1.3.1 Clinician-rated assessments

Most of the clinician-rated measures consist of structured or semi-structured interviews on the basis of which clinicians judge the patient's insight. This is then rated either in a dichotomous way with patients deemed as having or not having awareness (Loebel *et al.*, 1990; Lopez *et al.*, 1994; Seltzer *et al.*, 1995b) or on a categorical basis with generally three or four categories in recognition of 'partial' insight or 'mild' denial (Sevush & Leve, 1993; Verhey *et al.*, 1993; 1995; Weinstein *et al.*, 1994; McDaniel *et al.*, 1995). The divisions between categories are determined by criteria set by the researchers. For example, Sevush and Leve (1993), on the basis of their interview of patients with Alzheimer's disease, categorise patients into having *no insight*, i.e. no acknowledgement of memory impairment, or *partial insight*, i.e. showing some awareness of the presence of memory impairment but not its full extent, or *full insight*, i.e. acknowledgment of both the presence and severity of the memory impairment. On the other hand, McDaniel *et al.* (1995) using the Consortium to Establish a Registry for Alzheimer's Disease (CERAD) structured interview, have a slightly different emphasis in their categorisation: *normal insight* – total insight into the illness and implication, or *partial awareness* of disease or implications or *unawareness or denial* of symptoms of illness. Thus, there are differences in terms of detail and specificity of criteria to determine categories between different studies. Similar categorical divisions have been used to evaluate insight in patients with Huntington's disease (Caine *et al.*, 1978) and Parkinson's disease (Danielczyk, 1983). However, in addition to the differences between studies in terms of anchor points for categories, as with any categorical ratings, judgements will clearly be of a general nature. They cannot therefore address detailed qualitative aspects of insight and will depend very much on the subjectivity of the judger.

Other researchers have developed rating scales so that insight is assessed on a continuous scale. For example, Ott and Fogel (1992) devised a scale (Insight Rating Scale) consisting of four areas of questioning relating to four 'objects' of insight, namely, situation, memory impairment, ADL and progression of disease. Each of these are rated individually from 0 to 2 according to whether clinicians judged the patient as having good insight (0) up to no insight (2). Thus, a higher score on the scale indicates a lower degree of insight in the patient. A quite different measure, in terms of its content, was devised by Gil *et al.* (2001) whose Self-Consciousness

Questionnaire consists of 14 items relating to their particular 'objects' of awareness assessment (e.g. identity, prospective memory, etc., see above).

Further differences between such clinician assessments are also present in terms of how the evaluations take place. Thus, some clinician judgements are based on interviews with patients only (Sevush & Leve, 1993; Weinstein *et al.*, 1994; McDaniel *et al.*, 1995). Others are carried out in the presence of patient's relative or carer so that the judgement takes into account the latter's views (Loebel *et al.*, 1990; Ott & Fogel, 1992; Verhey *et al.*, 1993). On the other hand, some researchers have categorised patients' insight on the basis of information in case notes only (Reed *et al.*, 1993; Auchus *et al.*, 1994; Lopez *et al.*, 1994). It seems likely therefore that further differences in the elicited insight phenomenon will emerge depending on the source of the information obtained.

5.1.3.2 Discrepancy measures

A great many studies exploring insight in patients with dementia have developed insight assessments based on discrepancy measures. These measures determine levels of insight on the basis of discrepancies between the *patient's assessment* of abilities and either: (a) the *carer's (relative's) assessment* of the patient's abilities (De Bettignies *et al.*, 1990; Feher *et al.*, 1991; Michon *et al.*, 1994; Starkstein *et al.*, 1995a,b; Vasterling *et al.*, 1995; Smith C.A. *et al.*, 2000) or (b) *'objective' measures* of impairment, such as a battery of neuropsychological tests (Anderson & Tranel, 1989; Dalla Barba *et al.*, 1995; Wagner *et al.*, 1997; Barrett *et al.*, 2005) or (c) a combination of *both forms* of discrepancy assessments (McGlynn & Kaszniak, 1991a, b; Green *et al.*, 1993; Correa *et al.*, 1996; Clare *et al.*, 2002; Duke *et al.*, 2002). Such methods have been important in assessing awareness into neurological states, particularly traumatic head injury (see Chapter 4). Discrepancy measures of insight are based on the assumption that an 'accurate' assessment of an individual's functioning can be obtained either directly via another person's (one who knows the individual well) observations or indirectly by means of scores on performance in certain tasks. Such assessments are then compared with the patients' own assessments of their functioning and any discrepancy found between patients' ratings and carers' ratings or test scores are attributed to the patient's lack of awareness or insight into such functioning. Consequently, the greater the discrepancy that is obtained, the greater the degree of unawareness or insightlessness shown by the patient. Since the questionnaires or tests involved are scored (e.g. total score on questionnaire obtained from patient subtracted from total score obtained by carer, or ratios calculated in relation to test scores), the discrepancies have ranges of values and hence insight assessed by such methods is quantified along a continuum of scores.

As far as insight assessments using patient-carer discrepancy are concerned, the main differences between questionnaires used in the various studies relate to different 'objects' of insight and/or to different types of judgements contained in the contents. The issue around different 'objects' of insight has already been mentioned and relates to the questionnaires addressing different aspects of dementia in relation to which insight is assessed. Thus, some questionnaires focus on ADL, and patients and carers are required to rate patients' abilities in those particular areas (e.g. De Bettignies *et al.*, 1990; Mangone *et al.*, 1991). Other questionnaires focus on memory and/or other cognitive problems (e.g. Feher *et al.*, 1991; Michon *et al.*, 1994; Seltzer *et al.*, 1995b). Still others use questionnaires addressing both these areas (e.g. Seltzer *et al.*, 1997) and additional ones, such as mood changes, behavioural problems and others (e.g. Kotler-Cope & Camp, 1995; Starkstein *et al.*, 1995a; Vasterling *et al.*, 1995; Deckel & Morrison, 1996; Smith C.A. *et al.*, 2000; Snow *et al.*, 2004). In addition to these differences in 'object' of insight there are, however, also differences in the types of judgements that patients and carers are being asked to make. For example, some questionnaires focusing on evaluations of memory ask patients (with parallel questions for the carers) to rate the *degree of severity* of problems they perceive as having with their memory (Green *et al.*, 1993; Duke *et al.*, 2002). Other questionnaires, also focusing on memory evaluations, ask patients to rate their memory *as compared with some years previously* (McGlynn & Kaszniak, 1991a, b; Michon *et al.*, 1994) or even *as compared with others of a similar age* (Deckel & Morrison, 1996). On the other hand, some questionnaires ask patients to rate the *frequency with which they make mistakes* in various memory-related tasks (Migliorelli *et al.*, 1995; Starkstein *et al.*, 1996; Seltzer *et al.*, 1995b; Derouesné *et al.*, 1999). Some studies include various mixtures of such types of judgements (e.g. Feher *et al.*, 1991; Clare *et al.*, 2002). In other words, as with similar discrepancy measures used in, for example, head injury, the various measures demand different types of judgements from patients (and carers). This is important to highlight, not just because the overt content of such questionnaires may be different, but also because such specific judgements themselves may well be contributing to the elicitation of different phenomena of insight. Being asked to evaluate the severity of current problems with memory may involve quite different sorts of judgements from those made when comparing memory with that of other individuals or with memory from some years previously. Thus, whilst the various questionnaires elicit some aspects of insight, it is questionable whether in fact the same or similar aspects of insight are assessed in studies using different questionnaires even if all are purporting to measure insight into memory problems (Hermann, 1982).

Apart from such differences between individual questionnaires, questionnaire discrepancy measures raise a number of other important issues concerning their validity as measures of patients' insight. There is firstly the question concerning the extent to which a 'carer/relative' can be expected to provide an accurate evaluation of a patient's functioning in different areas. For various reasons, carers may both overestimate or underestimate levels of impairments in patients. For example, De Bettignies *et al.* (1990) examining discrepancies between patients and carers in evaluation of patients' independent living skills found that whilst patients' insight was not correlated with age, mental status, education or level of depression, it was significantly related to the degree of caregiver concern or burden. In other words, the higher the degree of burden perceived by the carer, the higher the discrepancy (i.e. lower patient insight) between patient and carer assessments. The authors suggested that the high discrepancy in this situation was not only due to the patients' overestimation of living skills but that carers with greater perceived burden were underestimating the capacity of patients. Other factors might also play a part in carers' underestimating patients' functioning including carers' mental states, physical health, relationship with patient, etc. Similarly, carers might equally overestimate patients' function in different areas again because such judgements will depend to some extent on individual factors relating to the carer, e.g. mental state of carer, extent of denial, motivation to keep patient 'well' (e.g. because of driving), level of knowledge concerning the patient, etc.

In general, studies exploring the 'accuracy' of carers' evaluations of patients in different areas have found reasonably good correlations between carers' assessments and other measures of patients' functioning. For example, in *memory assessments*, in contrast to patients' own evaluations, carers' evaluations of patients' memory difficulties have correlated significantly with neuropsychological tests of memory function in patients (McGlone *et al.*, 1990; Grut *et al.*, 1993; Koss *et al.*, 1993; Jorm *et al.*, 1994; McLoughlin *et al.*, 1996). Interestingly, the study by Jorm *et al.* (1994) also found that carers' ratings of patients' cognitive state were influenced by depression and anxiety experienced by carers. The type of carer involved (in terms of relationship of carer to patient or degree of contact with patient) has sometimes been found to relate to the 'accuracy' of carer evaluation. For example, McLoughlin *et al.* (1996) found that spouses' evaluation of patients' memory correlated more strongly with neuropsychology tests than first degree relatives' evaluations and that second degree relatives' evaluations of patients' memory function had no significant correlation with memory tests.

Similarly, in *assessments of daily living activities*, carers'/relatives' evaluations of patient function have been more strongly correlated with 'objective' tests of ADL than patients' evaluations (Kuriansky *et al.*, 1976). Interestingly, examining differences in the assessments of ADL of elderly physically ill patients, Rubenstein *et al.* (1984) found that, using structured scales, patients evaluated themselves as functioning significantly better compared with the evaluations by their relatives whilst nursing staff's evaluations fell intermediate between those of patients and carers. In other words, it is clear that individual factors are important in determining such assessments. The researchers highlighted the issue, inherent in any questionnaire discrepancy methods, that it may not be possible to distinguish between overestimations made by subjects and underestimations made by others.

In the case of evaluating *depressive symptoms*, the questionnaire discrepancy methods are beset by additional problems because of the problems involved in others judging the 'subjective experiences' of individuals. Studies have shown discrepancies between the evaluations made by patients, relatives and clinicians, with patients generally underreporting depressive symptomatology compared with carers or clinicians (Mackenzie *et al.*, 1989; Teri & Wagner, 1991; Logsdon & Teri, 1995; Snow *et al.*, 2005). However, Burke *et al.* (1998) showed that carers/relatives rated not only patients with Alzheimer's disease as more depressed, compared with patients' evaluations, but they also rated patients without cognitive impairment as more depressed. The authors suggested that the discrepancy reflected exaggeration of problems on the relatives' part and that this in turn might relate to their perceived burden of care. In other words, the study emphasised the importance of individual factors, both patient and carer related, that might contribute to discrepancies and the difficulty in distinguishing between such factors to determine to what extent a discrepancy measure can evaluate a subject's awareness or insight of problems.

Secondly, apart from the question of carer 'accuracy' in assessing patients' function, other issues concerning questionnaire discrepancy methods need to be considered. Sevush (1999) raised the problem (applied to both questionnaire and performance discrepancy measures) that carer assessments (and test performance) will inherently incorporate assessments of dementia severity itself. Thus, studies using discrepancy measures of assessing patients' insight to examine the relationship between patients' insight and severity of dementia may show inflated correlations because the 'severity of dementia' variable will be both a dependent and independent variable in the correlations obtained. Another problem concerning questionnaire discrepancy methods relates to the way the scores are calculated. These tend to be composite scores based on the totals derived from patients and carers. However, individual items on the measures could be discrepant in different ways and these could be lost when total scores are used. In addition, some discrepancy measures use cutoff points to determine patients with and without insight (Migliorelli *et al.*, 1995; Starkstein *et al.*, 1995a; 1997b, etc.) and thus again information might be lost as only patients at either extremes are included in the analysis (Lamar *et al.*, 2002).

Discrepancy methods using performances on 'objective' psychometric tests, rather than carers' assessment, as the gold standard against which patients' insight is derived, are complicated by other issues. Such neuropsychological tests are relatively detailed and specific, and have little in common with memory/cognitive problems that come up in daily life. Yet, patients' awareness of memory or cognitive problems is determined by the discrepancy in their scores on such tests and their subjective assessment on a global rating of how severe they believe their memory problem to be (e.g. Anderson & Tranel, 1989; McGlynn & Kaszniak, 1991a, b). As others point out (Hermann, 1982; Sunderland *et al.*, 1983; Larrabee *et al.*, 1991; Trosset & Kaszniak, 1996), the poor correspondence between what the tests are assessing and what the patients are being asked to assess makes it difficult to attribute the size of discrepancies solely to patients' impaired awareness of cognitive problems. Some researchers have attempted to reduce this particular problem by devising measures that are more practically relevant to the individual (e.g. Clare *et al.*, 2002) and by the use of prediction and/or postdiction discrepancy methods. In the former, specific neuropsychological tests (e.g. recall of word lists) are first explained to the patients and then they are asked to predict how they would perform on such tests. The discrepancies between patient predictions and actual performance are taken as a measure of patient awareness (e.g. McGlynn & Kaszniak, 1991a, b; Green *et al.*, 1993). In the latter, again, the tests are first explained to the patients, but in this case the patients are asked to rate how well they have performed only after completing the tests. The discrepancies between patient performance and their postperformance assessments are taken as reflecting their insight into their cognitive problems (Correa *et al.*, 1996).

Within the metamemory framework, focusing on self-monitoring (rather than awareness or insight), some studies have assessed patients' predictions on recall tests following practice (Moulin *et al.*, 2000). Others have differentiated between assessments based on patients' predictions of recalling and those based on patients' predictions of recognising (feeling-of-knowing) words from lists (Souchay *et al.*, 2002). However, the crucial point is that irrespective of the specific design of such discrepancy methods, the phenomenon of awareness or insight elicited by the different methods (test performance, prediction, postdiction) will vary accordingly. Thus, depending on the test's demands (both in content and design), it will incorporate different types of judgements into the discrepancy measure. Consequently, the different assessments will elicit different aspects of insight. Trosset and Kaszniak (1996) argue that discrepancy measures, based on psychometric tests, reflect not only patients' awareness of cognitive problems but also their judgements concerning the difficulties of such unfamiliar tests. They suggest that one way to distinguish between these types of judgements is to consider also patients' assessments of their relatives' performances on the tests as well as the relatives' assessments of themselves and the patients on the same tests. However, clearly all sorts of additional judgements would then complicate the ensuing assessment and it might be difficult to tease out individual aspects. Nevertheless, some studies have devised insight measures that have included a combination of patients' and carers' predictions (McGlynn & Kaszniak, 1991a, b), and postdictions of own and the others' functioning as well as predictions and postdictions of the performance of an unfamiliar person (videotaped interview) on memory tests (Duke *et al.*, 2002).

5.1.3.3 Composite measures

In recognition of the likely different aspects of insight elicited by the various approaches, some researchers have employed combinations of both clinician-rated assessments and discrepancy measures in an attempt to provide a more global and comprehensive picture of insight (Correa *et al.*, 1996; Ott *et al.*, 1996a; Derouesné *et al.*, 1999; Howorth & Saper, 2003). Similarly, acknowledging the assumptions involved when using carers' information as the gold standard against which patients' responses on questionnaires are assessed, Snow *et al.* (2004) devised a more composite instrument to assess deficits in awareness about dementia. This includes not only discrepancies between patients and carers but also discrepancies between patients and clinicians. Thus, they developed three parallel forms of their Dementia Deficits Scale to be independently completed by patients, carers and clinicians. They emphasised the need to consider the biases of the different proxies involved, and argued that the different perspectives thus collected added unique information to the capture of patients' self-awareness as a whole.

In addition, some studies have also included novel ways of assessing insight. For example, Giovannetti *et al.* (2002), apart from using discrepancy methods also included a clinician-rated evaluation of patients' insight that was based on directly observed behaviours (videotaped). Insight in the latter situation was inferred on the basis of patients' reactions to and attempts at self-corrections of mistakes occurring during the course of three set everyday tasks. Similarly, Bologna and Camp (1997) in a small study inferred the presence of insight in patients on the basis of self-recognition in a mirror reflection. Clare (2003), on the other hand, attempted a more in-depth assessment of insight by exploring patients' awareness in detailed interviews focusing on patients' understanding in the context of their individual and social backgrounds. The interviews were taped and interpretative phenomenological analysis was used to construct a model of awareness within a psychosocial context.

5.2 Relationship between insight, clinical and socio-demographic variables

Interest in the empirical exploration of insight in dementia particularly over the last 15 years seems to have arisen from various perspectives. As in relation to the research on insight in 'functional' psychiatric disorders, questions appear to converge predominantly on the nature of insight as a phenomenon. In contrast to the ideas on insight in psychoses, the debate on the nature of insight (or rather insightlessness) in dementia is, with a few exceptions (Clare, 2003), much more clearly polarised. In this sense, it is generally viewed either as a symptom inherent to the dementia process itself or as a psychological reaction inherent to the individual. Whilst these aspects of insight are likewise raised in general psychiatry (see Chapter 3), there is a less explicit division there. Furthermore, there is in addition a third position held in general psychiatry, namely that of insight conceived as an independent phenomenon or process, in the sense of being independent of both the disorder itself and of the psychology or reactivity of the individual. In dementia studies, the polarity between unawareness as intrinsic to the disease process and unawareness as a psychological denial seems to have been driven to a considerable extent by the work on anosognosia in non-progressive organic brain disorders (see previous chapter). Focus on insight in empirical studies has thus been aimed predominantly at two issues. Firstly, researchers have focused on developing understanding of the *dementia process* itself. In other words, studies attempt to relate insight with disease severity and to explore changes in insight in relation to different dementias or brain/neuropsychological dysfunction. Secondly, researchers have sought to examine the changes and *reactions of the person* with dementia. In other words, studies explore the relationship between insight and various moods and behavioural changes, such as depression/anxiety, etc. From a slightly different perspective, interest in the exploration of insight in dementia has also been generated from a wider consideration of the *patient and family* affected by the disease and its consequences. Hence, studies have attempted to consider the rehabilitation potential of insight (mirroring work on insight in relation to traumatic brain injury), its prognostic value and the effects of impaired insight on the family/carers looking after the patient.

It is perhaps not surprising that, in general, results of empirical studies exploring the relationship between insight, clinical and socio-demographic variables are as inconclusive in relation to dementias as they are in relation to functional psychiatric syndromes. Once again it is likely that the differences identified in the way insight is defined and conceptualised, the variable ways in which it is assessed, the range of 'objects' of insight involved as well as the fact that different outcome measures are used will all contribute to the mixed and inconsistent results. This makes it difficult to answer in a definite way some of the questions posed concerning the nature of insight as a clinical phenomenon and its relationship to both the individual and to the disease process.

5.2.1 Insight and socio-demographic variables

Searching for associations between insight and socio-demographic variables is a means of exploring only fairly general characteristics of insight that could be related to the individual and/or the disease. Overall there is more consistency between the studies reporting on such correlations than in other areas. Most studies report no significant correlations between the degree of patients' insight and variables, such as age (or age of disease onset) of the patient, education level or duration of illness (De Bettignies *et al.*, 1990; Feher *et al.*, 1991; Reed *et al.*, 1993; Auchus *et al.*, 1994; Starkstein *et al.*, 1995a; Vasterling *et al.*, 1995; 1997; Sevush, 1999; Gil *et al.*, 2001;

Giovannetti *et al.*, 2002). There are a few exceptions. For example, Sevush and Leve (1993), whilst finding no association between denial and age of onset of Alzheimer's disease, years of education or duration of illness, found, nevertheless, a significant correlation with gender, females showing more denial (less insight) than males. On the other hand, Migliorelli *et al.* (1995) reported in their study that males showed significantly more anosognosia (less insight) than females. Similarly, whilst most studies find no association between insight and the age of the patient, a few studies report a negative correlation between insight and age, i.e. the greater the age, the lower the patient's awareness (Verhey *et al.*, 1993; Weinstein *et al.*, 1994; Derouesné *et al.*, 1999). And, likewise, duration of illness has not been found to correlate with insight in most studies but a few have reported a negative correlation, i.e. less insight associated with longer duration of illness (Migliorelli *et al.*, 1995; Starkstein *et al.*, 1996; 1997a).

Given the few significant correlations between insight and socio-demographic variables, in the face of mostly non-significant findings, it is difficult to interpret very much. As is seen from Table 5.1, the studies vary in their methodologies, particularly, in their measures of insight and it is likely that different aspects of insight are elicited which, in turn, is likely to affect the correlation sought. Moreover, variables such as duration of dementia can be very difficult to ascertain given the lack of detailed understanding around the disease process.

5.2.2 Insight in different types of dementia

Exploring the relationship between impairment of insight and different types of dementia means, essentially, addressing the question of whether impaired insight is a symptom or process that is specific to the disease itself rather than to the individual. In other words, if patients were to show more impaired insight according to the type of dementia affecting them, then perhaps insight could be conceived as intrinsic to the particular pathological process associated with that dementia. Most work on insight has, in fact, been carried out in Alzheimer's disease (Table 5.1, most studies use the NINCDS-ADRDA (McKhann *et al.*, 1984) criteria for probable Alzheimer's disease) and there has been little systematic work undertaken in other types of dementia. In general, it is claimed that patients with cortical dementias (e.g. Alzheimer's disease, Pick's disease/frontal lobe dementia) show greater loss of insight than patients with subcortical dementias, e.g. Huntington's disease, Parkinson's disease, etc. (Kaszniak & Christenson, 1996; Lishman, 1998). Pick's disease and/or frontal lobe dementia have been noted particularly for a marked and early loss of insight (Gustafson & Nilsson, 1982; Neary *et al.*, 1986; Orrell & Sahakian, 1991). On the other hand, studies exploring insight in subcortical dementias such as Huntington's disease or Parkinson's disease have remarked on the relative preservation of insight in these patients (Aminoff *et al.*, 1975; Caine *et al.*, 1978;

Caine & Shoulson, 1983; Danielczyk, 1983). Caine *et al.* (1978) commented on patients with Huntington's disease showing not only insight into their cognitive problems but also into changes of temperament or disposition, and into difficulties in controlling their affect. However, most of these studies have not used any structured assessments of insight nor provided defined criteria for establishing the presence or absence or partial presence of insight.

Some studies using structured insight assessments (albeit of different kinds) have explored differences in insight between patients with Alzheimer's disease and vascular dementias. One of the issues to consider here is the validity of using the Hachinski criteria (Hachinski *et al.*, 1975) to distinguish between Alzheimer's disease and vascular or multi-infarct dementia which has been subject to some criticism (e.g. Dening & Berrios, 1992). Interestingly, studies have shown opposing results. Thus, some researchers have found no difference in the insight shown between patients with Alzheimer's disease and those with vascular dementias (Verhey *et al.*, 1993; 1995; Zanetti *et al.*, 1999; Giovannetti *et al.*, 2002). However, other studies report a significant difference in insight between the groups, with Alzheimer's disease patients showing greater impairment of insight than patients with vascular disease (De Bettignies *et al.*, 1990; Wagner *et al.*, 1997). Again, little can be concluded at this stage and the differences in methodologies of the studies are described in Table 5.1. More systematic work is needed to be able to address the question of differences in patients' insight in different dementias and such work continues to be additionally problematic in the face of practical difficulties around determining onset/stage of disease and its severity.

5.2.3 Insight in relation to severity, stage and progression of dementia

Questions concerning the relationship between patients' insight and the severity, stage and/or progression of their disease are, once again, aimed at determining to what extent impairment of insight is intrinsic to the disease process (and progression) and, hence, part of its 'pathology' as opposed to representing a psychological reaction to knowledge of the consequences of having dementia.

As can be seen from Table 5.1, studies exploring the relationship between patients' insight and the severity of their dementia also yield variable results. Many studies report a strong positive correlation between poor insight and more severe dementia (e.g. Mangone *et al.*, 1991; Verhey *et al.*, 1993; Lopez *et al.*, 1994; Seltzer *et al.*, 1995a, b; Vasterling *et al.*, 1995; Correa *et al.*, 1996; Harwood *et al.*, 2000; Duke *et al.*, 2002; Vogel *et al.*, 2005). Others report only a weak association between severity of dementia and poor insight (e.g. Feher *et al.*, 1991; Michon *et al.*, 1992; Ott *et al.*, 1996b; Sevush, 1999). Yet, others find no relationship between insight and severity of dementia (e.g. Loebel *et al.*, 1990; Green *et al.*, 1993; Reed *et al.*, 1993; Weinstein *et al.*, 1994; Dalla Barba *et al.*, 1995; Giovannetti *et al.*, 2002;

Table 5.1 Studies of insight in dementia: relationship with clinical/socio-demographic variables

Study	Patients	'Object' of insight	Insight assessment	Outcome variables	Main results Dementia	Ψ/behavioural	Other
Anderson and Tranel (1989)	CVA: 32 AD: 29 MID: 5 MD: 15 HT: 19	Cognitive and motor deficits	Discrepancy between patient assessment and performance on neuropsychology tests	Neuropsychology tests: 1–8 Computerised tomography (CT) and/or magnetic resonance image (MRI)	Poor insight associated with right hemisphere damage and lower intelligence quotient	–	No difference in insight across diagnostic groups
De Bettignies et al. (1990)	AD: 12 MID: 12 Elderly control: 12	Independent living skills	Discrepancy between patient and carer on questionnaire	PSMS IADL HDRS	AD patients had lower insight than VD and controls	No association between insight and depression	Poor insight associated with greater carer's burden
Loebel et al. (1990)	AD: 32	Memory problems	Clinician-rated structured interview of patient and carer	MMSE Fluency Rating Scale	No difference in severity of dementia between patients with and without insight	–	Poor insight associated with better speech fluency
Feher et al. (1991)	AD: 38	Memory problems	Discrepancy between patient and carer on questionnaire	MMSE GDS HDRS Neuropsychology tests: 4, 9,10	Weak correlation between poor insight and more severe dementia	Weak correlation between poor insight and less depression	–
McGlynn and Kaszniak (1991a)	AD: 8	Memory problems	1. Discrepancy between patient and carer on questionnaire	MMSE Neuropsychology tests: 11–22	Poor insight associated with more severe dementia	–	Patients over-estimated own function but accurate in

			2. Discrepancy between patient prediction and performance on cognitive tests				estimating carers' abilities
McGlynn and Kaszniak (1991b)	HD: 8	Memory problems Motor problems	As above and discrepancy between patient prediction and performance on motor tests	MMSE Neuropsychology tests: 10, 19, 22 Motor tasks: a–e	Poor insight associated with more severe dementia	–	Poor insight with questionnaire discrepancy Better insight on prediction tests
Mangone *et al.* (1991)	AD: 41	Physical self-maintaining activities Activities of Daily Living (ADL)	Discrepancy between patient and carer on questionnaire	MMSE, GDS, BDRS, BPRS Neuropsychology tests: 9, 23–30	Poor insight associated with more severe dementia Best predictors of poor insight: GDS, BPRS, tests: 23, 27	Poor insight more frequent in patients with paranoid delusions	–
Michon *et al.* (1992)	AD: 15	Memory problems	Discrepancy between patient and carer on questionnaire	MMSE Neuropsychology tests: 22, 31–34	Minimal correlation between poor insight and severity. Significant correlation between poor insight and 'frontal' tests	–	–

Table 5.1 (*cont.*)

Study	Patients	'Object' of insight	Insight assessment	Outcome variables	Main results		
					Dementia	Ψ/behavioural	Other
Ott and Fogel (1992)	AD: 37 VD and others: 13	1. Reason for clinic visit 2. Memory problems 3. ADL 4. Progress of deficits	Clinician rating on scale in the four areas based on information from patient and carer	MMSE, CDRS HDRS, COR, GerDS	Poor insight associated with more severe dementia	Mixed association – between insight and depression, depending on depression scale (see text)	
Green *et al.* (1993)	AD: 20	1. Remote memory 2. Recent memory 3. Attention 4. Daily activities	1. Discrepancy between patient and carer on questionnaire 2. Discrepancy between patient prediction and performance on cognitive test	Neuropsychology tests: 2, 35 DRS	No association between insight and severity of dementia	–	Least insight into recent memory and ADL. No correlation between the two insight measures
Reed *et al.* (1993)	AD: 57	Memory problems	Clinician rated from case notes. Scale identified four categories	MMSE, DSM-III (for depression) Neuropsychology tests: 35–38 SPECT (*n* = 20)	No association between insight and severity of dementia. Poor insight associated with poor recognition memory	No association between insight and depression	Poor insight associated with reduced perfusion in right dorsolateral frontal areas

Study	Sample	Construct	Method	Measures	Cognitive findings	Depression findings	Other
Sevush and Leve (1993)	AD: 128	Memory problems	Clinician-rated structured interview: three categories	ACAD Three-item scale for depression	Poor insight associated with more severe cognitive deficits	Poor insight associated with less depression	–
Verhey et al. (1993)	AD: 103 VD: 43 Others: 24	Cognitive deficits	Clinician-rated structured interview of patient and carer	GDS DSM-III-R (for depression), HDRS	Poor insight associated with more severe dementia	No correlation between insight and depression. Correlation between poor insight and less psychic anxiety (HDRS)	–
Auchus et al. (1994)	AD: 28	Cognitive deficits	Clinician rating from case notes	DRS Neuropsychology tests: 2, 9, 27, 36–39	No association between insight and severity of dementia. Correlation between poor insight and poor visuo-constructive skills (38, 39)	–	
Feher et al. (1994)	AD: 83 AAMI: 200 Conrols: 64	Memory problems	Self-report of memory problems on questionnaire	HDRS Neuropsychology tests: 4, 9, 10	Poor insight associated with more severe dementia	Poor insight associated with less depression	
Kiyak et al. (1994)	AD: 40 Control: 53 Follow-up study	1. Functional health 2. General health	Discrepancy between patient and carer on questionnaire	DRS	Insight worse over time, in association with decline of cognition	–	Longitudinal study: partial preservation of insight over time

Table 5.1 (cont.)

Study	Patients	'Object' of insight	Insight assessment	Outcome variables	Main results — Dementia	Main results — Ψ/behavioural	Main results — Other
Lopez et al. (1994)	AD: 181	Cognitive deficits	Clinician rating from case notes	Structured Ψ interview; DSM-III-R. Neuropsychology tests: 3, 5, 25, 31, 36, 40–45	Poor insight associated with more severe dementia. Poor insight associated with poor frontal tests	No difference in depression, delusions or hallucinations between patients with and without insight	–
Michon et al. (1994)	AD: 24	Memory problems	Discrepancy between patient and carer on questionnaire	MMSE, MADRS Neuropsychology tests: 22, 31, 32, 36, 38 Behavioural observations (Luria)	No correlation between insight and severity and most of tests. Significant correlation between poor insight and poor 'frontal' tests	No correlation between insight and depression	–
Weinstein et al. (1994)	AD: 41 Followed up also after 2–3 years	1. Memory problems 2. ADL	Clinician-rated structured interview: three categories	MMSE Neuropsychology tests: 39, 46, 47 Ψ history. Premorbid personality rating	No correlation between insight and severity or with any of tests	Poor insight associated with confabulation, delusions, misidentification, symbolic disorientation	Poor insight more often when AD presented initially with memory or behavioural changes
Dalla Barba et al. (1995)	AD: 12 DD: 12	Memory problems	Discrepancy between patient	MMSE, BDRS, MADRS	No correlation between insight	Depressed patients had less	–

Table (rotated). Column headers are truncated at the top of the page; visible header fragments include: "… rating of memory and performance on memory tasks", "… and frontal tests", "Neuropsychology tests: 22, 48–50 Occurrence of 'intrusions'", "insight into memory, and …".

Study	Domain assessed	Method	Tests	Cognition result	Mood / behaviour result	Other
Kotler-Cope and Camp (1995) AD: 13	nine objects – including cognitive, mood and behaviour	rating of memory and performance on memory tasks	Neuropsychology tests: 22, 48–50 Occurrence of 'intrusions'	Poor insight correlated with more intrusions	insight into memory, and overestimated memory more than AD, but not statistically significant	Better insight for Ψ and behavioural problems than for cognitive.
McDaniel et al. (1995) AD: 670 After follow-up: 1 year: 406 2 years: 148	Cognitive deficits	Clinician-rated direct questioning: three categories	MMSE, CDRS BDRS BDRS-short	Poor insight correlated with more severe dementia	–	Reduction of insight over time correlated with greater severity
Migliorelli et al. (1995) AD: 73	1. Cognitive deficits 2. Personality and interests	Discrepancy between patient and carer on questionnaire (AQ-D): cut-off point for those with and without insight	MMSE, CDRS HDRS, HAS FIM, STC, BMS, PLACS Neuropsychology tests: 4, 19, 32, 36–38, 43, 51–54	Poor insight correlated with more severe cognitive and ADL deficits No correlation with specific tests	Poor insight associated with more mania, pathological laughing and less dysthymia and anxiety. No correlation with major depression	–
Seltzer et al. (1995a) AD: 226	Memory problems	Clinician-rated set questions: two categories (with and without insight)	MMSE, CDRS BDRS: BMIC and BPEA Ψ interview	Poor insight associated with later stage and more severe dementia	Patients with insight had significantly more depressed mood (not disorder)	–

Table 5.1 (*cont*.)

Study	Patients	'Object' of insight	Insight assessment	Outcome variables	Main results Dementia	Ψ/behavioural	Other
Seltzer et al. (1995b)	AD: 36	Memory problems	Discrepancy between patient and carer on questionnaire (EMQ)	MMSE COR Three 5-point Likert scales to assess mood	Poor insight correlated with more severe dementia	Poor insight associated with less depression and more carer-rated irritability	–
Starkstein et al. (1995a)	AD: 24	1. Cognitive deficits 2. Personality and interests	Discrepancy between patient and carer on questionnaire (AQ-D)	MMSE, HDRS, FIM, STC Neuropsychology tests: 4, 19, 32, 36–38, 51–54 SPECT	No difference in severity or test scores between patients with and without insight	No difference in depression, ADL and social ties between patients with and without insight	Patients with no insight had reduced cerebral blood flow in right hemisphere
Vasterling et al. (1995)	AD: 43	Memory, general health, self-care, mood	Discrepancy between patient and carer on questionnaire (EMQ, GQ)	MMSE, CDRS	Poor insight associated with later stage and more severe dementia	–	Least insight in self-care and memory. Best insight in depression and general health
Verhey et al. (1995)	AD: 48 VD: 48	Cognitive deficits	Clinician-rated structured interview of patient and carer	GDS, BDRS DSM-III-R (for depression) HDRS	Poor insight associated with more severe dementia	–	No difference in insight or depression between AD and VD

Study	Groups	Domains assessed	Measures	Findings		
Correa et al. (1996)	AD: 20 MII: 18 Controls: 18	Memory problems	1. Discrepancy between patient and carer on questionnaire 2. Discrepancy between post-diction and performance on cognitive tests 3. Number of intrusions and self-corrections	MMSE Neuropsychology tests: 3, 4, 22, 55	Poor insight associated with more severe dementia	–	AD showed poorer insight into memory problems compared with memory impaired older adults
Deckel and Morrison (1996)	HD: 19 Controls: 14 (Neuro-impaired)	Cognitive and motor problems and emotions	Discrepancy between patient and staff ratings on questionnaire	Neuropsychology tests: 2, 5, 31, 32, 37, 43, 56	Poor insight associated with more impairments on tests	–	HD had less insight than neurological controls
Ott et al. (1996a)	AD: 26 Controls: 16	1. Reason for clinic visit 2. Memory problems 3. ADL 4. Progress of deficits	1. Clinician rated (Ott & Fogel, 1982, above) 2. Discrepancy between patient and carer on questionnaire for memory and ADL	MMSE COR Neuropsychology tests: 19, 36, 37, 39, 43, 57–59	Poor insight associated with poor performance on executive and visuo-spatial tests	No association between insight and depression	AD had less insight into memory and ADL than elderly controls
Ott et al. (1996b)	AD: 40	1. Reason for clinic visit	Clinician rated as above (Ott &	MMSE IADL, PSMS,	Poor insight correlated with	Poor insight correlated with	Patients with poor insight had

Table 5.1 (cont.)

Study	Patients	'Object' of insight	Insight assessment	Outcome variables	Main results Dementia	Ψ/behavioural	Other
		2. Memory problems 3. ADL 4. Progress of deficits	Fogel, 1982)	DBDS SPECT	worse ADL Small correlation between poor insight and severity	more apathy	lower perfusion in right temporo-occipital cortex
Starkstein et al. (1996)	AD: 170	1. Cognitive deficits 2. Personality and interests	Discrepancy between patient and carer on questionnaire (AQ-D)	MMSE, HDRS, HAS, AS, IS, BMS, PLACS, DPS, FIM Ψ interview Neuropsychology tests: 19, 32, 37, 38, 51, 53, 54, 60	Poor cognitive (but not behavioural) insight correlated with more severe deficit on NP tests	Poor insight (cog) correlated with more delusions, apathy and less depression. Poor insight (beh) correlated with mania and pathological laughing	Factor analysis yielded two factors: cognitive insight and behavioural insight
Seltzer et al. (1997)	AD: 40	Memory, self-care and social function	Discrepancy between patient and carer on questionnaire (EMQ, PCRS)	MMSE, CDRS BIZ	Poor insight in social and self-care (not memory) function associated with more severe dementia	–	Greater carer burden associated with poorer insight (into memory – not into self-care)
Starkstein et al. (1997a) Follow-up study	AD: 62 Follow-up study	1. cognitive deficits 2. personality and interests	Discrepancy between patient and carer on questionnaire (AQ-D)	MMSE, HDRS, Ψ interview DSM-III-R (SCID), HAS FIM, DPS,	Insight gets worse with progression of dementia	Insight associated with dysthymia but not with major depression (poor insight with	–

Study	Sample	Deficits assessed	Method	Measures	Findings		
Starkstein et al. (1997b)	AD: 55	1. Cognitive deficits 2. Personality and interests	Discrepancy between patient and carer on questionnaire (AQ-D)	MMSE Ψ interview Neuropsychology tests: 4, 19, 36–38, 43, 52–55, 61	Poor insight associated only with poor set shifting and procedural learning	–	–
Vasterling et al. (1997)	AD: 28 Follow-up study	Memory, general health, self-care, mood	Discrepancy between patient and carer on questionnaire (EMQ, GQ)	MMSE	Insight decrease not correlate with progress of dementia	–	Insight falls in relation to all 'objects' over time, no difference in size
Wagner et al. (1997)	AD: 73 VD: 23 Elderly Ψ controls: 17 Elderly controls: 19	Cognitive deficits	Discrepancy between patient rating of function and performance on cognitive tests	MMSE	AD had poorer insight than VD and others independent of severity	–	–
Cotrell and Wild (1999)	AD: 35	1. Remote memory 2. Recent memory 3. Attention 4. Daily activities	Discrepancy between patient and carer on questionnaire (Green et al, 1993, above)	MMSE, CDRS ADL, IADL 15-item questionnaire on driving	Poor insight correlated with more severe (MMSE) dementia	–	Only poor insight into attention predicted patients who no longer drove
Derouesné et al. (1999)	AD: 88 After follow-up of 21 months: 52	Cognitive deficits	1. Discrepancy between patient and carer on questionnaire	MMSE, ADL ZD, ZA, PBQ Neuropsychology tests: 22, 31, 54,	Poor insight correlated with worse MMSE at first visit but	Poor insight correlated mainly with more apathy	Poor insight correlated with lower perfusion in frontal

Table 5.1 (*cont.*)

Study	Patients	'Object' of insight	Insight assessment	Outcome variables	Main results		
					Dementia	Ψ/behavioural	Other
			2. Clinician rated 3. Carers' ratings	60, 66 Frontal behaviours SPECT	not at follow-up. Correlation with ADL at both visits. No correlation with tests	and with less anxiety. No correlation with depression.	cerebral regions
Sevush (1999)	AD: 203 Controls: 40 After follow-up of 15 months: AD: 106	Memory problems	Patient-rated questionnaire (AMIS) Also ratings by clinician and discrepancy measures used to compare	MMSE ACAD	A small correlation between poor insight and severity at first visit but no correlation with progress of disease	–	Greater correlation between poor insight and severity when using clinician or discrepancy measures
Zanetti et al. (1999)	AD: 37 VD: 32	Memory problems and objects from Ott and Fogel (1982, above)	1. Clinician-rated interview (Verhey et al.,1993, above) 2. Clinician-rated questions (Ott & Fogel, 1982, above)	MMSE, CDRS, ADL, IADL GerDS, NPI Neuropsychology tests (n = 36): 5, 9, 19, 22, 32, 36, 54, 67	Poor insight correlated with more severe dementia and cognitive impairment but complex (see text)	No correlation between insight and depression	No difference in insight between AD and VD
Harwood et al. (2000)	AD: 91	Cognitive and functional deficits	Clinician rated: Item 12 (inaccurate insight item) from NRS	MMSE, NRS BDRS-short	Poor insight associated with more severe dementia	Poor insight associated with less depression but more agitation No correlation with psychosis	–

Study	Sample	Deficits	Insight measure	Tests	Severity / frontal findings	Depression	Other findings
Smith C.A. et al. (2000)	AD: 23 Controls: 30	Cognitive, motor and affective problems	Discrepancy between patient and carer on questionnaire	MMSE, GerDS Neuropsychology tests: 8, 19, 37, 38, 43, 57, 68, 69	No correlation between insight and severity, except after controlling for depression (see text)	Poor insight associated with less depression	After controlling for depression, poor insight correlated with severity and with poor frontal tests performance
Gil et al. (2001)	AD: 45	Identity, cognition, affect, body, prospective memory, introspection, moral judgements	Clinician-rated questionnaire answered by patients (SCQ)	MMSE Neuropsychology tests: 70	Poor insight correlated with more severe dementia No correlation with frontal tests	–	Different 'objects' of insight affected to different extents Body and identity least affected
Koltai et al. (2001)	D: 22 Randomised controlled trial with Memory and Coping Programme (MCP)	Cognitive deficits	Clinician rated: two categories (with and without insight)	MMSE, GerDS, GerDS-rel., EMQ, EMQ-rel. Neuropsychology tests: 36, 57, 58	Patients with insight made greater gains in memory with MCP than those without	–	Relatives perceived greater gains with MCP independent of insight
Duke et al. (2002)	AD: 24	Cognitive deficits	Discrepancy between: 1. Patient and carer on (PCRS) questionnaire	MMSE, DRS Neuropsychology tests: 71	Poor insight correlated with more severe dementia	–	Patients and carers both overestimated performance of fictional patient

Table 5.1 (*cont.*)

Study	Patients	'Object' of insight	Insight assessment	Outcome variables	Main results Dementia	Ψ/behavioural	Other
			2. Patient rating, and prediction and postdiction on cognitive tests: of self, other and fictional patient				on video. Poor correlation between the insight measures
Giovannetti et al. (2002)	AD: 9 VD: 18 PaD: 10 MD: 17 Controls: 10	Cognitive deficits, ADL and naturalistic action errors	1. MLAT-S clinician rating of errors in tasks 2. Discrepancy between patient and carer on questionnaires (AQ-Dm, IADL)	MMSE, GerDS Neuropsychology tests: 22, 35, 36, 39, 60, 72–74	No correlation between insight and severity, number of errors or test scores	No correlation between insight and depression	Insight varied across error types. No difference in insight across diagnostic groups
Harwood and Sultzer (2002)	AD: 91	Cognitive and functional deficits	Clinician rated: Item 12 from NRS (inaccurate insight item)	MMSE HDRS NRS	–	Association between poor insight and less hopelessness	–
Robert et al. (2002)	AD: 60 MCI: 24 PaD: 12 Controls: 19	Apathy (components: emotional, initiative, interests)	Discrepancy between patient and carer on questionnaire (IA)	MMSE NPI IA	–	AD had less insight into emotional blunting and lack of initiative than MCI, PaD	–
Rymer et al. (2002)	AD: 41	Memory and functional	Discrepancy between patient	MMSE, CDRS FrSBe	Poor insight correlated with	–	Both poor insight and disinhibition

Study	Patients	Symptoms assessed	Measures	Instrument	Results		
		deficits	and carer on questionnaire (Green et al., 1993, above)	ADL BIZ	more severe dementia		contributed to carer burden, but disinhibition contributed more
Howorth and Saper (2003)	AD: 18 VD: 8 LBD: 2 MD: 4	Cognitive deficits, ADL, general: sense of self, behaviours	1. Clinician rated (Verhey et al., 1993, above) 2. Discrepancy between patient and carer on IADL and PSMS 3. Discrepancy in patient rating and prediction on memory tests 4. Interview with patient and carer	BDRS	No correlation between insight and severity of dementia. Only insight assessed by prediction correlated with cognitive test performance	–	Poor correlation between measures of insight (see text)
Vogel et al. (2005)	AD: 36 MCI: 30 Controls: 33	Memory problems	1. Discrepancy between patient and carer on questionnaire (Michon et al. 1994) 2. Clinician-rated categorical 4-point scale (Reed et al., 1993)	MMSE, CDRS, FBI, Neuropsychology tests: 22, 32, 36, 43, 55, 75–78, SPECT	Correlation between insight and dementia severity (MMSE). No correlation between insight and executive function	Performance on FBI (behavioural changes associated with lesions in prefrontal cortex) correlated with insight but only on discrepancy measure	No difference in insight between AD and MCI. Poor insight, but only on discrepancy measure correlated with reduced rCBF in right inferior frontal gyrus

Abbreviations:

Patients: AAMI: Age-Associated Memory Impairment; AD: Alzheimer's disease; Dep.: Depressive Disorder; HD: Huntington's Disease; HT: Head Trauma; CVA: cerebral infarction subjects; D: Dementia (aetiology not specified); LBD: Lewy Body Dementia; MCI: Mild Cognitive Impairment; MD: Dementias of

Notes to Table 5.1 (cont.)

Multiple aetiologies; MID: Multi-Infarct Dementia; MII: Memory-Impaired Individuals (not meeting criteria for AD); PaD: Parkinson's Disease; VD: Vascular Dementia.

Scales/Measures: ACAD: Assessment of Cognitive Abilities in Dementia; AMIS: Awareness of Memory Impairment Scale; AQ-D: Anosognosia Questionnaire-Dementia; AS: Apathy Scale; BDRS: Blessed Dementia Rating Scale; BIZ: Burden Interview (of Zarit *et al.*); BMIC: Memory–Information–Concentration component of the BDRS; BMS: Bech Mania Scale; BPEA: Performance of Everyday Activities component of the BDRS; BPRS: Behavioural Pathology Rating Scale; CDRS: Clinical Dementia Rating Scale; COR: Cornell Scale for Depression; DBDS: Dementia Behaviour Disturbance Scale; DPS: Dementia Psychosis Scale; DRS: Dementia Rating Scale; EMQ: Everyday Memory Questionnaire; FBI: Frontal Behavioural Inventory; FIM: Functional Independence Measure; FrSBe: Frontal Systems Behaviour Scale; GDS: Global Deterioration Scale; GerDS (-rel): Geriatric Depression Scale (-relatives version); GQ: General Questionnaire; HAS: Hamilton Anxiety Scale; HDRS: Hamilton Depression Rating Scale; IADL: Instrumental Activities of Daily Living Scale; IS: Irritability Scale; MADRS: Montgomery and Asberg Depression Rating Scale; MLAT-S: Multi-Level Action Test – Short form; MMSE: Mini-Mental State Examination; NPI: Neuropsychiatry Inventory Scale; NRS: Neurobehavioural Rating Scale; OAS: Overt Aggression Scale; PBQ: Psychobehavioural Questionnaire; PCRS: Patient Competency Rating Scale; PLACS: Pathological Laughing And Crying Scale; PSMS: Physical Self Maintenance Scale; RBMT: Rivermead Behavioural Memory Test; SCQ: Self-Consciousness Questionnaire; STC: Social Ties Checklist; ZA: Zung Anxiety Scale; ZD: Zung Depression Scale.

Neuropsychology tests: 1: Benton Orientation Questionnaire; 2: Wechsler Adult Intelligence Scale – Revised; 3: Rey Auditory–Verbal Learning Test; 4: Benton Visual Retention Test; 5: Rey–Osterrieth Complex Figure Recall Test; 6: Multilingual Aphasia Examination; 7: Test of Facial Recognition; 8: Judgement of Line Orientation; 9: Logical Memory from Wechsler Memory Scale (WMS); 10: Paired Associates from Wechsler Memory Scale; 11: Word Recall – immediate; 12. Word Recall – delayed; 13: Word Recognition – immediate; 14: Word Recognition – delayed; 15: Picture Recall – immediate; 16: Picture Recall – delayed; 17: Picture Recognition – immediate; 18: Picture Recognition – delayed; 19: Digit Span; 20: Verbal Span; 21: Spatial Span; 22: Verbal Fluency; 23: Continuous Performance Test; 24: Alternating Sequence Test; 25: Go–No-Go Paradigm; 26: Alzheimer's Disease Assessment Scale – ideomotor, ideational and constructional praxis tests; 27: Visual Reproduction; 28: Right–Left Differentiation Test; 29: Spatial Relationships Test; 30: Word List Generation; 31: WMS; 32: Wisconsin Card Sorting Test; 33: Graphic Series; 34: Frontal Behaviours; 35: California Verbal Learning Test; 36: Boston Naming Test; 37: Controlled Oral Word Association Test; 38: Block Design; 39: Clock Drawing; 40: Visual Form Discrimination and Face Recognition; 41: Simple Drawings; 42: 3-D Block Design; 43: Trail Making Tests (A and/or B); 44: Simple Reaction Time; 45: Letter Cancellation; 46: Face–Hand Test; 47: Short Story Recall; 48: Modified Card Sorting Test; 49: Sequencing Test; 50: Cognitive Estimates Test; 51: Buschke Selective Reminding Test; 52: Apraxia Subtest of Western Aphasia Battery; 53: Token Test; 54: Raven's Progressive Matrices; 55: Buschke Cued Recall Procedure; 56: Finger Tapping Test; 57: CERAD Word List Learning Test; 58: CERAD Constructional Praxis; 59: Mazes; 60: Similarities; 61: Maze Test; 62: CERAD Word List Recognition; 63: CERAD Verbal Fluency Test; 64: Vocabulary; 65: Information and Orientation from WMS; 66: Boston Diagnostic Aphasia Examination; 67: Corsi's Block Tapping Test; 68: Orientation–Memory Concentration; 69: Visual Span; 70: Frontal Assessment Short Test; 71: Hopkins Verbal Learning Test; 72: Boston Revision of WMS; 73: Goldberg Graphical Sequences Test; 74: Semantic Probe Test; 75: Danish Mental Status Test; 76: Danish Adult Reading Test; 77: Stroop Test; 78: Design Fluency.

Howorth & Saper, 2003). One study found a significant correlation between poor insight and severity of dementia only after controlling for depression (Smith C.A. *et al.*, 2000).

Given the vast amount of research carried out in this area (see Table 5.1), it is worthwhile considering some of the factors that are likely to be contributing to the continued lack of consistency in results. Most obvious of course is the employment of different insight measures in the studies. As detailed above and indicated in Table 5.1, such differences relate to how insight is assessed, who does the rating, how the rating is expressed (dichotomies or categories or continuous ratings), the level of structure and detail applied to the assessment as well as differences in the 'object' of insight, i.e., the aspect of the patient's illness addressed by the insight measure. Clearly, the range and types of differences that are involved would suggest that measures elicit somewhat different aspects of insight and that this may make a difference to the results of correlational studies. It is interesting that when studies employ a combination of different measures of insight, results vary according to the measure of insight used. For example, Sevush (1999) found only a small association between poor insight and more severe dementia when using a patient-rated questionnaire but the same study found a stronger correlation when using a patient-carer discrepancy questionnaire or when using a clinician-rated measure. Similarly (but with contrasting results), Howorth and Saper (2003) found no correlation between insight and severity of dementia when using a clinician-rated measure and a patient-carer discrepancy questionnaire. However, they found a correlation between insight and severity when using a discrepancy method based on the patient's prediction of cognitive test results.

When studies distinguish between various 'objects' of insight in their analyses, then different correlations have obtained again. For example, Starkstein *et al.* (1996) found that only poor insight into cognitive problems correlated with more severe dementia, whereas there was no such association between insight into personality changes/interests and severity of dementia. Interestingly, the opposite result was reported by Seltzer *et al.* (1997). They found that whereas there was no correlation between insight into memory problems and severity of dementia, there was a significant correlation between poor insight into social function, self-care and dementia severity. It seems therefore that many aspects around the insight measures are likely to be important contributors to the type of insight elicited and hence determine the correlations obtained.

Apart from different insight assessment measures used in the various studies, there are other likely factors contributing to the variability in results. Of particular note is the complicated issue concerning the assessment of the severity and/or stage of dementia. One of the most frequent measures used by studies to assess the severity of dementia is the Mini-Mental State Examination (MMSE) (Folstein *et al.*, 1975). Whilst clearly this is a useful screening measure of global cognitive function with high inter-rater reliability (Hodges, 1994), as a measure of dementia severity, there are two main factors that need to be considered. Firstly, it focuses solely on severity of cognitive dysfunction and consequently patients can have similar MMSE scores but, nevertheless, very different behavioural and functional problems. In other words, the severity of the disease may, arguably, relate not only to severity of cognitive problems but also to problems posed by behavioural and psychiatric disturbances. Secondly, because it is designed as a screening measure and one that can be carried out relatively quickly, the MMSE does not assess focal cognitive deficits. Consequently total scores may encompass a wide range of severity of actual cognitive impairments. Some studies have used other or additional measures of severity such as the Global Deterioration Scale (Reisberg et al., 1982) which attempts to stage the dementia on the basis of behavioural and functional changes as well as cognitive complaints. Thus severity or stage of dementia is measured according to assessed behavioural problems. But, cognitive function is measured on the basis of patient complaints and on difficulties in performing everyday tasks rather than on a formal cognitive assessment. Other measures of severity of dementia have included more detailed cognitive measures which capture focal as well as global deficits and other behavioural assessments (e.g. Neurobehavioural Rating Scale). The point, however, is that all these measures of severity pick out different aspects of problems in dementia with emphasis placed on different disease profiles. Consequently, patients with a range of 'severity' may in fact be represented in one category or by one (or a range) score. Such difficulties in assessing severity of dementia are also likely to be contributing to the variability of results found when correlating insight with severity of illness.

A few studies have attempted to examine what happens to patients' insight with progression of their disease. Results of these studies, too, are variable. Thus, while there is general agreement that patients' insight seems to get worse over time, there is less agreement concerning the interpretation of this in relation to progression of the dementia process. Some studies claim that patients' insight becomes worse with disease progression (Reisberg et al., 1985; McDaniel et al., 1995; Starkstein et al., 1997) in that insight deteriorates with cognitive deterioration over time (i.e. insight correlates with severity at both baseline assessment and follow-up review). Other studies, however, argue that whilst insight tends to fall over time, there is no specific relationship between patients' insight and the progression of their dementia as assessed by cognitive deterioration (Vasterling et al., 1997; Sevush, 1999). For example, Vasterling et al. (1997), found that although longitudinal progression of unawareness of deficits took place (over 16 months), this was not related to the degree of change in MMSE scores over time. Furthermore, the initial differences in the size of patients' awareness in relation to different aspects of the dementia process were not sustained over time as awareness seemed to deteriorate regardless of the disease domain. Other studies report mixed results suggesting that patients show partial preservation of insight over time (Kiyak *et al.*, 1994; Derouesné *et al.*, 1999). For example, in the study by Derouesné *et al.* (1999), a correlation was found between poor insight and more severe dementia as assessed by MMSE at baseline but not at the follow-up assessment 21 months later. On the other hand, patients did show a correlation between worse insight and more severe dementia at both time points when severity was assessed by ADL rather than cognitive deterioration. Several studies report that some patients seem to maintain their level of insight over time (Kiyak, *et al.*, 1994; Weinstein *et al.*, 1994) or even show increased insight over time (McDaniel *et al.*, 1995). Clearly the mixed results and the too few longitudinal studies make it difficult to conclude much about the relationship between patients' insight and disease progression. The same problems concerning different measures of insight in various studies apply also to interpretation of results. Likewise, the practical difficulties of measuring severity/stage of dementia and its longitudinal changes in a sensitive way are the significant problems in research of this kind (Vasterling *et al.*, 1997).

5.2.4 Insight in relation to specific brain dysfunction

In an attempt to explore possible neurobiological mechanisms underlying the impairment of insight in patients with dementia, studies have followed neurological research (Chapter 4) and tried to examine the relationship between poor insight and specific brain dysfunction, focusing particularly on possible frontal lobe pathology. Most work in this area has sought to correlate patients' insight with their performance on neuropsychological tests though a few studies have also examined patients' insight in relation to neuroimaging studies of brain function. In line with the research on anosognosia and frontal lobe pathology, some studies specifically examined the relationship between patients' insight and performance on tests of frontal or executive function. Table 5.1 shows that here again studies show some variability in results. Several studies found that poor insight was correlated with significant impairment on 'frontal' tests, such as the Wisconsin Card Sorting Test (see Table 5.1), (Mangone *et al.*, 1991; Michon *et al.*, 1992; 1994; Lopez *et al.*, 1994; Ott *et al.*, 1996a; Starkstein *et al.*, 1997b). Loss of insight in patients with dementia was thus proposed as being intrinsic to the pathological process underlying dementia when this affected frontal lobe function. The study by Weinstein *et al.* (1994) whilst not examining the relationship between patients' awareness and their performance on frontal tests, nevertheless, suggested that patients with poor awareness presented with more behavioural disturbances suggestive of frontal and paralimbic involvement rather than with impairments in reading, writing, calculation and visuospatial orientation indicative of posterior brain involvement. The study by Smith C.A. *et al.* (2000) found a correlation between poor insight and frontal tests only after patients were controlled for depression.

However, a number of other studies exploring the relationship between patients' insight and performance on neuropsychological tests, including 'frontal' tests, have failed to find such a correlation (Reed *et al.*, 1993; Dalla Barba, 1995; Migliorelli *et al.*, 1995; Starkstein *et al.*, 1995a; Derouesné *et al.*, 1999; Gil *et al.*, 2001; Giovannetti *et al.*, 2002; Vogel *et al.*, 2005). A couple of studies have suggested that poor insight in patients with dementia correlated with impairment of visuoconstructional skills (Auchus *et al.*, 1994; Ott *et al.*, 1996a) thus implicating a role for right hemisphere dysfunction as an underlying mechanism for unawareness. Some support for this has been proposed by the few neuroimaging studies showing decreased perfusion in the right hemisphere on single-photon emission computed tomography (SPECT) in patients with poor insight (Reed *et al.*, 1993; Starkstein *et al.*, 1995a; Ott *et al.*, 1996b). At the same time, these studies did not show any correlation between patients' insight and their performance on the appropriate neuropsychological tests. Likewise, Derouesné *et al.* (1999), using SPECT, found reduced perfusion in the frontal cerebral regions in their patients with poor insight but no such correlation between patients' insight and frontal neuropsychological tests. Similarly, Vogel *et al.* (2005) reported reduced perfusion in the right inferior frontal gyrus in patients with poor insight but no such correlation is found between patients' insight and frontal neuropsychological tests. Interestingly, they found this correlation only held when insight was assessed using a discrepancy measure rather than a clinician-rated categorical measure. Other studies have simply reported a non-specific association between poor insight and performance on a battery of neuropsychological tests (e.g. McGlynn & Kaszniak, 1991a, b; Correa *et al.*, 1996; Deckel & Morrison, 1996). The study by Starkstein *et al.* (1996) specified that only patients' insight into their cognitive problems correlated with impaired performance on neuropsychological tests whereas their insight into their behavioural and personality changes showed no such correlation.

As summarised in Table 5.1, the variations in methodologies, including differences in insight assessment, types and numbers of patients involved, and the range of outcome measures employed, all are likely to contribute to this mixed and inconsistent picture concerning the relationship between patients' insight and any possible brain dysfunction.

5.2.5 Insight in relation to psychiatric/behavioural syndromes

Much work has focused on examining the relationship between patients' insight and depression. The basis for this exploration relates to the question of whether impaired insight seen in patients, rather than being a manifestation of an intrinsic disease process reflecting damage to specific neuronal systems, is perhaps better understood as a psychological defence against the knowledge of having such a progressive destructive disease and its consequences. Thus, it could be hypothesised that patients with greater insight into their condition would show more depressive symptomatology whereas patients without insight would show little in the way of affective change. Studies exploring the relationship between patients' insight into their dementia and levels of depression once again yield variable results (see Table 5.1). Many of the studies find no association between patients' insight and depression (De Bettignies *et al.*, 1990; Reed *et al.*, 1993; Verhey *et al.*, 1993; Lopez *et al.*, 1994; Michon *et al.*, 1994; Cummings *et al.*, 1995; Starkstein *et al.*, 1995a; Ott *et al.*, 1996a; Derouesné *et al.*, 1999; Zanetti *et al.*, 1999; Giovannetti *et al.*, 2002). However, in contrast, several studies do report a significant correlation between patients' insight and depression, with greater insight being associated with more depression (Sevush & Leve, 1993; Feher *et al.*, 1994; Seltzer *et al.*, 1995a,b; Harwood *et al.*, 2000; Smith C.A. *et al.*, 2000). In addition, other studies present mixed results reporting either weak correlations between insight and depression (Feher *et al.*, 1991) or correlations that are specific in particular ways. Thus, the study by Starkstein *et al.* (1996) only found correlations between insight into cognitive problems and depression, whereas no such correlation was obtained between insight into behavioural and personality changes, and depression. Other studies have specified the type of depressive symptomatology correlating with insight. Migliorelli *et al.* (1995) and Starkstein *et al.* (1997a) did not find a correlation between patients' insight and the presence of major depression (DSM-III-R) but they did obtain a correlation between patients' insight and the presence of dysthymia. Similarly, Seltzer *et al.* (1995a) reported a correlation between patients' insight and depressed mood but not with a depressive disorder.

Exploring the relationship between patients' insight into dementia and depression is, however, complicated by additional problems which make interpretation of results particularly difficult and which are also likely to contribute to the variable outcomes outlined above (Table 5.1). Firstly, the question of the nature of depression in patients with dementia needs to be considered. The hypothesis that greater insight is associated with more depression in patients with dementia is based on the assumption (amongst others) that the depression in these patients is 'reactive' in nature, i.e. a consequence of the experienced disabilities resulting from having dementia. Thus, empirical findings of an association between levels of insight and depression could be interpreted as supporting the notion that impairment of insight was the result of psychological denial on the part of the patient. It might be argued that patients, unable to face the knowledge of having such a terrible condition, could deny (by means of various psychological processes) this knowledge. In turn, this lack of knowledge would prevent patients from experiencing the distress (and hence depression) that this knowledge would entail. The problem is, however, that there is little evidence to suggest that depression in patients with dementia is solely a reactive process. Most research indicates that depression, either as a disorder or as a constellation of symptoms, represents a range of heterogeneous conditions in relation to dementia and indeed to other neurological states, such as cerebro-vascular disease, head injuries, multiple sclerosis, etc. (Lishman, 1998). Depressive syndromes in the context of dementia may therefore represent not only individual reactions to having the disease but might be 'organic' manifestations of the disease process or lesion. They can also be coincidental (genetic or other vulnerability) manifestations or indeed can be behavioural phenocopies of multiple origins (Berrios & Marková, 2001). Thus, in the latter case, symptoms and signs whilst resembling depression may manifest as a result of the dementia disease process but without actually representing a depressive illness or syndrome. Furthermore, somatic symptoms such as anorexia, fatigue, weight loss, insomnia, etc. have been regarded as symptomatic of the dementia process rather than necessarily reflecting a depressive disorder (Troisi et al., 1996). At present, however, it remains difficult to discriminate between such syndromes on clinical or phenomenological grounds but, nevertheless, empirical findings of association or lack of association, between depression and patients' insight, must be interpreted in this context.

Secondly, measures used to rate depression in dementia are also likely to con-tribute to the variability of results. The issues here fall into several areas. Firstly, there is the question of the validity of using depression scales in patients with cog-nitive impairment given that cognitive dysfunction may affect the reporting as well as the manifestation of depressive symptomatology (Feher et al., 1992). Secondly, there is the issue concerning the choice of rating scales and, particularly, the deci-sion around whether clinician-rated scales or self-rated scales are used. Several studies have suggested that discrepancies in diagnosing depression arise when self-rating scales of depression are compared with clinician or carer ratings of patient depression. Most studies find that patients 'under-report' depressive symptoms (Mackenzie et al., 1989), but according to some studies patients report more depres-sive symptoms in comparison to clinician-rated diagnoses (Burns et al., 1990). Other studies suggest a more complicated relationship between clinician ratings and self-ratings depending on different patient groups (Sayer et al., 1993; Snow et al., 2005). This raises questions concerning the nature of the depression that is being elicited by the different instruments. Ott and Fogel (1992; Table 5.1), using both a clinician-rated instrument (COR) and a patient-rated instrument of depression (GerDS) found that as patients' dementia became more severe (in terms of cogni-tive dysfunction), then the clinician-based scale and self-rating scale showed more divergent results. The authors concluded that self-ratings tended to underestimate the presence and degree of depression in patients with dementia and that clinician-rated instruments of depression would have greater validity in this population. A similar result was obtained by Feher et al. (1992), who also compared results using a clinician-rated instrument (HDRS) and a self-rating measure (GerDS), finding that the latter was valid in mild to moderate dementia only. Nevertheless, like Burns *et al.* (1990), they found that patients with worse memory complained of more depressive symptoms. Most studies however report that patients complain less of depressive symptoms as their dementia progresses (Reifler *et al.*, 1982; Mackenzie *et al.*, 1989; Ballard *et al.*, 1991). Thirdly, there is also the issue concerning different contents included within various depression measures. Harwood *et al.* (2000), e.g., suggested that one of the reasons for inconsistent results was that the studies using measures which contained a significant focus on somatic or neurovegetative symptoms as inherent to depression (e.g. COR, HDRS, DSM-III-R diagnoses) reported negative findings, whereas studies using measures which included more subjective expressions of depression such as sad mood reported positive correlations between insight and depression. However, it is likely that there are additional factors involved for, as Table 5.1 shows, studies which have used measures including somatic items have also reported positive correlations (Feher *et al.*, 1994; Seltzer *et al.*, 1995b) and similarly, studies using more subjective measures have reported no correlations (Derouesné *et al.*, 1999; Zanetti *et al.*, 1999; Giovannetti *et al.*, 2002).

Given such variable results, as well as the complicated issues around the nature and assessment of depression in patients with dementia, some researchers suggest that, rather than searching for associations between patients' insight and a depressive *disorder*, it makes more sense to explore the relationship between patients' insight and depressive/anxious *symptoms* since these may be more representative of reactive states. As Table 5.1 shows, studies by Migliorelli *et al.* (1995) and Starkstein *et al.* (1997a) found that whilst patients' insight did not correlate with major depression, it did seem to correlate with dysthymia. Seltzer *et al.* (1995a,b) likewise found that whilst insight did not correlate with depressive disorder, it correlated with depressive mood. Several studies suggested that patients' insight was associated with more anxiety (Verhey *et al.*, 1993; Migliorelli *et al.*, 1995; Derouesné *et al.*, 1999) and one study found an association between patients' insight and feelings of hopelessness (Harwood & Sultzer, 2002). Other studies have found no correlation between patients' insight and anxiety (Seltzer *et al.*, 1995b). There are too few studies in this area, however, to draw firm conclusions.

Similarly, studies exploring other psychiatric and behavioural phenomena in relation to patients' insight in dementia have been few in number and again yield mixed results (Table 5.1). One of the more consistent results reported by a few studies is of a correlation between poor insight and greater apathy (Ott *et al.*, 1996b; Starkstein *et al.*, 1996; Derouesné *et al.*, 1999; Robert *et al.*, 2002). Nevertheless, in a study exploring the prevalence and clinical correlations of apathy and irritability in 101 patients with Alzheimer's disease, Starkstein *et al.* (1995b) found no correlation between apathy and insight. The association between insight and apathy has been based on the speculation that both poor insight and apathy may share a similar underlying pathophysiological mechanism involving either frontal or right hemispheric function. However, any conclusions concerning the relationship between insight and apathy would be premature particularly given the variable findings in relation to the correlations between patients' insight and measures of cognitive/brain function.

Likewise, attempting to link impairment of insight with brain mechanisms putatively underlying psychotic symptoms in dementia, some studies have explored the relationship between patients' insight into dementia and the presence of psychotic/behavioural symptoms (Table 5.1). These studies have also yielded mixed results with some researchers reporting an association between poor insight and the presence of psychotic symptoms (Mangone *et al.*, 1991; Weinstein *et al.*, 1994; Migliorelli *et al.*, 1995; Starkstein *et al.*, 1996; 1997a), and others finding no correlation between insight and psychotic phenomena (Lopez *et al.*, 1994; Harwood *et al.*, 2000). Starkstein *et al.* (1996) found that the correlations between insight and different psychotic symptoms varied according to the 'object' of insight assessed. Thus, poor insight into cognitive problems was associated with the presence of delusions whilst poor insight into behavioural/personality problems correlated rather with more mania and pathological laughter. Seltzer *et al.* (1995b) reported a correlation between carer-rated irritability in patients and worse insight, and similarly Starkstein *et al.* (1995b) found a correlation between patients with irritability and poor insight. Once again, the too few studies carried out in these areas preclude any definite conclusions. In addition, the variable methods used in assessing psychotic/other behavioural features and the different inclusions within these (e.g. delusions, misidentifications, mania, etc.) are also likely to contribute to the overall inconsistent results in this area.

5.2.6 Insight in relation to other variables

A few other associations have been sought by some studies exploring patients' insight into dementia. Of particular clinical importance has been the finding that impairment of patients' insight correlates with a greater perceived burden of care on the part of patients' carers (De Bettignies *et al.*, 1990; Seltzer *et al.*, 1997; Rymer *et al.*, 2002). Here again the results of these few studies are not straightforwardly endorsing poor insight as a contributor to carers' burden but they raise once more the likely complicated nature underlying the relationship concerned. For example, De Bettignies *et al.* (1990) reported on patients' poor insight into daily living skills as correlating with increased burden of care perceived by the patients' carers. This finding was not replicated by Seltzer *et al.* (1997) as they did not find a correlation between patients' insight into their self-care and carers' burden. On the other hand, they did obtain a correlation between patients' poor insight into their memory and greater carers' burden. Thus, it is not yet clear what aspect of insight may or may not be important in determining carers' perceptions of stress and burden. Rymer *et al.* (2002) found that whilst poor insight in patients (including insight into memory and functioning) correlated with more carer burden, disinhibited behaviour on the part of patients was a stronger contributor to such burden. Lastly, it should be mentioned that isolated case reports found an association between patients' insight and suicide risk (e.g. Rohde *et al.*, 1995; Ferris *et al.*, 1999), and one study reported that poor insight into attention was a predictor of patients who stopped driving (Cotrell & Wild, 1999). At this stage, such findings can only be considered as possible indicators for further work and exploration.

5.3 Impaired insight/awareness into function in dementia

For the sake of completion, a brief mention should be made concerning the notion of impaired insight or awareness into *function/knowledge* in patients with dementia. As already discussed in Chapter 4, the concept of implicit memory has been an area of research from the neuropsychology and cognitive psychology perspectives in healthy subjects and patients suffering from amnesic syndromes. To reiterate briefly, performance on cognitive tasks can be improved on the basis of specific experiences (e.g. priming or skill-learning tasks) of which individuals can remain unaware (Schacter, 1995). In other words, implicit memory focuses on the idea that learning specific tasks can be aided by mental processes of which the individual has no conscious awareness. Patients with dementia, like those with various amnesic syndromes, have been observed to show impaired explicit memory but, at the same time, to preserve their implicit memory (McGlynn & Schacter, 1989; Schacter, 1995). This demonstrates that dissociations can occur between possibly independent aspects of memory functioning. In other words, patients' performance on specific memory tests can be enhanced using priming without the patients being aware of, or showing insight into, the mechanisms by which they are able to recall set tasks. Similarly to patients with amnesic syndromes, researchers have reported that patients with Alzheimer's disease show dissociations between the various types of implicit memory that is preserved. Thus patients can exhibit different impairments in implicit memory which suggests that awareness at an *unconscious* level may be disrupted. For example, the commonest finding with respect to Alzheimer's disease has been that priming for word-stem completion tasks (lexical and pictorial priming) is impaired whilst priming for motor tasks is preserved (Shimamura *et al.*, 1987; Burke *et al.*, 1994; Russo & Spinnler, 1994; Schacter, 1995). The converse, i.e. deficits in procedural, motor-related tasks and sparing of verbal-related tasks, has been found in patients with Huntington's disease (Heindel *et al.*, 1989; Butters *et al.*, 1990). This difference in the specific type of preserved implicit memory observed between patients with Alzheimer's disease and those with Huntington's disease has been related to possible different psychologically and neurologically distinct implicit memory systems involved in the diseases. Thus, Butters *et al.* (1990) postulate that verbal and pictorial priming may be dependent on the integrity of neocortical association areas which are damaged in Alzheimer's disease. On the other hand, the motor skill learning is likely to be mediated by the corticostriatal system which in turn is damaged in basal ganglia diseases such as Huntington's disease. Similarly, Keane *et al.* (1991) reported further dissociation in priming deficits in their study of patients with Alzheimer's disease finding that verbal priming was impaired but perceptual priming was preserved. This they linked to possible neuronal mechanisms relating to dysfunction of the temporo-parietal lobe underlying the former and preservation of function in the occipital lobe relating to the latter, in keeping with the Alzheimer's disease process.

The question, however, of whether implicit memory not only represents a distinct memory system from an explicit memory system but is also itself constituted by a number of distinct implicit memory systems continues to be debated. Whilst the observations of dissociations between explicit and implicit memory and, particularly, the double dissociations observed in implicit memory is a powerful argument for the existence of multiple distinct memory systems (Heindel *et al.*, 1989; Schacter, 1995; 1999), the underlying assumptions behind the implicit/explicit memory research need to be understood (Chapter 4). At the same time, others have argued against a purely multiple memory systems view, proposing instead other possible explanations for the experimental dissociations in memory observed focusing more on the ways in which memory might be stored, retrieved and contextualised (see Bauer *et al.*, 1993).

Finally, the question still remains, as far as implicit memory or knowledge is concerned, where does awareness itself fit in the models proposed? Clearly, the distinction between explicit and implicit memory has been formulated as the absence of conscious awareness in the manifestation of the latter. This then raises further questions concerning the nature of awareness as a mental structure, the extent to which the different mental functions might be associated with different levels of awareness, the importance of awareness at different times, whether mental functions themselves are defined in some way by awareness, etc. As was emphasised in Chapter 4, the concept of implicit memory, or memory without awareness, has been defined and formulated in a neuropsychological and cognitive psychological framework in which mental functions are viewed in terms of independent/semi-independent albeit interacting modules. Within this structure, implicit memory is elicited on the basis of very specific cognitive tasks. The question, however, of how unconscious awareness or mental processing might relate to an overall structure or concept of insight remains to be explored.

5.4 Conclusion

Empirical studies on insight in dementia yield mixed and inconsistent results. As in other clinical areas this variability is in part the result of methodological differences between studies such as differences in patient groups, in measures used to assess insight, in evaluation of disease severity and in the assessments of other clinical variables. Measures developed to assess insight have been particularly numerous and diverse. These measures vary in a wide range of attributes, including content, perspective, level of detail, complexity, how they are scored, who does the ratings, etc. Consequently, they elicit phenomena or aspects of insight that are likely to be very different. It is interesting to note that where studies have employed various measures of insight concomitantly, different outcomes have been found in relation to the specific measures used, providing some empirical confirmation that different aspects of insight/awareness are elicited by the different measures (Green *et al.*, 1993; Derouesné *et al.*1999; Sevush, 1999; Duke *et al.*, 2002; Howorth & Saper, 2003; Vogel *et al.*, 2005).

In addition, however, factors specific to the study of dementia itself present further difficulties for the empirical exploration of insight. Firstly, dementia is an area of clinical and research interest for a number of professional disciplines, including, neurology, psychology, neuropsychology, psychiatry, medicine, etc. The study of insight in dementia is thus particularly influenced by differences in disciplinary approaches. Often, such differences relating to the specific conceptual framework of the discipline are not made explicit and this is likely to contribute to some of the confusion around the nature of the insight phenomenon under study.

Secondly, it is apparent from the reviewed studies that researchers refer to a multitude of related terms and concepts. Terms, such as unawareness, lack of insight, anosognosia, denial, etc. are used both in different ways and interchangeably. Concepts underlying these terms are correspondingly variable. The meaning of insight thus varies considerably in empirical studies and, again, such differences in meaning are generally not made explicit. Consequently, the phenomena of insight elicited on the basis of different concepts of insight will vary and likewise contribute to the mixed results of studies.

Thirdly, it is evident that there is a wide range of 'objects' of insight assessment used in studies exploring insight in patients with dementia. In other words, researchers are assessing insight in relation to various aspects of dementia. This carries significant implications for the meaning of insight in terms of the clinical phenomenon that is elicited in each case (Marková & Berrios, 2001). This is an important issue and is discussed in detail in Chapter 7. In brief, however, exploration of insight into '*dementia*' will elicit a different phenomenon of insight than exploration of insight into a '*specific cognitive impairment*'. This, in turn, elicits a different phenomenon from that elicited by the exploration of insight into '*ADL*' or '*depression*', and so on.

Part II

Conceptual

So far, the chapters in this book have explored how, in clinical psychiatry, the notion of insight has become conceptualised as an independent phenomenon, one that not only could be observed (to different extents) in patients with mental illness but one that could, moreover, be measured and related to other clinical and non-clinical variables. We have seen how, in Western cultures, this demarcation of insight as an independent variable became possible in the context of a number of factors including, a background of philosophical/psychological thought encouraging self-observation and self-understanding, changing ideas concerning the nature of mental illness itself, and, an environment that fostered close clinical observation. Then, reviewing the study of patients' insight in various clinical areas, we have seen that perspectives taken to understand and assess insight in clinical (and non-clinical) populations have been quite different. In part, this seems to have occurred as a result of diverse theoretical positions taken by the different professional disciplines. In addition, however, and closely interlinked with this is the fact that the different demands of the various clinical populations have determined to some extent the approaches taken. This issue will be discussed in more detail later. However, it is of interest to reiterate, that in general psychiatry it was the observation that patients with mental illness could have insight that led to further work exploring this phenomenon. In contrast, in patients with neurological/neuropsychological impairments, it was the converse observation that determined approaches exploring insight in this clinical group. In other words, the study of insight in patients in these areas was approached from opposite perspectives. In the former it was the surprising *presence* of understanding and in the latter it was the surprising *absence* of understanding that contributed to the different approaches taken in relation to these patients. Apart from the differences in approaches to the study of insight between the different clinical populations, we have also seen how within one clinical population differences are evident in the way insight is conceived and evaluated. And, common to all the clinical areas is the striking finding that studies exploring insight in these patient groups have yielded mixed and inconsistent results when attempting to relate levels of patients' insight with other clinical variables.

From the work examined thus far, a number of questions seem to emerge. The first question relates to the multiple approaches taken to the study of insight in patients. What does this mean in terms of understanding the concept or structure of insight? Can the different conceptions and measures of insight be related or unified in some way? Or is it simply the case that different phenomena are being invoked sharing only a superficial resemblance with each other? Secondly, how can the variable results of the studies on insight be explained? Why is it that despite extensive empirical work, it is still not possible to conclude much about the predictive validity of insight in relation to mental illness or its relationship to either the patients' illness or to individual/environmental factors? While some of the inconsistent results between studies exploring insight could be explained on methodological grounds, i.e. differences in study designs, different patient groups, different outcome measures, etc., I would argue that there has to be another important factor to consider here, borne out also by the other questions raised, and that has to do with the concept of insight itself. Throughout my arguments so far, I have emphasised the complexity of the concept, the difficulties in delineating its boundaries as well as its likely multidimensional structure.

Perhaps then, in order to start answering some of the questions raised so far, it is important to examine the concept of insight in detail, to look at its conceptualisation and to identify the crucial issues for clarification. This section of the book therefore focuses specifically on exploring the conceptual problems that arise in relation to the study of insight. Chapter 6 examines the concept of insight from the perspective of its likely nature. Specifically, it addresses the issues involved around the various meanings of insight and their determinants and discusses the implications these have for the empirical study of insight. Chapter 7 focuses on a crucial feature of insight, namely, its relational aspects. It explores the ways in which different 'objects' of insight influence the clinical phenomenon of insight that is elicited and examines the implications this carries for the structure of insight. Based on the issues identified in the preceding chapters, Chapters 8 and 9 go on to develop a model for a structure of insight. Firstly, Chapter 8 argues, on theoretical and empirical grounds, for a meaningful distinction to be made between *awareness* and *insight*. Then, Chapter 9, on the basis of this distinction, proposes a model of insight structure that accommodates the relational 'object' of insight assessment. Thus, a framework is presented which allows the identification and definition of specific insight phenomena for the purposes of future empirical work.

6

The conceptualisation of insight

In order to start unravelling some of the problems engendered by the mixtures of terms and conceptualisations of insight apparent in the literature, it would make sense to approach a concept of insight in terms of its possible structure and components. For this purpose it is useful at this point to first of all make an explicit distinction between (1) the *theoretical concept* of insight and (2) the *clinical phenomenon* of insight.

The former refers to insight as a whole, to a construct whose structure and components can be theoretically defined. As such, it can accommodate the range of meanings of insight that have so far been offered albeit within a complex, multidimensional structure whose boundaries are wide and blurred. The latter, on the other hand, refers to the clinical manifestation (or elicitation) of what necessarily can only be an *aspect* of the concept of insight. In other words, the concept of insight is wider than the phenomenon of insight but it provides the scaffolding against which specific phenomena of insight can be delineated and understood. Making this distinction is important for a number of reasons. Firstly, it helps to organise and clarify the various conceptual difficulties that are involved in the study of insight. Thus, it may help us to understand specifically where problems may lie and what type of problems we are dealing with. In turn, such understanding may help either by pointing towards appropriate ways of addressing the different problems or by providing a space in which the contribution of particular issues may be acknowledged. Consequently, this enables us to understand more clearly the limits to which problems can be resolved and the necessary underlying assumptions that may be involved. Secondly, whilst the distinction between insight as a concept and as a phenomenon is artificial since both the concept and phenomenon of insight are constructs and their relationship is not straightforward (see later), it allows us to translate in a more structured or systematic way from the concept to those aspects of insight that may be manifested or elicited empirically. In turn, this allows us to understand and devise measures of insight in terms of clearer ideas concerning which components of insight are explored, in what way they may be different from those assessed by other measures, and how individual components might relate to an overall structure of insight.

This chapter therefore shall first explore issues relating more specifically to the *concept* of insight, followed by those relating more specifically to the *phenomenon* of insight. As implied above, this distinction is made for ease of analysis and it should be understood that, in fact, in many respects the concept and phenomenon of insight are interdependent. Hence, much of what is said about the concept will apply to the phenomenon and vice versa. Throughout both sections, the chapter highlights the implications of the issues raised for both the structure of insight and for its empirical study.

6.1 The concept of insight: problem of meaning

The central question addressed in this section concerns the nature of the problems which contribute to the complexities surrounding the concept of insight. In other words, what is it about the concept of insight that gives rise to the difficulties we have seen in defining it in a consistent way? Evidently, the different approaches to the study of insight that have been reviewed share some things in common and, in various ways, refer to some understanding or knowledge the individual has concerning his/her condition. However, there are, as has also been clearly apparent, significant differences. Such differences seem to present at various levels and need to be examined in some detail in order to allow us to develop a putative structure for insight. The differences in meaning of insight can be usefully divided into two main types or groups, namely, (i) problems of content and (ii) problems concerning the nature of insight. Each of these will be explored in turn.

6.1.1 The meaning of insight: problems of content

We have seen how the content of the various definitions of insight offered in different clinical areas, as well as within a particular clinical area, varies in a number of ways including, specificity, breadth, complexity, type of judgements demanded, aspects of condition involved, and so on. One of the most obvious types of difference to emerge from the overall review, perhaps, lies in the breadth of definitions, i.e. the ways in which the meaning of insight ranges from a narrow content at one end to a broad or wide content at the other end.

In the narrow sense, insight refers to an awareness or recognition of a particular condition or its aspect. This narrowness relates to the issue that the content of insight is confined to a concept of knowledge in its most basic or unitary form, i.e. as a simple perception of something with no further elaboration concerning the nature or extent of this perception (Oxford English Dictionary, 2nd edition). It is in this sense that the notion of insight was originally understood in the early nineteenth century when it was first separated from the concept of madness and became, in its own right, a subject for observation. Insight was simply awareness of madness, a perception on the part of the patient that was given words in the acknowledgement 'I am mad' (e.g. Guislain, 1852). This narrow conception of insight changed, however, and broader views of insight are evident in the subsequent debates around the notion (e.g. Société Médico-Psychologique, 1870) and in much of the later work that focused specifically on this topic (e.g. Parant, 1888). Insight became more than a *perception* of a madness state but was conceived as a knowledge of a madness state, the knowledge that was understood in a wider sense than awareness or perception. Hence, patients could have some knowledge about different aspects of their illness and they could make judgements to varying extents about their condition and how it affected them. This wider conceptualisation of insight meant that it was possible to distinguish between various degrees of insight and patients, therefore, could be described as showing different amounts and types of knowledge in relation to their madness. In the context of increasing focus on quantitative research and the operationalisation of clinical variables, the empirical studies exploring insight in patients with mental disorders highlight very clearly a similar range of definitions of insight from the narrow to the wide (Chapter 3). Thus, the earlier studies view the patient's acknowledgement or recognition of being unwell as tantamount to having insight (e.g. Eskey, 1958; Van Putten *et al.*, 1976; Heinrichs *et al.*, 1985) paralleling the narrow conception of insight as awareness or perception of disturbance. At the same time, the meaning of insight in such studies, whilst narrow in the sense of the awareness or perception inherent in the definition, is broad in the sense of the lack of specificity relating to the mental disturbance itself (see Chapter 3). Most of the studies where insight is conceived in an all-or-none or categorical fashion imply a conception of insight as a basic awareness or perception of a mental disturbance. Many of the more recent studies, on the other hand, invoke a multidimensional conception of insight where clearly the meaning of insight is broadened to a wider understanding of the knowledge involved (e.g. Greenfeld *et al.*, 1989; Amador *et al.*, 1991; Marková & Berrios, 1992a). This knowledge is wider in that it includes not just the perception or awareness of some change in the patient but it also demands some judgements on his/her part concerning the nature and consequences of the experienced changes.

Perhaps some of the widest conceptions of insight have been offered in the psychoanalytic literature (Chapter 2). Here, insight has been conceived as a much 'deeper' knowledge of changes in the self – deeper, in several senses of the term. Firstly, the type or content of the knowledge itself is viewed as deeper, encompassing the understanding an individual has of his/her self in the context of life experiences and relationships together with the understanding of his/her motivations, the latter often couched in terms of unconscious mental processes. Secondly, the way in which such knowledge or insight is acknowledged is conceived as taking place at different levels of understanding. In other words, distinctions are made between the levels at which such knowledge is understood by an individual, e.g. cognitive, intellectual, emotional or dynamic level (Reid & Finesinger, 1952; Bibring, 1954; Richfield, 1954). Thirdly, possible reasons or motivations behind changes in insight are incorporated into the concept itself. Denial in this context is a psychological coping response designed to protect individuals from the consequences of having knowledge of their illness/ disabilities (Weinstein & Kahn, 1955). Thus, the concept of insight within this particular psychological framework is very much broader including knowledge not just of particular experiences but of the way in which the self relates to them, absorbs them and acts on them and understands underlying reasons and purposes.

In contrast, as has been emphasised in the work on insight in neurological states, insight in the narrowest sense of awareness or perception has been exemplified particularly by the original concept of anosognosia (Chapters 4 and 5). Perhaps it is because of its derivation from the opposite perspective, namely, as the study of the lack of insight or unawareness of a particular deficit/impairment (explored in detail in Chapter 7), that the meaning of insight in this context has persisted in the narrow, circumscribed sense of awareness, i.e. the perception (or lack of) that something is wrong. Even with some broadening of this concept engendered by the proliferation of empirical work, qualitative differences in awareness or knowledge have been limited to knowledge of different aspects of the impairment such as severity (Prigatano et al., 1986), change compared with previous ability (Sherer et al., 1998a) or prediction of ability (Schacter, 1991). In other words, the knowledge remains focused on different aspects of the actual impairment but does not refer (in a comparable way to the conceptions of insight in general psychiatry or psychodynamic psychology) to knowledge of what the impairment means for the self.

Captured within the range of breadths of meanings of insight are the other differences between contents of definitions that were noted above. For example, striking is the range of different types of judgements inherent to the various conceptualisations of insight, particularly as far as the more complex multidimensional definitions are concerned. Thus, in addition to an awareness of some change, concepts of insight include various judgements relating to the following:

1 an attribution of the change to pathology (e.g. Jaspers, 1948; David, 1990; Amador et al., 1991);
2 social consequences of illness (Amador et al., 1991);
3 views concerning aetiology and likely recurrence (Greenfeld et al., 1989);
4 perception of changes in the self and one's interaction with the world (Marková & Berrios, 1992a);
5 need for medical treatment (McEvoy et al., 1989a; David, 1990; Amador et al., 1991).
6 attitudes towards experiences (Soskis & Bowers, 1969; Cutting, 1978; Marks et al., 2000);
7 comparisons with previous function (Sherer et al., 1998);

8 predictions/postdictions of performance on specific tests (Schacter, 1991; Correa
   et al., 1996);
9 resemblance of own experiences to hypothetical cases (McEvoy et al., 1993b);
   and many more.

All of these judgements represent aspects of knowledge, elaborated from the
perception of change, about what might be happening to the individual. The issue
here, however, is that these judgements are *different* from one another and that the
resulting differences in content of the concept of insight in the various definitions
offered may be important in terms of the phenomenon of insight subsequently
elicited.

Having re-examined some of the main differences evident in the content of the
various conceptions of insight, the next question is: What does this mean? How can
knowledge of such differences help in the formulation of a coherent structure for
insight? Earlier, it was claimed that identifying specific problems at different levels
would help to clarify some of the complexities surrounding the concept of insight.
We have established that contents relating to the concept of insight vary considerably from narrow notions of knowledge or perception that something is wrong to
much broader knowledge incorporating a wide range of different sorts of judgements as to what might be wrong, what this means for the individual and how this
affects him/her. The crucial problem that clearly emerges raised by these issues,
however, is one that concerns conceptual boundaries or limits. In other words, it is
apparent that the concept of insight, as defined by awareness and knowledge, has
contents whose boundaries are difficult to define and fix. Knowledge in a general
sense, by definition, cannot be demarcated easily and here, knowledge in the specific
sense of understanding about a particular condition and how it affects an individual is further complicated by the problems pertaining to the condition itself (particularly as far as mental disorder is concerned and how it is understood generally)
as well as factors relating to knowledge of the self. This can be illustrated by taking
schizophrenia as an example. Thus, when examining what it means to have knowledge of schizophrenia, a multitude of questions arise, such as: To what extent might
a patient be expected to know about their mental disorder; even in fairly general
terms about its likely cause, course and prognosis (issues which may be difficult for
the clinicians themselves to answer)? What level of knowledge and information is
needed in order for an individual to be aware of having a mental disorder? Is it possible for a patient to have insight into having a mental disorder in a situation where
he/she does not actually have the relevant information concerning the mental disorder? What about awareness or knowledge concerning the individual components
or symptoms/signs that constitute the condition? Is it necessary for a patient to be
able to appraise accurately all his/her symptoms or is it enough to perhaps show

understanding of some? How many symptoms 'correctly' appraised would signify insight? (And who determines the constituting symptoms/signs of a particular mental disorder?) How 'correct' does the patient need to be in terms of judging the severity of the condition affecting him/her? What degree of certainty concerning his/her awareness or knowledge is necessary for an individual to have insight? To what extent should an individual be able to assess the consequences of having a particular condition or disability? Should this apply to all areas, or only some, of his/her life? How much change should an individual be able to judge and relate to his/ her self and functioning? How much knowledge should a person have of his/her self and in which contexts? Which implications of having a condition should be understood by the patient? Listing such questions may give the impression that more questions are raised than answered by examining the contents of meanings of insight. However, what these questions illustrate in common is the impossibility of drawing a line encompassing a finite content to the answers. The theoretical concept of insight *cannot* have a clearly demarcated border for the limits or extents of different aspects of awareness or knowledge relevant to the individual and his/her illness may simply not be possible to define.

6.1.2 The meaning of insight: problems concerning its nature

A fundamental question concerning the meaning of insight remains that surrounding its nature, i.e. irrespective of the contents of the concept, what sort of entity is it that is understood by the concept of insight? There are different, though interrelated, approaches to addressing this question. One way is to consider this question from a philosophical viewpoint and, specifically, examine the concept of insight from an ontological and epistemological perspective.

Thus, taking an ontological view of the concept of insight would be to conceive this as a 'real' entity, as something that has an existence which, given its definition in mental terms and captured as a mental phenomenon, would, by virtue of some form of brain–mind mapping, be underpinned by a physical reality. However, trying to then determine this existence in a meaningful way would entail exploration around the definition of such a physical reality – whether this can be understood in terms of brain circuits, receptors, molecules, etc., as well as attempting to address the old question concerning the nature of the relationship between mental and brain structures. Moreover, the question of the existence of insight as an independent entity, i.e. as an entity independent of a physical (brain) reality would also have to be raised. At this stage then, such an approach may not be particularly useful.

An epistemological perspective, on the other hand, would consider insight not so much in terms of its possible existence as some real entity but in terms of the legitimacy of the knowledge that is involved in its construction as a concept. In a second sense, an epistemological perspective will also consider insight in terms of what it can tell us about a particular aspect of the mind or the way in which individuals think and behave in regards to certain situations. In other words, taking an epistemological perspective would mean that the 'reality' of insight as a structure is defined not as an entity in itself but in terms of the validity of knowledge constituting it as well as through the way in which it helps to understand and organise mental phenomena. Whilst this book takes an epistemological perspective in general, this does not, at this point, help to clarify in a practical way the nature of the concept of insight.

A somewhat different though related approach, therefore, and one that I propose to take here, is to examine the nature of the concept of insight from the perspective of clinical meaningfulness. The above distinction between ontological and epistemological perspectives is mentioned mainly because these perspectives are in some ways reflected in the clinical approach. Specifically, I want to argue that the concept of insight refers to a *mental state* and not to a mental symptom. This is a significant claim because it carries important implications for understanding insight and for empirical research in this area. These implications will be discussed later. At this point, it is necessary to define the distinction between state and symptom.

By 'mental state' I am simply referring to a condition of the mind, or 'the mental or emotional condition in which a person finds himself at a particular time' (OED, 2nd edition). For example, a mental state may comprise of mixtures of emotions/feelings, thoughts, worries, daydreams, reflections, etc., any of which may assume prominence at a specific time. By 'symptom' I am referring to an indicator of disease, i.e. 'a phenomenon, circumstance, or change of condition arising from and accompanying a disease or affection, and *constituting* an indication or evidence of it; a characteristic sign of some particular disease' (OED, 2nd edition, my emphasis). For example, symptoms include a range of specific experiences which are perceived as being out of the ordinary, uncharacteristic or even unexplained, such as pain, low mood, fatigue, hallucination, etc. In other words, the main distinction between the concepts I want to emphasise, and without making any assumptions concerning ontology, lies in the crucial link with some form of pathology in the concept of symptom. To repeat then, I would argue that it makes more sense to conceive the nature of the concept of insight as a mental state and not as a symptom. Firstly, however, are there grounds to this argument, i.e. is it the case that insight, or rather lack of insight, is generally considered as a symptom, a phenomenon indicating disease, in the context of the empirical work that has been examined in this book?

6.1.2.1 Insight as a symptom?

It is of interest that, whilst a great deal of effort has focused on defining insight in terms of contents of meaning, on the development of new multidimensional models of insight and on the devising of instruments designed to capture those meanings empirically, there has been little work specifically exploring the possible *nature* of insight as a concept or phenomenon. In general psychiatry, there is some direct reference to the view that poor insight represents a symptom or feature of the mental disorder itself but otherwise most of the evidence substantiating this view is indirect. In terms of the direct evidence, the most obvious source, as has already been mentioned, has been the large study described in the *Report of the International Pilot Study of Schizophrenia* (World Health Organization, 1973), in which 'lack of insight' is reported as the most frequent *symptom* found in schizophrenia. This finding, contained in a table depicting relative frequencies of symptoms found in patients with schizophrenia has, since then, been reproduced not only in various textbooks of psychiatry (e.g. Gelder *et al.*, 1996) but also in numerous subsequent articles exploring insight in patients. Thus, much of the empirical work examining insight in general psychiatry has been based explicitly on this assumption that poor insight is a symptom (or sign) of schizophrenia (e.g. Carroll *et al.*, 1999; Weiler *et al.*, 2000; White *et al.*, 2000; Pyne *et al.*, 2001; and many more). In addition, some researchers have themselves been explicit in articulating this view, e.g. Cuesta and Peralta (1994) suggest that 'lack of insight could be a primary symptom resulting directly from the schizophrenic process' (p. 359) and reinforce this view in subsequent work (e.g. Peralta & Cuesta, 1994; Cuesta *et al.*, 1995). Similarly, Amador *et al.* (1994) reiterate that 'poor insight is best viewed as a symptom (or sign) comprising multiple components' (p. 827). Cuffel *et al.* (1996) consider poor insight to be an 'important manifestation' of schizophrenia, and, Kim *et al.* (1997) refer to lack of insight as 'an inherent trait of schizophrenia' (p. 117). Perhaps one of the most explicit expressions of the idea that poor insight is conceived as a symptom of the disorder is seen in the study by Mohamed *et al.* (1999) where they say, 'poor insight can be conceptualised as an expression of the disorder [schizophrenia], much as hallucinations or delusions' (p. 525). Similar assumptions concerning the notion that poor insight is a symptom of the disease can be found, to varying degrees of explicitness, in studies exploring insight in organic brain disorders (e.g. Green *et al.*, 1993; see Clare, 2004 for review) and other conditions (Chapters 3–5). There are some exceptions (and qualifiers, see below) to this general view concerning the nature of insight. One obvious exception is the perspective taken within psychoanalytic psychology where insight is viewed as a mental state, one which, moreover, explicitly colligates emotions and thinking into a whole specifically relevant to the person. However, in general as far as empirical studies of insight into general psychiatric disorders and organic brain syndromes are concerned, it becomes apparent that poor insight is 'treated' as a symptom of the patient's condition.

Moving on to some of the indirect evidence for this claim, this can be inferred from a number of points arising from both the theoretical and empirical work on insight reviewed in this book. First of all, as already mentioned, it is clear that there has been little specific focus on examining the *nature* of insight as a concept/ phenomenon. In whatever way defined, insight has been referred to in general terms as a concept, a phenomenon or a construct. However, these terms, whilst providing a particular frame for the contents of the definition, do not say anything about the nature of these contents in the sense of what sort of entity they might represent. Thus, apart from the claims explicitly viewing poor insight as a symptom as described above, little else has been said directly. In fact, it is fair to say that this issue has tended to be disguised somewhat by some confusion engendered through deployment of various allusions relating to this point. For example, the concept of insight is discussed in terms of *aetiology* or *mechanisms*, i.e. focusing on processes that might result in poor insight (e.g. Arduini *et al.*, 2003; Drake & Lewis, 2003; Rossell *et al.*, 2003) or *models/theories*, i.e. structures or frameworks that might help to explain poor insight (e.g. Birchwood *et al.*, 1994; Lysaker *et al.*, 2003; Thompson *et al.*, 2001) or *perspectives*, i.e. different ways of conceiving poor insight (David & Kemp, 1997). In terms of such mechanisms or models or perspectives described, the nature of the concept of insight is indirectly addressed. As we have seen in Chapter 3, in general psychiatric disorders these mechanisms/models tend to fall predominantly into three groups so that poor insight is explained in terms of: (i) organic/neurocognitive dysfunction (e.g. Lysaker *et al.*, 1998a; Young *et al.*, 1998; Larøi *et al.*, 2000) or (ii) psychological/motivational response to illness or (iii) symptomatic, i.e. intrinsically linked to a disease process and hence associated with psychopathology (e.g. Collins *et al.*, 1997; Smith *et al.*, 2000) and many researchers suggest that poor insight is a product of a combination of such mechanisms (e.g. Vaz *et al.*, 2002). In addition, some have suggested further possible models or perspectives, including personality factors and cultural or socially determined attitudes (e.g. Johnson & Orrell, 1995; David & Kemp, 1997; White *et al.*, 2000; Clare, 2004). In the main, however, the underlying explanations for poor insight have focused on the disease process itself either in terms of the psychopathology of the illness or in terms of neurocognitive dysfunction. As Amador *et al.* (1991) state clearly, 'some forms of unawareness may stem directly from the pathophysiology of the disorder' (p. 128) and this view has been the principle one on which the postulated mechanisms underlying poor insight are based. These suggested models/theories underlying poor insight assume the link between insight and disease and hence the nature of insight in these cases is construed as a symptom or indicator of the disease process. Clearly, there are some qualifications to this claim in that psychological defence mechanisms (or coping/motivational factors) have also been invoked as possibly underlying poor insight and this would then be counter to the notion that poor insight is a symptom of the condition and instead would be seen as a response to the condition. Similarly, the suggestion that social/cultural determinants may underlie the concept of insight would likewise go against the idea that poor insight is simply a symptom of the patient's condition. Furthermore, there has been the occasional suggestion that insight is viewed as an independent phenomenon from psychopathology or neurocognition (e.g. Jørgensen, 1995). Nevertheless, overwhelmingly, it is apparent that the research on insight in general psychiatry has, in terms of the underlying models proposed, considered poor insight in patients as a symptom or indicator of disease. Much the same has been evident in work on insight in organic brain syndromes where, as we have seen, the polarity between poor insight as intrinsic to the disease process itself and poor insight as a psychological response has been more explicitly discussed (see Chapters 4 and 5). Here again, however, the main assumption underlying the models proposed for unawareness of illness has been based on the view that poor insight results from impairment of neurological or neurocognitive processes, i.e. poor insight is a function of the disease process itself (Clare, 2004).

Apart from the types of models or theories proposed to underlie poor insight, further indirect evidence suggesting that the concept of insight is generally viewed and treated as a symptom comes from the general direction and methodology of research taken in this field. As has already been alluded to in the earlier chapters, much of the rationale behind studies examining the relationship between patients' insight and clinical variables, such as severity or stage of illness, is dependent on the view that poor insight is symptomatic of the condition (White et al., 2000). In addition, much of the more recent focus of research on insight is in determining brain structures underlying lack of insight by means of structural brain imaging (e.g. Flashman et al., 2000; 2001) or correlating lack of insight with specific cognitive dysfunction (e.g. Young et al., 1998; Drake & Lewis, 2003; Lysaker et al., 2003). Rationale for this is clearly based on the view that lack of insight might represent some sort of deficit or pathology and generally this has been linked to the illness affecting the individual. Likewise, focus on exploring associations between poor insight and specific neurocognitive dysfunction and neuroimaging in patients with dementia (e.g. Ott et al., 1996b; Derouesné et al., 1999) has been based on the view that poor insight is caused by the disease process itself. Finally, other indirect evidence indicating that poor insight is considered as a symptom of the patient's condition can be seen in the way it is frequently evaluated. We have seen in the studies reviewed that many different ways of assessing insight in patients have been developed. However, it is apparent that many of the studies employ rating scales in which poor insight is simply one of the 'symptoms' or variables assessed (e.g. Positive and Negative Syndrome Scale (PANSS), *Manual for the Assessment and Documentation of Psychopathology* (AMDP), Hamilton Depression Rating Scale (HDRS), etc.). There are two points to consider about this. Firstly, there is no distinction between the way in which the intensity or severity of poor insight is rated and the way in which the intensity or severity of the other symptoms are rated. Secondly, the overall severity of the condition is assessed by the total score on such instruments and consequently, it is clear that poor insight contributes to the severity of the condition in an analogous fashion to that of the other 'symptoms'. In other words, whatever the theoretical notion of insight might be, the issue is that in practical terms, the concept is handled as another symptom.

6.1.2.2 Insight as a mental state?

In light of the above, the question is, whether it makes sense to consider poor insight as a 'symptom' or neuropsychological deficit? Here I would argue for a number of reasons that, in fact, it makes little sense to construe insight as a symptom and that it may be more useful to view the concept of insight as referring simply to a mental state.

In the first place, it is difficult to reconcile the view of insight as a symptom with some of the conceptualisations of insight as a multidimensional construct. Part of the problem is that, in whatever way insight is framed, there has not yet been put forward a theory of how these variously postulated components might relate to each other. For example, David (1990), proposes a construct of insight that is based on three distinct but overlapping dimensions (awareness of illness, the capacity to re-label psychotic experiences as abnormal and treatment compliance). The question is, what does overlapping dimensions actually mean? How do these proposed components of insight overlap (i.e. in what form is this envisaged, is it that they are part of a single structure or are they different components which share some properties, etc.?) and to what extent? Similarly, the multidimensional models of insight put forward by others (e.g. Greenfeld et al., 1989; Amador et al., 1991) include a number of component dimensions but again it is not clear how these dimensions might relate to or interact with each other in a structural sense. In a telling statement, Vaz et al. (2002) define insight as a 'multidimensional phenomenon that includes elements of a psychological, psychopathological, neurocognitive, and interactional nature' (p. 311). Clearly, the complexity of different dimensions underlying insight is highlighted but the nature of the interaction, or overlapping, between the dimensions has not yet been addressed. Likewise, David and Kemp (1997) describe various distinct perspectives from which insight can be considered and which may reflect different underlying mechanisms. However, the way in which these perspectives may or may not relate to each other still needs to be examined. Undoubtedly, there are major difficulties in trying to do so. The problem relates directly to the complexities around the concept of insight itself and this has crucial implications for understanding insight and for its empirical study. In other words, there is simply no theory available to bring together the possible structural elements of insight and, consequently, while a conceptual definition of insight is possible, the *nature* of insight as a whole remains obscure. However, as is demonstrated by the range of perspectives from which insight can be explored (David & Kemp, 1997), by the different types of dimensions that may constitute insight (Greenfeld *et al.*, 1989; Amador *et al.*, 1991), and by the different forms of judgements that may be involved (Marková & Berrios, 1995a, b), it is difficult to conceive how all these elements together could be understood in the nature of a symptom. This is not to take away any inherent complexity from symptoms themselves but to argue that the different forms or perspectives in which the possible components of insight are conceived, i.e. their disparateness, suggest that, as a whole, they relate more to a mental state than to a symptom signifying a disease process or dysfunction.

It is possible of course that some specific aspect of the structure of insight may be more directly linked to a disease process, and, theoretically, this can be envisaged more clearly as regards the narrower concept of anosognosia or circumscribed unawareness of a specific deficit (see Chapter 4). Indeed the same point is made empirically by Freudenreich *et al.* (2004) who, on the basis of using the Scale to Assess Unawareness of Mental Disorder (SUMD) in their study, suggest that, in schizophrenia, symptom unawareness is most likely to reflect illness pathology compared with other components of insight as determined by the SUMD, namely, the judgements made around attribution of symptoms or willingness to accept treatment. Similarly, recognition that social and cultural factors are important to the views held by individuals concerning beliefs around mental disorders (Johnson & Orrell, 1995; Lam *et al.*, 1996; Chung *et al.*, 1997), i.e. representing another perspective or dimension of insight, is much more indicative of reflecting a mental state rather than being part of a disease process. Thus, the wider notion of insight as knowledge and judgements or attributions concerning what is happening to the individual cannot easily fit into a symptomatic picture of the concept. Again, however, this highlights the need for a theory to bring together the components of insight into some form of structure that can help clarify insight as a whole.

Secondly, apart from the fact that the components or dimensions of the concept of insight are so different from one another, the types of contents of many of the proposed judgements also are suggestive as reflecting more of a particular mental state than a specific symptom of illness. For example, judgements relating to knowledge of a condition and of its consequences to the individual are composite in nature and themselves dependent on a wide range of subsidiary judgements affected by social, cultural and personal factors most of which are difficult to conceive as determined purely by illness/pathology. Moreover, as was established above, the problem of setting specific or defined limits to the contents of such judgements again would be more fitting with reflecting particular mental states rather than particular mental symptoms. This can be illustrated by even cursorily comparing conventional symptoms with the sorts of judgements that are involved in defining insight. Thus, a complaint of feeling anxious or suffering pain or experiencing a hallucination are symptoms which can be defined in terms of direct experiences on the part of the individual. The patient may perceive a change in his/her state and the ensuing symptom is an expression of the patient's judgement concerning this change, his/her description of the experience. In contrast, insight brings together a range of different and disparate judgements in order to define the phenomenon; i.e. as we have seen in metacognitive parlance, it involves judgements *vis-à-vis* the individual's experience as opposed to judgements involving the description of the experience. I suggest that this would fit more with a mental state view of insight rather than a mental symptom. There is, in addition, a further, more specific, point to consider here and one that will be examined in more detail in the next chapters. Here, it is sufficient to say that, by definition, any subjective experience described by an individual is dependent on his/her awareness of this as a phenomenon for it would not be possible otherwise to mark this out and apart from the underlying mental state. Consequently, it follows that the experience of subjective phenomena is itself intrinsically linked with aspects of the processes which constitute insight. This again implies that the concept of insight has a wide, outreaching structure, one that would more easily be viewed as underpinning a mental state than a symptom in the conventional sense.

Thirdly, the empirical work that has been reviewed both in general psychiatric disorders and in organic brain syndromes shows convincingly the very mixed pictures of outcomes between patients' insight and clinical variables (Chapters 3–5). Thus, some studies show an association between poor insight and more severe disease (e.g. Verhey *et al.*, 1995; Rymer *et al.*, 2002; Vaz *et al.*, 2002; Rossell *et al.*, 2003) but other studies disagree (e.g. Green *et al.*, 1993; Lysaker & Bell, 1994; Chen *et al.*, 2001; Howorth & Saper, 2003). Similarly, some studies report an association between poor insight and neurological lesion or neurocognitive dysfunction (e.g. Ott *et al.*, 1996a, b; Young *et al.*, 1998; Lysaker *et al.*, 2002) but, again, others find no such association (e.g. Weinstein *et al.*, 1994; Goldberg *et al.*, 2001; Mintz *et al.*, 2004). The relationship between poor insight and disease factors can therefore at best be described as variable. In other words, the rationale behind such studies, in terms of viewing poor insight as an intrinsic feature of the illness itself, cannot be properly sustained given the inconsistency of results. Again, this is suggestive of a wider conception of insight as a mental state rather than a symptom.

Lastly, there is the issue of considering insight in so-called healthy individuals. Is it the case, e.g. that healthy subjects are always insightful concerning experienced events? Do such individuals always have full awareness and understanding about their experiences and behaviours? It is difficult to argue for this being the case. In fact, there is a great deal of evidence to suggest that in regards to 'normal' experiences and behaviours, individuals show a range of insight or knowledge (Nisbett & Wilson,

1977; Wilson & Dunn, 2004). Leaving aside the question of value, i.e. whether full insight is necessarily always beneficial to the individual, much work concerning 'healthy' individuals has focused on exploring possible mechanisms underlying the different levels of insight or knowledge individuals have at different times and in relation to different experiences. Just like in the work on insight in pathological states, it has been postulated that both *motivational* and *non-motivational* processes are important; the former are conceived in terms of both conscious and unconscious mental processes and can be understood in various frameworks, e.g. psychoanalytic or self-deception (Fingarette, 1969; Haight, 1980); the latter are conceived in more cognitive psychological approaches where unconscious mental processes are viewed as intrinsic to the structure of the mind and consequently inaccessible to introspection (Wilson & Dunn, 2004). The issue here, however, is that, irrespective of possible reasons and mechanisms underlying individuals' insight into their experiences, so-called lack of insight can be viewed as a common and normal and sometimes adaptational phenomenon in healthy subjects. In this case, the question of a link between lack of insight and pathology or illness simply does not arise. This leaves us with the option that lack of insight in patients, conceived as a *symptom*, represents a different phenomenon from lack of insight in healthy people. Alternatively, and more plausibly I would argue that insight, is more usefully viewed as a mental state whether this is in a healthy subject or in a patient with a particular illness. Pathology or illness is only one factor that may affect an individual's insight (or aspect of insight) but clearly many other factors will also be important. In other words, as a mental state, insight will be independent from the disease as such but interdependent with various factors, including disease, affecting mental processes.

6.1.2.3 Insight as a dynamic mental state?

Viewing the nature of insight as a mental state rather than a symptom indicative of disease carries a number of important implications. A mental state by its nature is a dynamic process and will therefore fluctuate according to internal and external changes. This means that some aspects of insight as a mental state may be more stable or resistant to changes whilst other aspects may vary more readily. Consequently, insight as a mental state will entail the consideration of a structure for insight that would allow for such changes and that could generate hypotheses concerning the likely stable aspects of the concept. This could be an important area of empirical work. In addition, conceiving insight in terms of a dynamic mental state can help to understand some of the results of empirical studies. For example, longitudinal studies examining patients' insight in relation to progression of dementia report that patients' insight generally seems to reduce over time (see Table 5.1). Nonetheless, the same studies report that a proportion of patients show improved insight over the time of the study (e.g. McDaniel *et al.*, 1995; Derouesné *et al.*, 1999) and yet this finding tends not to be discussed, presumably because this would be counter to the notion that poor insight is a symptom intrinsic to the disease process. Viewing insight as a dynamic mental state, however, could help to explain such findings as the disease would only be one factor affecting insight and other changes, such as for example increased information given to patients about what they are experiencing, might contribute to insight held at a particular time. The other main implication for empirical work, arising from the view that insight may more usefully be considered a mental state, lies in the design of studies searching for relationships between lack of insight and disease variables. This will be explored in more detail later but essentially the issue lies in the question of localisation of lack of insight with brain changes or cognitive dysfunction. As a mental state, it would make little sense to attempt to correlate this with structural brain lesions. Efforts made at examining possible neurobiology underlying poor insight are unlikely to be successful in relation to the mental state as a whole. Instead, it would make sense to determine first perhaps those aspects of poor insight that might be more directly related to a pathological process such as unawareness/anosognosia in the narrow neurological sense and concentrate on likely associations there. Similar principles would apply to studies exploring poor insight as inherent to the disease process. In turn, this would depend on revising the methods developed for assessing insight and addressing explicitly the specific aspects of insight to be explored.

6.2 The phenomenon of insight: problem of interpretation

Earlier, for ease of analysis, the distinction was made between the *concept* and the *phenomenon* of insight, the former referring to the theoretical structure or meaning of insight and the latter referring to that aspect of the concept that is elicited in a clinical or empirical situation. It was emphasised that the concept of insight was wider than the phenomenon as it would be unrealistic to expect to be able to elicit in a clinical event the totality of what insight as a whole might encompass. However, it was also stressed that this distinction is artificial and made simply to organise the arising theoretical issues around insight and its empirical study. Therefore, it is important to reiterate that the problems of meanings of insight, as discussed above, likewise apply to the phenomenon of insight. If, as was argued, insight is most usefully viewed as a specific mental state with wide, undefined borders to its content, then similarly, the phenomenon of insight can be viewed as a particular aspect of such a mental state. In addition, however, the phenomenon of insight raises other more specific issues and problems which also need to be examined. Whereas the focus of the problems raised in relation to the *concept* of insight was seen as problems of meaning, here in this section, the focus of problems in relation to the *phenomenon* of insight can be best described as problems of interpretation.

Problems of interpretation emerge by definition. Thus, by virtue of defining the phenomenon of insight as that aspect of insight that is elicited clinically, the question of interpretation necessarily arises because of the participation of judgement on the part of another individual with respect to the patient. This is important because of the contribution of this external judgement to the phenomenon of insight itself. In other words, while, as was stressed earlier, the concept of insight is wider than the phenomenon of insight, nevertheless, the phenomenon of insight will include extra or additional elements relating to different forms of external judgements that are involved in determining the phenomenon itself. There are several aspects to consider in relation to this and it is worthwhile to briefly examine these and the implications they carry for understanding the phenomenon of insight.

6.2.1 Interpretation in translation from concept to phenomenon

Interpretation is involved at one level in the translation of the concept of insight into an empirical measure designed to capture this, or rather aspects of this. The numbers and varieties of measures for assessing patients' insight in general psychiatric disorders and organic brain syndromes have been illustrated in the previous chapters and the differences between them highlighted. There are two issues that are important here. Firstly, there is the question of the extent to which the measures actually reflect the underlying concept of insight held by the researchers and, as was seen in the earlier chapters, this varies considerably and seems to be partly dependent on the degree of operationalisation employed. Secondly, however, it is evident that researchers differ in their judgements concerning both the components of insight (i.e. contents of measures) and the ways in which such components are elicited (i.e. questionnaires, interviews, discrepancy measures, etc.). The phenomenon of insight that is captured by these instruments will thus vary accordingly. The crucial point here is not simply that there are differences between the phenomena obtained on account of the variability in measures used but that the *source* of these differences has to do with the way in which the concept of insight has been conceived. Consequently, the phenomenon of insight elicited will carry to some extent the particular judgements and preconceptions of the measure's originators. For example, a measure of insight that determines insight on the basis of patients' appraisals of and comparisons with hypothetical vignettes (e.g. McEvoy *et al.*, 1993b; Chung *et al.*, 1997; Startup, 1997) demands different sorts of judgements on the part of the patients than a measure of insight that is dependent on patients judging their own mental states (e.g. Amador *et al.*, 1994; Marková *et al.*, 2003) or than a measure of insight that is dependent on degree of correlation between patient and carer on views concerning various abilities (e.g. Green *et al.*, 1993; Vasterling *et al.*, 1997). In each case, the types of judgements elicited from the patients have been influenced by the specific conceptualisations of insight by the researchers and by the particular ways these should be translated into an empirical measure.

6.2.2 Interpretation in clinician's judgement

At a more explicit level, interpretation plays a special role in the direct elicitation of patients' insight. There are various ways in which this takes place. In the clinical situation where the patient's insight is elicited by the clinician during an interview, by means of structured or unstructured questions, there are three aspects to consider. Firstly, there is the patient who interprets and articulates his/her experiences in a particular way, i.e. there is the phenomenon of insight which emerges as the patient's construct. Secondly, there is the clinician who interprets the patient's utterances and behaviours, i.e. there is the clinician's construct of the phenomenon of insight. Thirdly, there is the interview situation itself, the dynamic interaction between patient and clinician that is likely to contribute to the phenomenon of insight that is elicited. The phenomenon of insight as the patient's construct and the factors that are likely to be important in this will be discussed more fully in Chapters 8 and 9 when the structure of insight is specifically addressed. Here, I just want to raise and emphasise the likely contribution of the clinician and the clinician–patient interaction in determining the phenomenon of insight. In terms of the clinician, evaluation of patients' insight will be based on interpreting patients' speech and behaviours either in response to direct questions and/or indirectly, i.e. in the context of the psychiatric interview as a whole. Unless the evaluation consists of a simple transcription of patients' answers to a pre-set scale or measure, then such interpretation will in turn depend, to varying degrees, on specific individual clinician factors. These factors would include, e.g. the extent of the clinicians' experience, their level of knowledge, their own conception of insight, their professional backgrounds, their attitudes, biases, etc. Thus, the phenomenon of insight that is elicited will be constituted in part by these individual judgements. For example, the same words spoken by a patient may be interpreted by one clinician as the patient showing insight in that the patient acknowledges he/she is mentally ill and willing to accept treatment, but by another clinician as the patient showing little insight in that the patient is simply repeating statements for motivational reasons in the knowledge that these will help enable him/her to leave medical care. Much depends on the sort of rating of insight that the clinician employs. Clearly the more 'open' such a rating is, e.g. where insight is assessed as part of the normal mental state examination, or in some of the categorical ratings seen in the empirical studies (e.g. Van Putten *et al.*, 1976; Heinrichs *et al.*, 1985; Neary *et al.*, 1986; Starkstein *et al.*, 1993b) or where wide anchor points are used in relation to structured evaluations (e.g. the insight items on the Present State Examination), then the greater will be the contribution of individual clinician factors to the actual phenomenon of insight that is elicited.

6.2.3 Interpretation in the clinician–patient interaction

In addition to the individual factors relating to the clinician which help to determine the particular phenomenon of insight elicited, factors relating to the clinician–patient interaction are also going to play a part in contributing to the end-of-line construct. Such factors can only be speculative but are likely to shape the phenomenon of insight in different ways. For example, the degree to which rapport is established, the extent to which patient and clinician relate to one another and the mutual understanding that is experienced may determine the particular phenomenon of insight elicited. Thus, patients may in one situation feel able to express some of their worries and concerns that relate to their understanding and knowledge of what is happening to them but in another situation that same trust may not have developed and their beliefs concerning their experiences may remain inaccessible to the clinician. In addition, the clinician–patient interaction may have a more direct contribution towards the constitution of the phenomenon of insight. In other words, in the act of communication itself between the two individuals, patients' subjective experiences, particularly when these are inchoate and difficult to describe, may be to some extent named and defined via the clinician (or whoever is communicating with the patient). Thus, for example, half-expressed descriptions on the part of the patient may be 'helped' to fit into the clinician's terminology and in that sense become crystallised into the 'symptoms'. Making sense of these experiences therefore becomes an interactive process and the phenomenon of insight will contain elements of this interaction.

6.2.4 Interpretation in comparative judgements

Ultimately, determining the phenomenon of insight in the clinical or research situation, directly or indirectly and irrespective of the measure chosen, will always involve another important interpretative aspect, namely, the comparative judgement that constitutes the final definition of the phenomenon. In other words, as others have also emphasised (e.g. McGorry & McConville, 1999), the phenomenon of insight is, in the end, a relative judgement, i.e. it is determined on the basis of the *difference* between the clinician's and the patient's judgement concerning what is happening to the patient. At its simplest, therefore, it is a measure of concordance between the clinician and patient about the patient's condition. Interpretation at this level relates not just to the clinician's perception of the patient's condition but depends on the clinician's judgement of any discrepancy and is based on the assumption that the clinician has the 'correct' appraisal. As was demonstrated from reviewing the empirical studies exploring insight in patients with mental disorders and organic brain syndromes, a wide range of measures have been developed to evaluate patients' insight. The extent to which the judgement of discrepancy is exercised by the clinician thus also depends, *inter alia*, on the type of measure used. For example, measures of insight based on answers to general questions as to whether patients consider themselves mentally or emotionally ill will demand different sorts of interpretation of concordance from the clinician than measures which address a range of specific aspects of the patient's condition which perhaps narrow down some of the interpretative elements. On the other hand, measures of insight which already rely on discrepancies between patients and carers (e.g. Green *et al.*, 1993; Smith *et al.*, 2000) will introduce additional interpretative factors, not only from the clinician who evaluates the results but also from the family/carers who judge patients on various problems/abilities. As was shown earlier, such judgements on the part of carers are likely to be influenced by many factors, both individual and contextual, and may not necessarily represent accurate appraisals (De Bettignies *et al.*, 1990). The issue here, however, is not so much about the accuracy or inaccuracy of such external judgements of patients but about the fact that the final phenomenon of insight that is captured becomes a complex of subjective and 'objective' judgements and interpretations whose individual components may not be easy to define. Similarly, where measures of insight rely on discrepancies between patients' appraisals of problems and performance on specific tests (e.g. Anderson & Tranel, 1989), the assumption again is that performance on the tests provides the 'correct' evaluation of patients' abilities. Nevertheless, the issue concerning the extent to which such tests actually reflect a subjective experience of problems (generally couched in very broad terms) is a matter of another type of interpretation. Different again is the interpretation of discrepancy required in assessing insight on the basis of patients' behaviours. In fact, as was seen earlier (Chapters 3–5), there have been very few measures of insight focusing on patients' behaviours rather than speech but an interesting measure of insight in patients with dementia was designed by Giovannetti *et al.* (2002) who observed patients' reactions to mistakes on ordinary tasks and on this basis made a judgement of patients' awareness. Clearly, the sorts of interpretations involved in this type of appraisal will depend on different types of judgements and comparisons (i.e. judgements concerning how a healthy subject might respond in a similar situation).

Apart from the type of measure of insight used, interpretation of discrepancy between clinician and patient perception of problems will also depend on the 'object' of insight chosen for evaluation. In Chapter 5, the term 'object of insight' was introduced to refer to the different aspects of dementia in relation to which insight was examined (e.g. memory problems, activities of daily living, behavioural problems, etc.). 'Object of insight' as a general term referring to the relational aspects of insight will be the focus of examination in Chapter 7. Here, the term is used to briefly illustrate that different judgements are involved in the interpretation of discrepancies between patients and clinicians according to which aspect of a patient's condition is being assessed. For example, a clinician evaluating patients' insight into their ability to dress themselves or into their hemiplegia will be able to make such a judgement based on the discrepancy between patients' claims and their abilities by means of direct observation of that function or disability. On the other hand, a clinician evaluating patients' insight into their subjective experiences, such as depressed mood or hallucinations, will have to make such a judgement based on an indirect or inferred assessment of their experience. In other words, interpretations in these cases are made on different types of data and consequently will involve different sorts of judgements which in turn are likely to be influenced to greater extents by individual factors.

6.2.5 Phenomenon of insight: general implications

It can be seen from the above that the phenomenon of insight, referring to that aspect of the concept of insight that is elicited clinically, presents some additional problems that need to be considered in relation to its structure. Whilst, in definitional terms, the phenomenon of insight can be viewed as the clinical manifestation of an aspect of patients' understanding concerning their condition, in structural terms that understanding will be in part constituted by the interpretative factors belonging to the clinician as well as, in an interview situation, by the interactive process itself. The question is, however, what are the implications of understanding the phenomenon of insight in this way for empirical research exploring insight in patients? Firstly, it is important in terms of helping to appreciate more clearly the differing capacities of measures of insight to capture different aspects of the phenomenon of insight. In other words, even if all the possible external judgements likely to influence the phenomenon of insight cannot be taken into account, the relative contribution of different types and levels of interpretation involved when different insight measures are used can at least be estimated. Secondly, understanding the clinical phenomenon of insight in these structural terms (i.e. as a complex of patient–clinician interacting judgements) will help in devising or choosing insight measures for specific purposes in research. For example, it may make more sense to use measures of insight which capture relatively more of the patient construct than the complex patient–clinician construct in studies which attempt to address possible neurobiology underlying poor insight. Thirdly, much of the variability in empirical research outcomes can also be explained more clearly in the light of this understanding for it becomes evident that differences between instruments evaluating insight are more than simply differences in the contents of some defined mental substance owned by the patient. Instead, these differences reach out into a range of spheres external to the patient. Consequently, the phenomena of insight captured by these different measures are likely to contain quite diverse elements.

6.3 Conclusion

In order to address some of the complexities that have been raised around the study of insight in the previous chapters, it is essential to examine in some detail issues relevant to the conceptualisation of insight. For this purpose and reasons of analysis, a distinction has been made between the *concept* of insight and the *phenomenon* of insight. The concept of insight is defined as the theoretical structure of insight as a whole whilst the phenomenon of insight refers to the clinical manifestation of insight and, hence, reflects only an aspect of the concept of insight.

Examining the meaning of the concept of insight identifies two main areas of difficulties. Firstly, analysis of the range of definitions of insight in clinical and empirical work indicates that it is the lack of defined boundaries to the various contents that poses the main conceptual difficulty. In other words, the extent of the patient's knowledge or understanding of a condition that is required for insight, in terms of detail of information, degree to which it affects oneself, the level of certainty, etc., is difficult to demarcate clearly. Secondly, from a clinical perspective, exploring the possible nature of the concept of insight shows that there is some confusion about this in the literature. Most studies suggest that the concept of insight (or poor insight) is viewed as a symptom or intrinsic feature of the condition affecting the patient. On the basis of evidence provided here, however, I argue for a view of the concept of insight as a particular mental state. In this sense, the concept of insight is, to some extent, independent of the condition affecting the patient though its aspects are likely to be affected by disease factors as well as by other non-disease-related factors. Many of the multidimensional constructs of insight proposed in the literature would fit in better with a mental state view of insight rather than a symptom view, particularly, since so far there has not been a theory put forward to help understand the relationship of the various dimensions of insight to one another.

The view of the concept of insight as a mental state carries a number of important implications including its conception as a dynamic process and one that is likely to fluctuate under the influence of various internal and external factors. Most importantly though, it carries implications for the way in which future studies on insight need to be directed, especially as far as research on possible neurobiology is concerned where more specified aspects of the concept of insight would need to be determined.

Examining the phenomenon of insight identifies the main conceptual problem as one of interpretation. In other words, as the phenomenon of insight is manifested or elicited in a clinical situation, there will always be another participant/clinician involved in making a judgement. Interpretation can be identified at different levels including at the level of translation from concept to empirical measure, at the level of clinician judgement and in relation to an interactive communicative context.

In the end, a judgement of patients' insight is determined by the level of agreement between patient and clinician (whether this is by interview, by questionnaires, or discrepancy methods, etc.) and hence this is another form of interpretation. In consequence of the interpretations that take place at different levels, the clinical phenomenon of insight incorporates *additional external* elements that are not within the concept of insight itself. The types and extents of such external components will vary according to the measure of insight that is employed. What seems to emerge from the analysis is that the phenomenon of insight cannot be considered simply a particular identified 'section' of the concept of insight or cross-section of a theoretically derived mental state. (The relationship between the concept and phenomenon of insight is represented diagrammatically in Chapter 9.) Instead, it must be viewed in the context in which it is determined, and, the external factors that are likely to be contributing to its formation need to be acknowledged. These factors themselves do raise practical problems because of their inherent nature. Hence, whilst in theory factors relating to individual judgements (knowledge, experience, attitudes, biases, preconceptions, mood states, etc.) and interactional processes can be postulated as contributing to the determination of the clinical phenomenon of insight, in an empirical situation they would be difficult to manage. Nevertheless, this should not detract from understanding that the phenomenon of insight carries these extra elements and is best conceived as a complex or composite of the particular mental state of the patient, the various judgements on the part of the clinician/interlocutor and their interaction.

The relational aspects of insight: the 'object' of insight assessment

Following on from the previous chapter, in terms of examining some of the conceptual problems underlying the meaning of insight, the focus in this chapter is on another highly important aspect of insight, namely its relational nature. So far, problems of meaning of insight have concentrated simply on the term itself. The differences in the meaning of insight in regards to definitions varying in breadth, detail, components, and otherwise, have been highlighted and difficulties around specifying boundaries of the content of the concept have been identified. Likewise, it has been argued that the nature of the *concept* of insight is most usefully regarded as a mental state and consequently determined by multifarious elements of which the mental disorder or condition affecting the patient is only one. Additional problems relating to the meaning of the *phenomenon* of insight have been raised on account of the specific issues involved in the interpretation of a clinical state necessary to the determination of the phenomenon of insight.

It has been apparent, however, both with respect to the exploration of insight in different clinical disorders and with respect to the exploration of insight in a particular clinical disorder, that insight cannot be explored in isolation as some sort of independent entity. Instead, the phenomenon of insight is always manifested or elicited in relation to some aspect of the condition affecting the patient. In other words, insight is a *relational* concept – or an 'intentional' concept in the sense of Brentano (1874/1995). It can only be understood or expressed in terms of its relation to something, be that a pathological state or a non-morbid experience. Thus, one cannot have insight without there being something to have insight about and this 'something' has already been referred to as the 'object' of insight assessment (Marková & Berrios, 2001). The 'object', therefore, refers to the particular mental/physical state (e.g. mental symptoms, illness/disorder, neurological abnormality, neuropsychological deficit, etc.) in relation to which insight is being assessed. The essential point that will be argued in this chapter is that this relationship between the phenomenon of insight and the 'object' of insight assessment is *bi-directional* (and interactional). This means that, when exploring insight empirically, not only is it the case that the 'object' of insight assessment needs to be specified but, and crucially, the 'object' of insight assessment will, to a significant extent, determine the phenomenon of insight that is elicited. This latter point forms the central issue in this chapter and carries important implications for understanding the structure of insight as well as for interpreting empirical studies on insight and for determining future research in this area. In effect, this is saying that, different 'objects' of insight assessments (e.g. delusions/hallucinations as opposed to mental disorder as opposed to memory impairment, etc.) will determine phenomena of insight that are characterised by essentially different clinical features. In other words, the phenomena of insight elicited or manifested in relation to different 'objects' of insight assessment will be *structurally* different from each other. Structure, in this context, refers to the constitutive framework underlying insight, in terms of numbers and types of components, their interrelationships and the rules (historical, theoretical, language based, etc.) governing their interrelationships.

Before moving on to explore how different 'objects' of insight assessment might exert their effect on the clinical phenomena of insight, the chapter first looks at the importance of this claim in the context of current research work and in further developing understanding around the meaning of insight at both the conceptual and phenomenal levels. Next, the definition of 'object' of insight assessment will be examined in more detail and, finally, different ways in which the 'object' of insight assessment may shape the clinical phenomenon of insight will be discussed.

7.1 Significance of the relational aspects of insight

At first glance it might seem that any discussion around the importance of, and implications underlying, the relational aspects of insight is somewhat misplaced at this point and would better belong at the end, after explication of the ways in which objects of insight assessment may shape clinical phenomena of insight. However, there is a two-fold purpose in dealing with this now and the second aspect relates to presenting a rationale behind the examination of insight as a relational concept. In other words, the significance of the relational aspects of insight is tightly bound up in both the current assumptions made in empirical research as well as in the implications that are carried for future research and understanding of insight, and these are difficult to disentangle cleanly from one another. Hence, from an explanatory perspective, it is more useful to discuss the importance of the relational nature of insight here.

What then is the significance of the relational aspects of insight? The fact that clinically or empirically insight is explored in relation to different 'objects' of insight assessment is not particularly surprising given the range and variety of conditions affecting individuals. We have thus seen that, for example, insight has been elicited in relation to different *disorders* (e.g. schizophrenia, bipolar affective disorder, depression, obsessive-compulsive disorders (OCD), dementia, head injury, cerebrovascular accident, etc.), in relation to different *symptoms* or groups of symptoms (e.g. delusions, hallucinations, positive/negative symptoms of schizophrenia, depressed mood) and in relation to different *disabilities* (e.g. hemiplegia, blindness, memory impairment, behavioural disturbances, etc.). The various insight measures employed in studies focus to different extent on the particular 'object' of insight assessment chosen by researchers. What is being claimed here, however, is that such different 'objects' of insight assessment themselves determine, in part, the clinical phenomenon of insight elicited. Therefore, it would follow that the phenomena of insight elicited in relation to different 'objects' are likely to be different, and, furthermore, that these differences between the phenomena of insight may be important in theoretical and practical ways. Taking the various parts of this argument separately and concentrating first on the point that different insight phenomena will be elicited in relation to different 'objects' of insight assessment, it could be argued that this is a self-evident claim. In other words, it makes sense for the relationship between the phenomenon of insight and the 'object' of insight assessment to be viewed as bi-directional in this way and that changes in the 'object' will necessarily affect the manifestation of the phenomenon that is dependent on it.

In fact, however, it is clear from the research reviewed in this area that this issue is not self-evident. Whilst, in general, studies may acknowledge that different phenomena of insight are elicited on the grounds that different assessment measures are used, there has been little serious consideration given to, firstly, the role of the 'object' itself in determining differences and, secondly, to the importance and implications of such differences. In practical terms, equivalence between insight phenomena in relation to different 'objects' is, therefore, frequently assumed. This is perhaps most obvious in the analogies made between anosognosia or unawareness of specific neurological impairments on the one hand and poor insight into general psychiatric disorders on the other (Chapter 3). Thus, as was seen earlier, the rationale behind many of the studies searching for correlations between frontal lobe and/or right hemispheric dysfunction and poor insight in schizophrenia and/or schizoaffective disorder (e.g. Young *et al.*, 1993; Lysaker & Bell, 1994; Flashman *et al.*, 2000; 2001 or mania (e.g. Ghaemi *et al.*, 1996) or dementia (e.g. Michon *et al.*, 1994; Ott *et al.*, 1996a, b; Vogel *et al.*, 2005) is based on the finding that anosognosia in relation to neurological states has been linked to frontal lobe dysfunction and right-hemisphere damage (e.g. Bisiach *et al.*, 1986; Starkstein *et al.*, 1992). In other words, it is assumed that 'anosognosia' as assessed in relation to an 'object' such as 'hemiplegia' and 'impaired insight' as assessed in relation to an 'object' such as 'mental illness', both refer to a similar phenomenon. For example, Young *et al.* (1993) whilst acknowledging the difficulties in determining a clear definition of 'unawareness' in schizophrenia, unequivocally base their study on the possible association between such unawareness and anosognosia. They define 'unawareness' in schizophrenia as: 'the phenomena in which individuals with long-standing schizophrenic symp-tomatology state upon intensive questioning that they are not ill, do not have symptoms or have no difficulties or abnormalities which they attribute to psychi-atric illness' (Young *et al.*, 1993, p. 118). They view this as analogous to anosog-nosia in neurological disorders and reiterate some years later: 'in schizophrenia, lack of awareness of illness may well derive from an organic substrate and may itself be a neurocognitive deficit ...' (Young *et al.*, 1998, p. 44). Mullen *et al.* (1996) are particularly explicit in equating these phenomena: 'The ability to re-label certain mental events as pathological *corresponds closely* to the concept of anosognosia. ... The recognition by a patient of neurological symptoms is *conceptually identical* with the recognition of psychiatric symptoms' (p. 645, my emphases). Similarly, amongst others, Amador *et al.* (1991), Amador and Gorman (1998), and Flashman *et al.* (2001) argue for a strong resemblance between poor insight in schizophrenia and anosognosia or unawareness of illness in neurological disorders.

Therefore, it is evident that much of empirical research on insight assumes that the phenomena of insight elicited in relation to such different 'objects' as 'neuro-logical impairment' and 'mental disorder' are, if not equivalent in form, then at least sufficiently similar to warrant theoretical and empirical generalisations between studies. On this assumption, therefore, it would follow that the phenom-enon of impaired insight or unawareness in schizophrenia and the phenomenon of unawareness in neurological impairments would share a common structure and a common underlying mechanism. Similarly, the phenomena of insight elicited in patients with dementia, where 'objects' of insight assessment tend to be particu-larly variable (Chapter 5), tend, nevertheless, to be viewed as broadly equivalent and hence as sharing a common structure and mechanism with those of insight phenomena elicited in relation to other 'objects'. It is this latter consequence from the assumption of equivalence between insight phenomena in relation to dif-ferent 'objects', i.e. the idea that common structures and mechanisms are likely to underlie the insight phenomena, that is particularly important and that is challenged here by the view that insight is inherently relational and hence the phenomenon of insight will be directly shaped by its relational 'object'. If it is the case that the 'object' of insight assessment determines in part the clinical phenom-enon of insight, it follows that phenomena of insight in relation to different 'objects' will be different accordingly. Depending on the nature of the clinical features delineating the insight phenomenon in each case, differences between insight phenomena could vary from minor surface characteristics to major clinical differences. In the case of the latter, it is likely that such different insight phenom-ena, consequently, would be underpinned by correspondingly different structures. This, in turn, carries implications for different mechanisms or processes under-lying insight in each case.

Clarifying the relational aspects of insight is, therefore, of theoretical and practical importance. From a theoretical perspective, understanding the relationship between insight and the 'object' of insight assessment should help to further determine the structure of insight both in terms of its overall structure as well as in terms of structures underlying specific individual insight phenomena. From a more practical viewpoint, clarifying the relationship between insight and the 'object' of insight assessment may again also help to explain some of the inconsistent research results and, furthermore, suggest appropriate methodological strategies for future empirical work. In addition, from the research perspective, clarifying the insight–'object' relationship is essential in order to address the assumption concerning equivalence between insight phenomena. In particular, given the current focus on brain localisation, it is vital that when exploring possible neurobiology of insight, whether this is by means of neurocognitive function or neuroimaging or any other way, the phenomena of insight chosen for investigation are of a similar structure.

7.2 The meaning of 'object' of insight assessment

Before moving on to discuss the ways in which the 'object' of insight assessment might shape and determine the phenomenon of insight, it is important to examine in a little more detail the sense in which the 'object' of insight assessment is meant. There are three aspects to this that need to be emphasised.

7.2.1 'Object' and 'domain'

First, the 'object' of insight assessment has been defined as that aspect of the patient's condition in relation to which insight is assessed. We have seen that, according to this definition, there is a wide range of 'objects' in relation to which insight is evaluated. Thus, as demonstrated in previous chapters, patients' insight is assessed variously in relation to, for example, 'mental illness', 'mental symptoms', 'neurological impairment', 'neuropsychological deficit', 'behavioural changes', 'functioning capacity', and a great many more. The crucial issue here is that these 'objects' of insight assessment are not just different in terms of their content but they are different in type. In other words, these 'objects' refer to different sorts of aspects of the patient's condition and, importantly, these aspects are not always comparable in meaning. For example, 'mental illness' cannot be considered as referring to a similar *type* of phenomenon as 'memory impairment' or as 'ability to carry out daily tasks' or as 'hemiplegia', etc. This is, in part, a *semantic* distinction and, in part, a *natural* distinction. The former relies on the fact that such 'objects' of insight assessment belong to different categories of meaning (Ryle, 1949/1990). The latter distinguishes such 'objects' of insight assessment on the grounds of basic differences between the kinds of 'objects' or entities these represent. These distinctions will be made clearer in the next section when the ways in which the 'objects' of insight determine phenomena of insight are examined in the light of such differences in semantic category and specific kind. Here, it is necessary to simply make the point that 'objects' are different in type. This also serves to distinguish from another term frequently used in relation to insight assessment, namely 'domains' of insight or awareness.

The term 'domain' of awareness has been used particularly frequently in the empirical work on insight in dementia (Chapter 5). We saw how, in dementia, researchers tended to distinguish much more specifically the different aspects of dementia in relation to which insight was elicited (e.g. Kotler-Cope & Camp, 1995; Vasterling *et al.*, 1995; 1997; Starkstein *et al.*, 1996). Domain, however, in this context refers to the particular feature of dementia that is being accessed. For example, domains of awareness are delineated in relation to memory problems, problems with activities of daily living, mood changes, etc. all of which are viewed as common characteristics of dementia as a disease. Thus, the domain can be considered an area or particular function affected by the disease and, as such, different domains contain different contents but will share the common feature of being a characteristic of the disease. The 'object' of insight assessment, on the other hand, refers to a wider notion for it includes not just characteristics of the condition affecting the patient but also the condition itself and indeed any non-disease-related areas. For example, in studies exploring insight in dementia where insight is explored into patients' experience of the condition as a whole, rather than specific features such as memory problems or language difficulties (e.g. Schneck *et al.*, 1982), the term 'domain' would not apply but 'dementia' would be the 'object' of insight assessment. Thus, the 'object' of insight assessment embraces anything in relation to which insight is assessed. Whilst it will include 'domains' of the particular disease affecting the individual, it also refers to other and different aspects of the specific condition experienced by the individual as well as to any states (not necessarily morbid or specific to a condition) chosen by clinicians or researchers.

7.2.2 'Object' and phenomenon of insight

The second aspect, from which the 'object' of insight assessment needs to be understood, is its intrinsic relationship with the phenomenon of insight. Indeed, it is this intrinsicalness that forms the argument (see below) for the claim that phenomena of insight are to some extent determined by the 'objects' of insight assessment. So, what is meant by this intrinsic relationship between the phenomenon of insight and its 'object'? Earlier, it was pointed out that insight is a relational or intentional concept, and that it is not possible to have insight without there being something to have insight about. In other words, whatever the contents of the concept of insight as a whole, i.e. the types of perceptions and judgements involved in the structure of the concept, the mental state represented by the concept of insight is always directed at something. This something or 'object' becomes the focus around which the perceptions and judgements are formed. Thus, when patients' insight is explored in a clinical or empirical situation, an 'object' of insight assessment is necessarily chosen, usually, though not always, by the clinician, in order that the phenomenon of insight is manifested. Without the 'object' there simply would be no phenomenon of insight to elicit. Consequently, in the manifestation or elicitation of the clinical phenomenon of insight, the 'object' of insight assessment becomes inherent or intrinsic to the structure of the phenomenon. The separation that is being made here, in this chapter, between the 'object' of insight and the phenomenon of insight, has to be understood, therefore, as a clarificatory device to help emphasise the direction from which the insight–object relationship is being explored and is not meant to signify a 'real' separation as far as the structure of the phenomenon of insight is concerned.

7.2.3 Patients' and clinicians' 'object' of insight assessment

The third aspect of the 'object' of insight assessment that needs to be mentioned is the issue of whether the clinician and patient are actually referring to the same 'object' when insight is being explored. In the previous chapter, problems of interpretation were raised in relation to understanding the phenomenon of insight elicited clinically. There, the focus was specifically on the phenomenon of insight as a whole (i.e. without considering the relational 'object' independently) and the interpretative issues involved were directed at ways in which the phenomenon of insight was constructed through the contributing judgements of clinicians (and others) as well as the different influences of the types of measures used in determining patients' insight. The 'object' of insight assessment was only mentioned with respect to the point that different types of 'objects' (e.g. 'hemiplegia' compared with 'mental illness') presented different types of 'data' to the clinician and hence involved different levels of interpretation when judgements were made concerning patients' insight. (This particular point is discussed in some detail in the next section.) However, the 'object' of insight itself (in a sense separate from the phenomenon) is also a matter of interpretation and may not be assumed, necessarily, to be a point of correspondence between the clinician and the patient.

For example, if we consider patients with dementia, they might be questioned about their views concerning their memory problems. Whilst it is possible that both patient and clinician consider the 'memory problems' as the 'object' of insight, it is also conceivable that there may be a covert discrepancy in that patient and clinician refer to different 'objects' of insight assessment. In this case, the clinician might, in his/her head, have 'dementia' as the 'object' of insight assessment whereas the patient might be focusing on 'memory problems'. In perhaps a less obvious way, even when clinician and patient both understand 'mental disorder' to be the 'object' of insight assessment, then differences between clinician and patient in their understanding of what 'mental disorder' actually means may result in consideration of different 'objects' of insight assessment. It is likely that the degree to which the 'object' is made explicit, as well as the individual understanding of what the 'object' means or represents, will both determine the extent to which there is agreement on this between the patient and clinician. As was discussed earlier in regards to the interpretative issues involved in the determination of the phenomenon of insight, this is likewise an issue that carries implications for the empirical assessment of insight particularly in relation to research. Again, this is something that simply needs to be understood, or taken into some account, when the structure of the phenomenon of insight is considered.

7.3 The phenomenon of insight as determined by the 'object' of insight assessment

Having highlighted some of the implications underlying the relational aspects of insight, as well as having looked at the perspectives from which the 'object' of insight assessment needs to be understood, this section, which forms the greater part of this chapter, now addresses the claim itself, namely, that the 'object' of insight assessment determines to some extent the clinical phenomenon of insight. The questions therefore are, how can the 'object' of insight assessment exert this effect on insight structure? And, in what ways will different 'objects' of insight assessment determine different sorts of insight structures? Three possible ways are proposed here: (i) 'object' as determined by discipline, (ii) 'object' as a semantic category and (iii) 'object' as a specific kind, and each of these will be explored in turn.

7.3.1 'Object' as determined by discipline

The 'object' of insight assessment is, by definition, different in relation to different professional disciplines. Within clinical psychiatry, for example, the 'object' of insight assessment generally refers to 'mental illness' and/or 'mental symptoms', although, as was reviewed earlier, often the distinction is not made (Chapter 3). In neurological disciplines, the 'object' of insight assessment tends to refer to neurological abnormalities; for example, 'hemiplegia' or neuropsychological deficits such as 'amnesia', 'dysphasia', etc. In psychodynamic psychotherapy, the 'object' of insight may refer to 'motivations' and 'behaviours' as well as other 'mental processes', and, in cognitive (Gestalt-influenced) psychology, the 'object' may be defined in terms of specific problem-solving routines, and so on. The important issue here lies in the nature of the differences between 'objects' as determined by discipline. This is because the differences in the 'object' of insight assessment do not simply only reflect differences of content representing the 'object', i.e. the content inherent to the subject matter of the disciplines, but also reflect more profound differences in structure. In other words, the 'objects' of insight assessment (and concomitantly, because of the nature of the insight–'object' relationship, the conceptualisation of insight with respect to the objects) are embedded in a theoretical background that itself is only understandable in terms of the historical development of the discipline. It is in virtue of this particular difference between 'objects' of insight assessment in relation to different disciplines that the 'objects' will exert their differential effect on the phenomenon of insight. This is best illustrated by looking at some examples.

7.3.1.1 General psychiatry

In general psychiatry, current thought conceives mental disorders as arising from a combination of individual (brain pathology, personality factors, psychological processes) and external (social pressures, environmental stressors, cultural issues) factors. The clinician's diagnosis of a mental disorder is based on an assessment of the patient's mental state in terms of identifying mental symptoms, signs and behaviours, contextualising these within the patient's personal and background history, and formulating this against the likely aetiological or triggering factors that may contribute to both the development and the manifestation of the mental disorder. The lack of clarity concerning pathogenesis of mental disorders (and consequently the reliance on a classification of mental conditions that is based on arbitrarily determined patterns of symptoms/behaviours whose updating is governed by the particular theoretical and social drives of the time (Cooper, 2004)), however, together with the lack of any biological markers comparable to those present in medical disorders, means that the diagnosis of mental disorders is particularly complicated in the sense of the types of clinical judgements that have to be involved. It is not the purpose here to explore these but only to emphasise that these judgements are problematical at different levels. Such levels include the elicitation of individual psychopathological phenomena, the ways in which symptoms, signs and behaviours are expressed, captured, conceptualised and named, the factors involved in putting these together into diagnostic categories as well as the epistemic validity carried by the ensuing symptoms and disorders (Berrios et al., 1995; Berrios, 2000; Berrios & Marková, 2002). It is these same symptoms, signs, behaviours as well as mental disorders as a whole that constitute the 'objects' of insight assessment in general psychiatry. They are therefore bound up in the same issues specific to this discipline in terms of the ways in which judgements are formed and psychopathology is understood. Thus, they incorporate a wide range of experiences, ones which vary in *nature* (e.g. subjective experiences such as feelings of anxiety, uncertainty or complaints of fatigue, of being watched, etc. and objective signs such as psychomotor retardation, thought disorder, etc.) and *content* (e.g. abnormal perceptions, affective disturbances, passivity phenomena, impairments/interferences with thinking, etc.). This variety of experiences, forming these 'objects' of insight assessment, demands a broad view of insight, and this is evident in the research reviewed earlier. Thus, whether referred to in terms of 'mental disorder' (e.g. Wing et al., 1974; Kay et al., 1987), 'mental experiences' (McEvoy et al., 1989; Marková et al., 2003) and/or 'mental symptoms' (David, 1990; Amador et al., 1993), the 'object' of insight encompasses a broad structure which in turn determines a broad conceptualisation of insight.

For example, taking 'mental disorder' as the 'object' of insight would entail conceiving insight in terms of the particular way the disorder is conceived at the time. This could thus include knowledge which ranges from notice of a change in the self to some understanding of a few individual symptoms/signs to understanding of the totality of the changes experienced as a result of the disorder and/or to understanding of the details of the disorder and its likely causes, precipitants and effects. In other words, 'mental disorder', however it is framed, whether this is in terms of an illness, a change in the self or a sum of a number of symptoms/signs etc., will demand patients' judgements that are wide or far reaching and of varying complexity. Similarly, when a symptom such as 'delusion' is the 'object' of insight assessment, this will demand a conceptualisation of insight that has to be based on judgements which reach beyond the awareness of some pathological experience and spread widely to form complex assessments concerning the nature of the experience. Therefore, in general psychiatry the 'object' of insight assessment itself determines a phenomenon of insight that is broad because it demands judgements which are wide and complex involving not only assessment of the subjective experience but also determining its meaning in the light of general knowledge, past experience, personal biases, etc. We have seen from the research in this area (Chapter 3) that, in theory at least, insight has indeed been conceptualised in this broad sense that encompasses, firstly, an awareness of patients' varied experiences and, secondly, some form of secondary elaboration of those experiences. The latter has been variously defined by researchers as judgements (Jaspers, 1948), attitudes (Lewis, 1934), re-labelling (David, 1990), attributions (Amador et al., 1991), self-knowledge (Marková & Berrios, 1992a), etc. Such conceptualisations of insight reflect the broad judgements that are determined by the likewise broad nature of the 'object' of insight assessment as a medley of mental and behavioural disturbance understood in a context of socio-cultural factors.

However, the 'object' of insight assessment determines the phenomenon of insight in an additional, more specific way. Mental phenomena and behavioural states thought to represent mental disorders are identified and captured by means of certain rules developed over time and themselves dependent on particular lines of thought, beliefs about the nature of the 'mental' and the relationship with the 'physical', conceptualisation of psychological processes, definitions of morbidity or pathology, assumptions concerning classification of mental functions, and many more.

This structure underlying the rules of the diagnostic process forms the framework of the clinical psychiatric discipline. Eliciting patients' mental and behavioural phenomena on the part of the clinician is dependent, therefore, amongst other things, on a particular way of conceiving such mental and behavioural phenomena, and their disturbances. This sort of understanding is, in turn, dependent on a taxonomy of mental function (and dysfunction) which is assumed *a priori* but is one that has developed within the discipline, and, in the context of other influences, over time. The question of whether such a taxonomy is 'valid', i.e. whether there is correspondence between the conventional mental taxonomy with brain mechanisms or functions, is not the issue here. Instead, the point here is that it is governed by the concepts developed specifically in the context and function of clinical psychiatry as a discipline and its antecedents. Mental and behavioural phenomena are identified, classified and prioritised on the basis of such concepts. And it is thus that the 'object' of insight assessment, necessarily enmeshed within this framework, will elicit a phenomenon that is likewise structurally bound to the same frame. Related disciplines, whilst sharing some of the conceptual background, are, by reasons of diverse histories, foci, and functions, underpinned by different theoretical structures constituted by different concepts and assumptions.

7.3.1.2 Psychoanalytic psychology

As was evident from the work examined in Chapter 2, in psychoanalytic psychology, the concept of insight and its 'object' are much more firmly integrated within the focus of the discipline itself. In other words, without necessarily being invoked as such, insight in the sense of 'deeper' self-knowledge has formed the basis of psychoanalytic theory. ('Deeper' here refers to gaining access to whatever hidden or 'unconscious' knowledge is deemed relevant to explaining the patient's psychopathology.) The attainment of such insight is one of the therapeutic objectives of psychoanalytic theory (Freud, 1973a, b). In contrast with general psychiatry, the concept of insight, and the corresponding phenomenon, hold a much more prominent position within psychoanalytic thought. The 'object' of insight here, tightly interwoven in the specific language and conceptual background forming the framework of the psychoanalytic discipline, refers, therefore, to some form of deeper knowledge of the self – irrespective of whether or not this is couched in terms of 'unconscious' mental processes. Consequently, the ensuing phenomenon of insight will require a different conceptualisation – one that needs to articulate such deeper knowledge. As was reviewed earlier, much of psychoanalytic work has focused on addressing the problem of trying to capture such deeper knowledge. Insight in this context has been conceptualised in terms of the ways in which this deeper knowledge is either *acquired* – e.g. descriptive versus ostensive insight (Richfield, 1954), insight through clarification versus insight through interpretation (Bibring, 1954), or *understood* – e.g. neutral versus emotional versus dynamic insight (Reid & Finesinger, 1952), or *manifested* – e.g. structured and/or re-created (Abrams, 1981; Sternbach, 1989; Blum, 1992). The 'object' of insight in psychoanalytic theory, therefore, determines a structure of the phenomenon of insight in ways that are different from those shaped by the 'object' of insight assessment in general psychiatry. Furthermore, apart from these differences determined by content, theory (i.e. the particular conceptual framework underlying psychoanalytic theory) and focus, the very nature of the 'object' of insight assessment (i.e. the 'deep' self-knowledge) makes it difficult for the phenomenon of insight to be elicited directly. Hence, the phenomenon has to be elicited indirectly through the exploration of likely mechanisms or effects of attaining insight in the individual. This carries specific implications for research in this area particularly as far as developing insight measures is concerned (Chapter 2).

7.3.1.3 Neurosciences

Different from general psychiatry and psychoanalytic psychology is the conceptual framework underlying the neurological and neuropsychological disciplines. Apart from the differences in terms of content and focus of the work undertaken, and the language and theoretical/conceptual frame on which this is based, one striking difference, already mentioned several times, is the perspective from which neurosciences have developed interest in insight and awareness. For example, in contrast to general psychiatry, it has been the dramatic loss of awareness or insight in the face of prominent neurological abnormality that has stimulated interest and research on insight in these disciplines. Consequently, conceptualisation of insight has been, from the very beginning (apart from some qualified exceptions where motivational theories have been proposed (Chapter 4, Weinstein & Kahn, 1955)), strongly linked to the neurological abnormality itself. This has resulted in a phenomenon of insight that has, analogously, a narrower content and much more clearly demarcated borders. Putting this another way, the 'objects' of insight within the neurosciences disciplines refer to the particular neurological deficits or neuropsychological impairments that are evident to the clinicians. These neurological deficits and neuropsychological impairments are themselves enveloped in the theoretical backgrounds of these disciplines. Therefore, in simplified terms the neurological and neuropsychological understanding of such impairments and deficits (e.g. hemiplegia, amnesic syndromes, dysphasia, etc.) is framed in a language (and concepts) relating to the *brain* and to putative *brain processes*. Thus, neurological impairment and deficits are explained in terms of brain localisation theories, either in structural (specific brain lesions) or functional (neuropathology or neuropharmacology of specific brain systems) terms or structured on modular and information-processing models in which neuropsychological processes are viewed as independent or semi-independent functions loosely superimposed on brain structure (e.g. Mesulam, 1986; Schacter, 1990;

Stuss, 1991). The point here is that the 'object' of insight assessment, represented by the neurological and neuropsychological impairments and deficits, is understood, within these disciplines, in this particular 'brain processes' language. In turn, this 'object' of insight assessment determines a phenomenon of insight that is likewise understood within this same theoretical structure. Hence, the phenomenon of insight elicited in relation to the 'object' determined by the neurosciences disciplines, is a structurally much narrower and more encapsulated phenomenon than that elicited in relation to the 'object' of insight assessment in general psychiatry or psychoanalytic psychology.

7.3.1.4 Cognitive (Gestalt) psychology

Gestalt-influenced cognitive psychology, in turn, focuses predominantly on cognitive processes deemed to underlie intelligent behaviour (Chapter 2). As such, insight has been conceptualised as a form of intelligent behaviour and the 'object' of insight assessment consists of various specific problem-solving routines (Sternberg & Davidson, 1995). In virtue of the different conceptual framework underpinning this discipline, the phenomenon of insight determined by the 'object' of insight assessment has to be very different from the phenomena of insight in relation to the different 'objects' from other disciplines. Interestingly, comparing Gestalt-influenced cognitive psychology with cognitive neuropsychology offers another example of the way in which the disciplinary background of the 'object' helps determine the phenomenon of insight. In this instance, the 'object' of insight assessment, embedded in Gestalt theory, determines a phenomenon of insight that represents, in a sense, the opposite of the phenomenon of insight elicited by the 'object' of insight in cognitive neuropsychology. This can be seen with respect to the phenomenon of 'feeling of knowing'. This phenomenon (implying some form of knowledge albeit at an inchoate or unconscious state), within cognitive neuropsychology, is representative of some degree of insight (Shimamura & Squire, 1986; Shimamura, 1994). On the other hand, in Gestalt cognitive psychology, this 'feeling of knowing' is, within the context of this discipline's framework, specifically defined as a solution which is not insightful (Metcalfe, 1986). This serves to illustrate how the concepts and foci underpinning a particular discipline will structure the way in which 'objects' of insight are conceived within it and these, in turn, will shape the specific clinical phenomena of insight elicited therein.

7.3.1.5 Dementia

Whilst dementia does not refer to a particular discipline, it is mentioned briefly here because of the special position it occupies in terms of crossing several professional disciplines and the implications this carries for the exploration of insight in this area. In other words, in clinical work and research in dementia, many of the clinical disciplines (e.g. general psychiatry, psychology, neurosciences, etc.) converge. This has consequences for research carried out on insight in patients with dementia. For example, it is likely that the mixture of disciplinary influences, in defining the 'object' of insight assessment and eliciting the ensuing clinical insight phenomenon, will be an additional factor contributing to some of the variable outcomes produced in this area (Chapter 5). We have seen that, in research on insight in dementia, many more 'objects' of insight assessment have been explicitly specified (e.g. dementia as a whole, memory impairment, independent daily living skills, affective symptoms, behavioural/personality changes, etc.). In turn, such 'objects' determine phenomena of insight which are in line with the framework of their particular disciplines. This is, to some extent, reflected in empirical studies through both the terminology used in referring to insight (e.g. lack of insight, unawareness, anosognosia, impaired self-awareness/self-consciousness, etc.) and the diversity of approaches taken to evaluate it (e.g. structured interviews, questionnaires, discrepancy methods, direct observation, etc.). The issue here is that the contribution of the disciplinary conceptual framework in determining the 'object' of insight assessment and hence the phenomenon of insight elicited is particularly important to consider in an area where different disciplines mix.

7.3.2 'Object' as a semantic category

Another important way in which the various 'objects' of insight are different from one another is that they belong to different 'semantic' categories. This feature also influences the way in which 'objects' shape the phenomenon of insight. Above, it was argued that 'objects' of insight assessment could be different on the basis of structural differences relating to the theoretical backgrounds specific to individual disciplines. Hence, the 'objects' would determine phenomena of insight that were likewise bound up in the discipline's conceptual frame. Here, the argument is that the 'object' of insight assessment may be different by virtue of the difference carried by the semantic category to which the 'object' belongs. In other words, the 'objects' of insight assessment may refer to different sorts or types of terms, i.e. belong to different categories of meaning in the sense of Ryle (1949/1990), and will, consequently, determine phenomena of insight that will be structurally different. This again is best illustrated by example.

The issue hinges on the validity of making comparisons between entities or objects belonging to a different order of meaning. It has been noted in several places, that some studies assume equivalence between the phenomena of insight elicited in relation to different 'objects' of insight assessment. Of particular relevance and importance in this regard has been the equivalence assumed between the phenomenon of insight elicited in relation to 'mental illness' and the phenomenon of insight elicited in relation to 'neuropsychological' or 'neurological deficit'

(Mullen *et al.*, 1996; Amador & Gorman, 1998; Young *et al.*, 1998; Flashman *et al.*, 2001, see above). As has already been demonstrated, this assumption has had important consequences for the direction of research taken in these areas, particularly, in terms of searching for a neurobiological explanation for impairment of insight. This assumption of equivalence between insight phenomena in relation to different 'objects' of insight assessment is, therefore, an important issue. Whereas above this assumption was challenged on the grounds that 'objects' of insight assessment, embedded in the specific conceptual backgrounds underlying different disciplines (in this case, general psychiatry versus neurosciences), determined phenomena of insight that were correspondingly structurally different, here the argument against this assumption lies in the different order of meanings presented by the 'objects'. The terms 'neuropsychological deficit' and 'mental illness' are simply different with respect to the categories of meaning they represent. A similar analogy can be made, for example, with the terms 'flower' and 'nature'. The former refers to a specific entity, directly observable and relatively easily demarcated with clear boundaries. The latter may incorporate flower within its definition but refers to much more than a collection of flowers and other such objects, and is not directly observable nor easily demarcated. Perhaps another more relevant analogy would be the difference between terms such as 'nurse' or 'doctor' and 'the National Health Service (NHS) system'. Whilst the former terms refer to specific entities or subjects, directly observable and relatively easily described and defined, the latter is clearly very much more than the sum of all the health professionals and resources (and patients, etc.) contained within it. Instead, it includes within its meaning the ways in which different parts of it work and interact, the politics involved, the social issues, the hierarchies, and all possible structural elements and their functional interrelationships. It is not directly observable and nor is it easily demarcated.

Returning then to the terms 'neuropsychological deficit' and 'mental illness', we are faced with similar categorical differences. The former refers to something that is 'objectively' ascertainable in the sense that it is in principle determinable by a third person either through direct observation or by means of specific tests and can be relatively sharply demarcated. There is a one-to-one relationship between the 'object' (neurological or neuropsychological deficit, e.g. amnesia, hemiplegia, dysphasia, etc.) and its determinable manifestation (e.g. poor memory, inability to move limb, difficulty with speech). The term 'mental illness', on the other hand, refers to a much broader *construct* and again, like 'nature' or 'the NHS system', does not simply consist of a number of like subcomponents but embraces a wider structure that, in the case of 'mental illness', includes not only the signs and symptoms of abnormal psychopathology (and the pathological aetiological factors) but also the social, cultural, environmental and political determinants of the construct.

Direct observation and/or specific tests might not necessarily elicit it and boundaries of the construct are far from clear. There may be a one-to-one relationship between *some* aspects of the construct (such as specific psychopathological signs) and their determinable manifestation (e.g. psychomotor retardation, hallucinations) but there is no clear one-to-one relationship between the construct as a whole and its determinable manifestation. Indeed, as a construct in this wider sense it would be illogical for it to have such a direct manifestation. Like 'nature' or 'the NHS system', it is simply not 'observable' in this sense and is only elicited or determined (in the technical sense) by means of the specialised clinical judgements exerted by health professionals. Moreover, many of the psychopathological, social, cultural, political, etc., determinants fluctuate over time. Hence, this is not a fixed concept and, as is clear from historical accounts, concepts of mental illness have changed over the years and will continue to change (Berrios & Porter, 1995). Signs and symptoms taken to indicate mental illness in one decade may not necessarily apply in another decade. Similarly, they may differ from one culture to another or even from one clinician to another.

In addition, whilst referring to a wide construct, the term 'mental illness' may, from the perspective of the sufferer questioned about his/her insight, be confusing or misleading in another sense, namely, with respect to the 'illness' component of the term. Thus, although the clinician or observer are in a position where they may be able to conceive 'mental illness' widely in terms of its theoretical determinants and understand 'illness' in terms of morbidity, the patient may not experience 'illness' in the conventional meaning of the term. This means that there has to be further distortion of the relationship between 'mental illness' as the 'object' and its overt manifestation. This serves to highlight in another way the contrast between the more direct one-to-one relationship between the 'object' of insight assessment and its determinable manifestation that is present when the 'object' refers to a 'neurological' or 'neuropsychological deficit' and the lack of such a direct relationship when the 'object' of insight assessment refers to a construct such as 'mental illness'.

It seems, therefore, that there are important differences between terms such as 'mental illness' and 'neuropsychological impairment'. These differences are not simply those of content but relate to the way in which the referent is understood. In other words, they belong to different categories of meaning. When 'objects' of insight assessment refer to such terms, then likewise, they refer to different semantic categories and in that sense they cannot be considered comparable (Ryle, 1949/1990). The phenomena of insight that are elicited in relation to such different 'objects' of insight assessment, consequently, will be structurally different. Thus, as is evident above, the phenomena of insight determined by these 'objects' must be constituted from different sorts of judgements, which are different not just in terms of their content but in the types and complexities of judgements involved.

It follows from this that the phenomenon of insight elicited in relation to mental illness may not be equivalent to the phenomenon of insight elicited in relation to neurological or neuropsychological impairment.

7.3.3 'Object' as a specific kind

Apart from the influence of the disciplinary conceptual background and the semantic category to which the 'object' of insight assessment belongs, 'objects' of insight assessment will exert their effect on the phenomenon of insight in yet another way, namely, one which depends on the *type* or *kind* of 'object' that is involved. Whereas the previous line of reasoning is based on the distinction between the semantic categories to which 'objects' of insight assessment belonged, here the argument is that even when 'objects' of insight assessment belong to the same category of meaning, an essential difference in the *kind* of 'objects' that they represent, can determine important differences in the phenomena of insight. In other words, 'objects' of insight assessment can refer to signs and symptoms of a particular disorder (such signs and symptoms, therefore, belonging to a common order of meaning, namely, characteristic features of a condition) and yet the nature itself of these 'objects' (or signs/symptoms) can shape, in specific ways, the phenomena of insight elicited in relation to them. It is useful to illustrate this point.

One of the most striking examples can be observed when comparing the sorts of 'objects' of insight assessment referred to by 'neurological impairment' or 'neuropsychological deficit' and 'subjective mental symptoms', and examining the respective phenomena of insight to which they relate (i.e. which they determine). Both these kinds of 'objects' of insight assessment refer to characteristics of a disorder that might affect a patient. Neurological deficit could refer to hemiplegia and constitute a sign of a cerebrovascular accident and neuropsychological impairment could refer to something like memory loss and this, in turn, might be a feature of dementia or focal amnesic syndrome or a cerebrovascular accident, etc. Subjective mental symptoms, on the other hand, could refer to, for example, hallucinations, delusions, anxiety or depressed mood which in turn might represent features of a mental disorder such as schizophrenia, schizoaffective disorder, bipolar affective disorder, organic brain syndrome, etc. Both of these sorts of 'objects' of insight assessment thus refer to particular features or signs and symptoms of a disorder. However, there is an important difference in the kind or nature of the features they represent. In the case of neurological/neuropsychological impairment, the nature of the features referred to is that of an observable *deficit* or *loss of function*. Something that was previously present as a normal or healthy function or ability is now gone or simply not 'working' at its previous level. This applies to the ability to walk, to move one's limbs, to remember current and/or past activities, to be able to speak and articulate clearly, etc. By contrast, in the case of subjective mental symptoms, the nature of the features referred to is not that of a loss of function/ability but that of an *added or new experience*. In other words, something that was previously not present in the normal or healthy mental state is added to it such that there is an experience of change. Even where that 'addition' results in a subjective experience of loss of ability or function (e.g. loss of interest, enjoyment, motivation, etc.), the point is that there is, by definition, an experienced change, which, whilst it may be qualitative or quantitative in nature, still represents an 'addition' to a mental state experience. What then does this mean for the phenomenon of insight elicited in relation to each of such 'objects' of insight assessment?

When the 'object' of insight assessment refers to an observable loss of function or ability, the phenomenon demanded by such an 'object', has as its primary focus the direct awareness of this loss or deficit. This seems to be the result of a combination of two factors, namely, the nature of the 'object' in this 'loss of function' sense together with the traditional perspective from which this is explored (i.e. as has been emphasised already, from the perspective of insightlessness or anosognosia) in neurological states. In other words, because interest in patients' insight into such problems arose following the observations that patients seemed to be oblivious to major impairments (Chapter 4), and because the impairments concerned are of a relatively clearly defined and objectively evident kind, in terms of loss of ability (e.g. loss of movement, loss of memory, loss of speech, etc.), this drives the insight phenomenon to focus purely on awareness of the impairment in the narrow sense. If a neurological loss of function/ability is clearly present, then awareness of not being able to function in the normal way has to be the imperative focus. If a patient is not aware of a deficit or disability, then that patient cannot make other judgements about this. Consequently, the elicited phenomenon of insight has to be structured in the narrow sense of awareness of the problem. Further judgements concerning the nature and effects of the problem become irrelevant if the patient is simply not aware of the loss of function in the first place. Clearly, as was also seen, with further clarification around the different natures of the various neurological or neuropsychological deficits, the phenomena of insight have widened somewhat to include judgements concerning severity of deficits, impact on functioning, etc. (Sherer *et al.*, 2003a, b), but the core of the phenomenon determined by such 'objects' has necessarily remained tightly bound to awareness in its narrow sense.

When the 'object' of insight assessment refers to 'subjective mental symptoms', the phenomenon of insight demanded by such an 'object' has, by definition, a different structural focus. It is a truism to say that individuals will be aware of 'subjective mental symptoms' (e.g. hallucinations, delusions, depressed mood, preoccupations with worries, etc.) because that is inherent to the definition of 'subjective'. Patients may either complain spontaneously of hearing 'voices', of being filmed by the government, of feeling low in mood or sad, of being constantly worried by something, etc., or these subjective phenomena may be elicited following direct or indirect questioning. Whichever way such phenomena become apparent, the issue is that awareness of them is to some extent part of their manifestation as symptoms. Clearly, however, the phenomenon of insight in relation to these mental symptoms is not considered to consist simply of their presence as elicited or spontaneously offered. Instead, the phenomenon of insight in relation to these mental symptoms is considered on the basis of the sense that patients make of such symptoms. In other words, insight is focused on whether, for example, patients consider the voices in their head to be pathological or normal, or represent some form of external influence. Similarly, insight is focused on whether patients consider their low mood to be pathological, a normal state they have always been in, the result of some real or imagined misdemeanour and whether it has any consequence to their ability to function or relate to others, etc. Thus, awareness of the presence of these mental symptoms cannot be viewed as a phenomenon of insight in a comparable way to that of awareness of the presence of a neurological deficit. Instead, 'subjective mental symptoms' as 'objects' of insight assessment demand a different focus for the phenomenon of insight. This focus has to do with the *sense* that individuals make of these subjective symptoms, i.e. the judgements that are made concerning their nature and meaning, the understanding that is held about their morbidity as mental experiences and wider assessments concerning their effects on the individual. As an 'object' of insight assessment, therefore, 'subjective mental symptoms' demand a level of awareness and judgement beyond that demanded by the 'object' of insight assessment when this is a 'neurological/neuropsychological deficit'. Consequently, 'unawareness of a mental experience' in an analogous sense to 'unawareness of a neurological deficit' has to be conceptually different from 'unawareness of the nature or morbidity of a mental experience'.

The 'object' of insight assessment, in terms of its nature or kind, therefore, is also important in shaping the clinical phenomenon of insight. The way in which this seems to happen, or means by which the phenomenon of insight is driven or determined by the specific nature of the 'object', is, however, clearly complicated by the interplay of various dichotomies relating to the manner in which the nature of the 'object' is characterised. These have been raised at different points but it may be helpful, for the sake of clarity, to identify them explicitly.

7.3.3.1 Subjective–objective dichotomy

This is perhaps the most important dichotomy, which makes a distinction between 'objects' of insight assessment that are primarily identified by the patient (e.g. complaints of pain, fatigue, low mood, hallucinations, fears, etc.) and those that are primarily identified by an external individual, professional or other, by means of observation or tests (e.g. psychomotor retardation, thought disorder, disinhibition, inability to move limbs, comprehension difficulties, etc.). This is a qualified distinction in that the two polarities are not mutually exclusive. For example, patients who complain of hearing voices may be 'observed' to be talking to someone in an empty room, or patients who complain of low mood may appear sad and tearful, and those worrying about persecutors may surround themselves with weapons, and so on. Thus, all such subjective experiences may result in 'objective' inferences made by clinicians that patients are hallucinating, are depressed or suffer from persecutory delusions. Similarly, patients unable to move their limbs or showing psychomotor retardation or having problems with their speech and thoughts may well also complain of these difficulties and thus incorporate a 'subjective' element to the 'objective' signs. The issue here, however, is that some symptoms (to which 'objects' of insight assessment refer) are generated by the individual/patient concerned and are not accessible in the direct sense by another person while other symptoms/signs are manifested indirectly (irrespective of how these may be interpreted by the patient), in an 'objectively' identifiable manner.

As we have seen, when the 'object' of insight assessment refers to symptoms which are primarily 'subjective', the resultant phenomenon of insight will have a very direct relationship with the 'object' or symptoms themselves. Thus, to reiterate, in the articulation of *subjective* complaints, individuals are, by definition, forming judgements on the basis of whatever it is they are experiencing. In the process of expressing such 'symptoms' (or 'objects' of insight assessment), individuals make basic judgements concerning the nature of such experiences and, therefore, these are intrinsically connected to the core processes involved in the formation of insight itself. When, on the other hand, 'objects' of insight assessment refer to '*objective*' symptoms/signs, then the resultant phenomenon of insight will not have this same direct relationship with the 'object'. Instead, the phenomenon of insight will be dependent, firstly, on the extent to which the patient experiences the 'objective' sign in a subjective manner (i.e. a core awareness on the part of the patient), secondly on the clinician's judgements and thirdly to a much greater degree on the discrepancy between patient and clinician judgements. The structures of the insight phenomena determined by 'subjective' mental states and those determined by 'objective' signs must, therefore, have important differences in core constituents.

7.3.3.2 Negative–positive dichotomy

Another distinction between different kinds of 'objects' of insight assessment is based on whether the 'object' refers to a *negative* symptom/sign, i.e. an *absence of a normal* experience, such as loss of function or ability in hemiplegia or amnesia, etc., or whether it refers to a *positive* (in the sense of something added rather than in the sense of positive content) experience, i.e. a *presence of an abnormal* experience such as depressed mood, hallucinations, pain, disinhibited behaviour, etc.

The phenomena of insight determined by 'objects' of insight with respect to this distinction will be shaped in different ways. Thus, the phenomenon of insight that issues in relation to a *negative* 'object', i.e. in relation to an absence of a normal function or experience, will necessarily be focused on awareness (in the narrow sense) of this loss. Where loss of function is concerned, this will determine a phenomenon of insight that has to be primarily concentrated on awareness or knowledge of that loss. Such a phenomenon will, therefore, be constituted of judgements which are limited in numbers and scope, and which give rise to a phenomenon that is correspondingly narrow and fairly sharply encapsulated in structure. Even when there is some awareness of the particular deficit on the part of the patient, further judgements concerning this knowledge will be limited to possible assessments of severity of the deficit and, rarely, impact of the deficit on functioning. For example, in patients with dementia, where memory problems are taken as the 'objects' of insight assessment, the phenomenon of insight that is elicited becomes structured in terms of judgements mainly concerned with how severe the memory problem is regarded by the patient (e.g. compared with some time ago, or compared to other people, or in terms of mistakes made or frequency of problems, etc., see Chapter 5).

In contrast, the phenomenon of insight issuing in relation to a *positive* 'object', i.e. in relation to the presence of an abnormal experience, determines a phenomenon of insight that has to rely on much wider judgements. The focus here is on the presence of something that is not normally there and, consequently, judgements need to reflect this not only in terms of acknowledging the presence of this state but also in terms of evaluating what this actually means (given that this is not the normal state), in what way this is abnormal and how it affects the individual. For example, a patient with schizophrenia may complain of 'voices' interfering with his/her thoughts. If the 'object' of insight is taken as 'auditory hallucinations', the phenomenon of insight that will be elicited in relation to this will incorporate not only the awareness of hearing voices, but equally, since these may be offered as complaints, they will also incorporate what these represent for the individual in terms of their meaning, sense and effects. The phenomenon of insight in this situation, constituted by such judgements, has to be wider and less circumscribed than a phenomenon of insight whose core structure is focused on an awareness of loss.

7.3.3.3 Insight–insightlessness dichotomy

Whilst this dichotomy does not distinguish between the natures or kinds of 'objects' of insight assessment, it does distinguish between perspectives from which the 'objects' are viewed. It is relevant to consider this here because, in conjunction with the other dichotomous factors, this distinction affects the shape of the phenomenon of insight that is elicited. Thus, when the 'object' of insight assessment is approached from the perspective of *insight*, e.g. insight into mental symptoms, or awareness of activities of daily living, or insight into behavioural changes, etc. the phenomenon of insight that ensues will naturally include additional judgements relating to the degree or extent of insight held. This will occur irrespective of how narrow or wide the elicited phenomenon becomes. In other words, from the perspective of 'insight' (or 'awareness'), the 'object' of insight assessment will demand a phenomenon that, whether or not taken up in research or empirical terms, incorporates judgements that involve ratings of the insight. For example, exploring insight into mental symptoms or awareness of memory problems, etc. will determine a phenomenon of insight based on judgements which can include the *extent* of knowledge individuals will have concerning their mental symptoms or their memory problems. Again, the issue is not whether in empirical terms such knowledge is actually sought. The point is, however, that the phenomenon of insight elicited in relation to this perspective has the potential in terms of its structure to include such judgements.

On the other hand, when the 'object' of insight assessment is approached from the perspective of '*insightlessness*', for example, unawareness of mental symptoms, or anosognosia in relation to hemiplegia or amnesia, etc., the phenomenon of insight that ensues is generally much more limited or narrower in structure simply because the other judgements do not follow in the same sort of way. Thus, and as was mentioned earlier, if an individual has no insight into his/her inability to move a leg or no insight into the fact that he/she has memory problems, then judgements concerning degree or extent to which the individual does not know cannot develop. If a patient does not 'know' that he/she is unable to walk, then he/she cannot judge the effect of this inability. In fact, as we have seen, speaking empirically, judgements have been incorporated into measures purporting to evaluate 'unawareness' or 'anosognosia' but in those situations, what is actually being assessed is degree of awareness and it becomes a purely semantic point. From the theoretical perspective, however, and borne out by the historical origins of the conceptualisations of insight (in general psychiatry) and insightlessness (in neurosciences), respectively, the following observation can be made. The phenomenon of insight determined by the 'object' of insight assessment will be narrower and more circumscribed in structure when approached from the perspective of *insightlessness* than when elicited from the perspective of *insight*.

It has to be acknowledged that, the dichotomies identified here with respect to the 'object' of insight assessment are not operating independently but interact in terms of their effects on the phenomenon of insight. Separating them as has been done in this section, however, helps to demonstrate the various different ways in which the nature of the 'object' of insight assessment will influence the structure of the phenomenon of insight elicited.

7.4 Conclusion

Insight is a relational or 'intentional' concept, i.e. it is only understood in terms of its relation to something. It makes little sense to talk about a person's insight without there being something to have insight about. This 'something' has been referred to as the 'object' of insight assessment and, in clinical practice, includes any chosen state relating to the individual: mental or physical, pathological or non-pathological. It has been argued that the 'object' of insight assessment has a crucial role in determining and shaping the clinical phenomenon of insight. In contrast to the previous chapter where the clinical phenomenon of insight was explored in terms of some of the definitional problems around the conceptualisation of insight itself and the interpretational issues inherent to the elicitation of the phenomenon, here the clinical phenomenon of insight is explored in the context of its relational aspects, namely from the perspective of its 'object'.

Three separate ways in which the 'object' of insight assessment can shape the clinical phenomenon of insight have been identified. Firstly, the 'object' of insight assessment is itself embedded within the conceptual framework guiding or underlying a particular professional discipline. This same conceptual framework will impose a similar structure (in terms of rules, concepts, assumptions, language, etc.) on the phenomenon of insight elicited within that discipline. Secondly, the semantic category to which the 'object' of insight assessment belongs (i.e. the type of term to which the 'object' refers) will exert its specific structure on the phenomenon of insight. This is particularly apparent when considering the difference in order of meaning between 'objects' referring to a wide multifactorial construct such as 'mental illness' and those referring to a narrower 'objectively' determined concept such as 'neurological' or 'neuropsychological impairment'. Thirdly, the specific nature of the 'object' of insight assessment itself will determine to some extent the sort of insight phenomenon that will be elicited. In this context, it is shown that various dichotomous factors can play a part in the shaping of the insight phenomenon. Among those, of particular importance is the subjective–objective dichotomy, i.e. whether the nature of the 'object' of insight assessment refers to a subjective state as opposed to a so-called 'objective' state. Where, in fact, the 'object' of insight assessment refers to subjective states (e.g. depressed mood, hearing voices, feeling persecuted, etc.), the core structure of the phenomenon of insight elicited must, by definition, share the structural components of the 'object', i.e. the subjective state, itself. In other words, in the articulation of subjective complaints, individuals are making judgements of their experiences based on awareness of those experiences. Consequently, a core aspect of the phenomenon of insight will be inherent to the subjective complaints themselves. This necessitates the phenomenon of insight in relation to such states to form a broader structure, one which includes wider judgements concerning the nature, meaning and effects of such experiences on the self.

The relational aspects of insight carry important implications for understanding and research on insight. Most importantly, since clinical phenomena of insight are determined to some extent by the 'object' of insight assessment, then phenomena of insight in relation to different 'objects' of insight assessment will vary in structure and, consequently, will likely involve different underlying mechanisms. This means that assumptions held concerning equivalence between insight phenomena in relation to different clinical studies will need to be qualified. Similarly, results of different studies will need to be interpreted in the context of the particular insight phenomenon under investigation.

8

Towards a structure of insight: awareness and insight, an essential distinction?

Various conceptual issues arising in the study of insight have now been identified and their likely role explored with respect to providing some explanation for the variable results obtained in empirical work on insight. It is evident that empirical research on insight faces many difficulties most of which relate to the ways insight is treated theoretically and to the sense that is made of the clinical phenomenon elicited. These, in turn, reflect the complexities inherent to the nature of insight as a concept. It remains crucial, however, notwithstanding the difficulties involved, to continue with efforts focused on clarifying and understanding the conceptual problems surrounding the study of insight. The meaningfulness of empirical studies, i.e. their theoretical significance and clinical importance as well as their limitations, is necessarily dependent on the level of such conceptual understanding. While the previous chapters focused on unpacking some of these conceptual problems, these last two chapters aim to bring together the identified points and issues with a view to developing a basic preliminary structure for the concept of insight. This chapter focuses on exploring the distinction between awareness and insight, and determines this as theoretically important and clinically relevant. The next chapter explores the relationship between awareness and insight in the context of a proposed overall structure for insight.

In Chapter 1, and following Berrios (1994a; 1996), it was pointed out that terms, concepts and behaviours do not inevitably correspond in a one-to-one manner to an object of inquiry. Thus, in order to understand the historical origins and development of the object in question, it is necessary to deal with the histories of the terms, concepts and behaviours independently, before points of convergence can be considered. This method was followed in the historical Chapter. It is of interest, however, how the subsequent reviews of empirical studies on insight in different clinical conditions bring this lack of correspondence to a particularly overt focus, although clearly from a different, i.e. non-historical perspective. This is evidenced mainly through the use of a range of related terms to variably defined concepts. As was shown in the previous chapters, the *same term* could be used to refer to different sorts of concepts (e.g. 'lack of insight' could refer to both a lack of perception of a deficit/problem as well as to a lack of an understanding of the nature and consequences of the problem). Equally, *different terms* could be used to refer to a similar sort of concept (e.g. 'unawareness', 'poor insight', 'anosognosia', 'denial', 'impaired self-awareness', etc. used interchangeably to refer to one particular concept of lack of recognition of problems). The interchangeable use of related terms ostensibly referring to one concept is particularly apparent in studies exploring insight in organic brain syndromes (e.g. Verhey *et al.*, 1993; Chapter 5). Occasionally, in such studies, conceptual distinctions are made between the uses of the different terms (e.g. Reed *et al.*, 1993; Weinstein *et al.*, 1994; Vasterling *et al.*, 1995) but in the main such distinctions are infrequent and, moreover, tend to be inconsistent in regards to the content of the ensuing conceptual categories. For example, Reed *et al.* (1993) use the terms 'anosognosia' and 'unawareness of memory impairment' interchangeably but distinguish these from 'denial' which they view as referring to a different concept, one incorporating affective changes. On the other hand, Weinstein *et al.* (1994) use the terms 'anosognosia' and 'denial' interchangeably but distinguish these terms from 'loss of insight' which they conceive as a different concept.

However, despite this source of confusion from the terminology and conceptual referents, I would argue that one distinction has emerged particularly, clearly and consistently in both the empirical research reviewed and in the conceptual analyses carried out. This is the general *conceptual* distinction between insight as a concept in the *narrow* sense (i.e. solely concentrated on awareness or perception of a problem, henceforth termed 'awareness') and insight as a concept in a *wide* or broad sense (i.e. involving other sorts of judgements in addition to the awareness of a problem, henceforth termed 'insight'). The important question, however, lies in whether this distinction in concepts is a valid distinction, in the sense of being meaningful from the perspective of understanding the structure of insight and in terms of its usefulness for the further exploration of insight empirically. This chapter, therefore, is concerned with addressing this question by firstly, clarifying the theoretical grounds for the distinction and secondly, by providing some empirical justification for the distinction.

8.1 Theoretical grounds for distinguishing between awareness and insight

As mentioned above, setting aside the variable terminology, the literature and research that was examined in the earlier chapters provide grounds for making a conceptual division between 'awareness' and 'insight' as a narrow and wide conceptualisation of insight, respectively. In other words, despite the interchangeable use of *terms* (including awareness, insight, etc.), two distinct *concepts* relating to insight can be identified as running in parallel, albeit, also converging and interacting. The distinguishing point between these concepts, I will argue, revolves around the narrowness or breadth of the concept involved and, as already stated, the terms 'awareness' and 'insight' will be used, respectively, from now on, to refer to these specific senses. The immediate question that arises with respect to this claim, must be what are the grounds for making this particular distinction? After all, we have seen throughout the book that in fact, there appear to be numerous distinctions between the various ways in which insight is conceived and, indeed, this fact has been continuously discussed and emphasised. However, the point I want to make here is that, whilst there are many different distinctions proffered in the conceptualisation of insight, the distinction between 'awareness' and 'insight' is of unique importance firstly, because this has direct implications for the structure of insight and, secondly, because this is essential for understanding the clinical phenomena elicited in relation to these concepts. In order to substantiate this claim we first need to understand what specifically is meant by a narrow and a wide concept of insight in the context of the sorts of conceptual distinctions that can be identified. Therefore, it is important to revisit some of the distinctions that have been made in the literature between concepts of insight in order to then identify and focus on the features that differentiate the nature of this particular distinction, i.e. on the 'narrow' (as 'awareness') and 'wide' (as 'insight') concept, from other types of distinctions.

Chapter 1 referred to some of the distinctions formulated by the earlier alienists. For example, amongst patients who seemed to show some insight into their condition, i.e. those who were aware of the pathological nature of their experiences, Billod (1870) distinguished between those who, despite this awareness, judged their psychotic symptoms as 'real' and those who judged their psychotic symptoms as 'false', albeit still experiencing distress as a result. Parant (1888) made several additional distinctions between different forms of insight that patients could show. These were based on other types of judgements, e.g. judgements concerning the morality of their actions, judgements that their experiences were pathological, discrepancies between patients' judgements, their behaviours and so on. Pick (1882), using the term 'awareness of illness' (*Krankheitsbewußtsein*) conceived a broad concept of understanding that patients had concerning the pathological nature of their experiences and divided this further into 'awareness of feeling ill' (*Krankheitsgefühl*) and 'insight into illness' (*Krankheitseinsicht*). In other words, his distinction was based on changes in *feeling* in the case of the former and processes of *reason* or *reflection* in the case of the latter. On the other hand, Arndt (1905) argued for this same distinction (i.e. between awareness of feeling ill and insight into illness) to be based on the degree of clarity with which the feeling/knowledge was experienced. Influenced to some extent by Pick, Jaspers (1948) made a distinction between 'awareness of illness' (*Krankheitsbewußtsein*) and 'insight proper' (*Krankheitseinsicht*). He conceived the former concept as referring to experiences of feeling ill and changed but without this capturing all symptoms or the illness as a whole. The latter, on the other hand, referred to a concept which encompassed a correct assessment made by the patient of the nature and severity of all symptoms together with the illness as a whole affecting him/her. Therefore, it can be seen that various types of distinctions between concepts of insight were made. Divisions have been drawn, e.g. between thoughts and feelings (Jaspers, 1948; Pick, 1882), between thoughts and behaviours (Parant, 1888), between degrees of clarity/detail in knowledge (Arndt, 1905; Aschaffenburg, 1915) and between specific types of thoughts/judgements (Billod, 1870; Parant, 1888), etc.

If we move on to the clinical areas of general psychiatry and psychoanalytic psychology, we find that again various distinctions between the concepts of insight have been made. In general psychiatry, it was pointed out that views of insight ranged from the more narrow, such as recognition of illness (Wing *et al.*, 1974; Heinrichs *et al.*, 1985), to much wider concepts which included further judgements demanded in relation to a variety of aspects of the patient's experiences (Greenfeld *et al.*, 1989; David, 1990; Amador *et al.*, 1991; Marková & Berrios, 1992a). The distinctions contained within these various conceptions of insight thus lie around the numbers and types of judgements involved concerning the patients' experiences. In some cases the judgement or acknowledgement of being 'ill' was sufficient in itself to constitute insight and in other cases, additional elaborations concerning views about the nature of illness or symptoms, the social consequences of the illness, need for treatment, etc. were necessary to determine insight (Chapter 3). In psychoanalytic psychology, we have seen that insight has been conceived even more broadly so that the judgements demanded of individuals in the elicitation of the phenomenon have been more complex. Here, distinctions between such judgements have been made not only with respect to the different *types* of judgements, i.e. extent of understanding patients have of different aspects of their experiences, but also of the *ways* in which such judgements might be assimilated. Thus, distinctions are made according to whether knowledge is attained in a relatively more superficial sense (e.g. intellectual, cognitive or descriptive insight) or whether it is in a relatively deeper sense (e.g. ostensive or emotional insight, etc.) and according to the extent to which judgements relate to more 'hidden' knowledge including unconscious processes underlying motivations and actions (Reid & Finesinger, 1952; Richfield, 1954; Chapter 2).

In neurological states (Chapters 4 and 5), we saw that there was a much more explicitly described polarity between *awareness* (or unawareness) of neurological impairment in the narrow sense and *denial* of impairment in the wider sense. The former referred to insight as the perception or awareness of the specific impairment and the resultant phenomenon of awareness was thus simply based on judgements acknowledging the presence of the impairment. On the face of it, this particular conception of insight is striking in its immediate contrast to the views of insight seen in the psychiatric literature where even the relatively narrow conceptions of insight lacked the clearly-defined and circumscribed boundaries of the 'neurological' concept. As was demonstrated, instruments for assessing the clinical phenomenon of awareness or unawareness have become increasingly sophisticated in terms of their attempts at characterising awareness. However, this core concept has remained focused on the narrow sense of awareness and subsequent distinctions have revolved around judgements concerning the specific features of the *impairment* (i.e. severity, frequency of problems caused, etc.). Denial, on the other hand, referred to a concept in which awareness of the impairment was viewed as implicit, or present at some level. Nevertheless, this was prevented from becoming overtly manifest through the patient's psychological processes acting to 'protect' the patient from the distress engendered by the knowledge (Weinstein & Kahn, 1955). Thus, this broader concept includes within its definition a postulated reason for the manifested phenomenon.

Therefore, it is apparent that various types of distinctions have been made in studies of insight in the different clinical areas and disciplines. It can be argued that they all range in different ways from 'narrow' to 'wide' concepts. However, amongst the various distinctions, there does seem to be a more prominent and consistent difference between views of insight in the *narrow* sense as in the neurosciences and the views of insight in the *broader* sense as in general psychiatry and psychoanalytic psychology. Whether some of the additional distinctions proposed within this latter broad concept of insight (such as the distinctions mentioned above made by the earlier alienists and those seen in the studies within general psychiatry and psychoanalytic psychology) are theoretically important and/or clinically useful remains to be answered and may form empirical questions of the future. However, the important issue here is that those latter distinctions are still bound within a broad concept of insight and there is not the clear separation of concepts that there seems to be when *awareness* as the narrow concept and *insight* as the broad concept are contrasted. This is evident not only in the explicit definitions used in the neurosciences and psychiatric clinical areas but also in the ways in which the respective phenomena of insight are elicited/manifested and evaluated.

Before focusing more specifically on the difference between awareness and insight, further grounds for this distinction are also evident from the exploration of the relationship between the phenomenon of insight and its relational 'object' (Chapter 7). Disciplinary backgrounds were found to be important in this respect and it was shown how 'objects' of insight assessment embedded in different theoretical backgrounds could determine phenomena of insight that differed in their narrowness or breadth. However, more significant was the influence of the kind or nature of the 'object' of insight assessment itself in shaping the phenomenon of insight elicited. Here, it became particularly apparent how, according to their nature, 'objects' could determine the narrowness or breadth of the phenomenon of insight. In this regard, the features of 'objects' of insight which were found to determine a broader phenomenon of insight, in terms of the complexity of judgements demanded and their relationship to the self, were those relating to *subjectivity* (where insight is explored into an experience that by definition incorporates some awareness), *positivity* (where insight is explored into the presence of an abnormal experience) and where the 'object' of insight was explored from the *perspective* of insight as opposed to insightlessness. Furthermore, where 'objects' of insight assessment referred to a more complex construct (such as 'mental disorder'), the phenomenon of insight determined by this 'object' was correspondingly broader in terms of its contained judgements. It is of important note that all these features relating to the 'objects' of insight assessment are those most characteristic of 'objects' as defined mainly in psychiatric disciplines. In the neurosciences, on the other hand, the 'objects' of insight assessment are more likely to be *objective* in nature (referring to the issue of being determined specifically by tests or a clinician), *negative* in type (referring to the absence or impairment of normal function) and approached from the *perspective* of insightlessness. In turn, such 'objects' as was demonstrated earlier, determine a phenomenon of insight that has to be much narrower and circumscribed in structure.

8.1.1 Nature of the boundary between awareness and insight

Therefore, so far we have seen from the literature that the broad distinction between awareness and insight is suggested by the way in which insight has been conceptualised and clinically evaluated within the different clinical disciplines. We have seen how the neurosciences have tended to favour the narrower conception of awareness, driven by their particular theoretical framework together with the nature of the 'object' of insight assessment encountered by their disciplines. Likewise, the psychiatric disciplines have tended to favour the wider conception of insight, driven in turn by their particular theoretical framework together with the specific types of 'object' of insight assessment met with in general psychiatry. Therefore, the next question concerns the nature of the specific distinction between awareness and insight that is being claimed above. How can narrowness and width be defined in this sense? In other words, where is the line that, it is argued, demarcates the narrow concept of awareness from the wider concept of insight? When exactly do judgements become of the sort and complexity that would indicate insight rather than awareness?

As already emphasised, this crucial distinction seems to emerge most clearly from the comparison of conceptions of insight between the neurological/neuropsychological clinical areas on the one hand and the psychiatric/psychoanalytic psychological clinical areas on the other. Determined, as was shown in the previous chapter, by the nature of the 'object' of insight as a neurological or neuropsychological deficit or loss of function, the conception of insight in the neurosciences has focused on awareness in its most narrow sense, i.e. perception of, or knowledge at its simplest level in relation to, a particular stimulus (or in this case loss of stimulus). However, we have seen that 'narrow' conceptions of insight have also been found in the work of the earlier alienists as well as in the empirical research reviewed in general psychiatry. Therefore, why is the line being drawn between awareness as construed in the neurosciences and awareness or insight as presented in the various psychiatric clinical areas?

The answer appears to lie once again in the crucial difference between the 'objects' of insight assessment in these respective areas. Even when the most narrow views of insight within psychiatry are examined (narrow in the sense of being presented as unitary definitions with no further explication), e.g. 'awareness of emotional problems' or 'recognition of mental illness', the phenomenon of insight/awareness demanded by the 'objects' in these cases, i.e. 'emotional problems' or 'mental illness', will always be wider than the phenomenon of insight/awareness determined by the 'objects' focused on in the neurosciences (i.e. neurological deficits or neuropsychological impairments). In other words, and for reasons that were explored in the previous chapter, whether termed 'awareness' or 'insight', the phenomenon sought and elicited within psychiatry (and psychoanalytic psychology) will be constituted of judgements which reach beyond that of an awareness or perception of 'impairment'. In a sense, awareness or perception of change must, to some extent, be a given in the conceptualisation of insight within psychiatry (with some qualifications, see later) but it is, in effect, the subsequent judgements based on this awareness that constitute insight. This is the case because, again as was demonstrated in the previous chapter, insight or awareness of, e.g. 'mental symptoms', in reality refers to more than the awareness of the *presence* of the symptoms (in an akin manner to the presence of a neurological impairment). In addition, it refers to awareness of the *sense* the mental symptoms make to the patient, i.e. of the judgements he/she makes concerning the nature and/or morbidity of the experiences. Likewise, insight or awareness of having a 'mental illness' refers to the *judgements* the patient makes in the context of awareness of a variety of subjective experiences. It is thus these judgements that are determined by the 'objects' of insight in psychiatry that constitute the difference between *awareness* and *insight*. In turn, it is the nature of the differences in 'objects' (with respect to the relevant discipline, the category type and the relative position along the dichotomous dimensions identified earlier, Chapter 7), determining the presence of such judgements, that fixes this distinction between awareness and insight. Distinctions between various concepts of insight identified by the early alienists or those identified in the empirical exploration of insight in general psychiatry are based on the types of subsequent *judgements* made on, already assumed, awareness of experiences. On the other hand, the distinction between the concept of insight in the neurosciences and the concept of insight in psychiatry is based on the focus on awareness in the former and focus on judgements based on awareness in the latter. Awareness may be a necessary component of insight but it is not a sufficient component in the conceptualisation of insight as explored in psychiatry.

Having provided some grounds for making the specific distinction between awareness and insight both in terms of reviewing the sorts of conceptual distinctions that have been made within different clinical areas and by arguing for the crucial role that the 'object' of insight assessment has in determining the narrowness and width of the phenomenon elicited, the question remains as to where, in practical terms, this boundary between awareness and insight lies. One way to address this question is to compare the clinical phenomena that are elicited in relation to each of these concepts, i.e. in relation to *awareness* and *insight* and thus examine in clinical terms the sorts of features representative of both.

8.1.2 Awareness and insight: similarities and differences

8.1.2.1 Phenomenon of awareness

Taking first the phenomenon of awareness as elicited or manifested in relation to neurological deficits or impairments, we have stressed that the phenomenon is based on a narrow conception of awareness as a simple perception of the deficit/impairment. Thus, measures to assess this awareness have focused on, firstly, determining whether awareness of the impairment is present or absent and, secondly, provided that awareness is present, then on characterising this in terms of the specific impairment (or 'object') itself. In other words, degrees of awareness are evaluated with respect to the perception or judgement on the part of the patient of the severity of their problem, or the frequency with which the problem interferes with something, or how it compares with 'before' or with 'healthy' people, etc. This gives a *quantitative* measure of awareness (a patient is said to have no awareness, full awareness or a measure/score in between) but, at the same time and somewhat confusingly, gives an impression of a qualitative assessment. However, this impression of a qualitative assessment comes from the fact, that it is the qualitative aspects of the impairment itself that are being sought by the awareness measure rather than the qualitative aspects of awareness. In other words, *it is not the nature of the awareness in relation to the 'object' (impairment) that the patient is being asked about, but, the awareness in relation to the nature of the 'object' (impairment).* Thus, in a sense, so-called qualitative aspects of awareness are elicited only on the basis of qualitative aspects of the impairment, i.e. the 'object' itself, as far as these can be gauged by the external individual (e.g. types of memory problems experienced as assessed by a range of psychometric tests, types of activities of daily living the patient is unable to carry out independently, etc.). Awareness, *per se*, is therefore evaluated principally quantitatively. In fact, this makes sense given the nature of the 'object' of awareness assessment explored in the neurosciences, namely its *negative* (i.e. loss or impairment of function) and *objective* qualities (i.e. directly evident on observation or tests). Consequently, as far as awareness is concerned, the focus has to be on the patient's understanding of the impairment in terms of the actual observable effects. And, because these observable effects can only be assessed by means of quantitative measures (frequency of problems experienced, degree of severity of problem, etc.), then awareness as a phenomenon is elicited in a quantitative way. Qualitative aspects of awareness are simply not accessible to the external person (clinician/carer). Hence, no comparisons between patient and another individual can be made for the purpose of determining the patients' 'knowledge' or perception of what is happening to them. The only qualitative features that are accessible for the purpose of such comparison are those features that characterise the impairment itself. As already emphasised previously, the intrinsic relationship between insight and the 'object' of insight assessment means that as far as the phenomenon of insight or awareness is concerned, the focus of qualitative features will lie on the 'object' of awareness in this case rather than on the 'awareness' itself. This is not to say that qualitative features of awareness are never elicited within the neurosciences disciplines. There are many different areas of clinical experiences where qualitative aspects of awareness are sought specifically, as in delineating abnormal sensory experiences e.g. phantom limb, or even in characterising various pains. However, the issue in these situations is different. The qualitative changes in awareness that are explored in these contexts are not carried out from the perspective of examining the understanding the patient has about a particular experience but from the perspective of describing and presenting the particular symptom concerned.

8.1.2.2 Phenomenon of insight

Looking in turn at the phenomenon of insight as elicited or manifested in relation to mental illness or mental symptoms, we have stressed that the phenomenon is based on a wider conceptualisation of insight in that it is constituted of a complex of both awareness of change and, significantly, on further judgements concerning the perceived nature and/or morbidity of the change. As argued previously, it is the *nature* of these further judgements that makes the concept of insight in this sense much wider. Even when termed '*awareness of mental illness*' or '*awareness of mental symptom*', the concept referred to is necessarily more than 'awareness' simply because of the *types* of judgements determined by the 'objects' of insight contained in each term. This is reflected in the phenomenon of insight elicited/manifested.

For example, the sorts of judgements that might be involved in making the decision relating to having a 'mental illness' will have to reach out to diverse aspects of knowledge and experience. This will include the individual's own views on the definition of 'mental illness', which, in turn, is likely to be based, amongst other things, on several kinds of knowledge. Among these, is the general knowledge (e.g. information from books, media, peers, etc.), and the personal knowledge held by the individual (e.g. past experiences in relation to self/others, the degree to which subjective experience is thought to match the theoretical knowledge/past experiences, etc.), as well as the way such knowledge is shaped and affected by the individual's own attitudes (i.e. in terms of general views of the world, personal biases, cultural perspectives, etc.). Similarly, the sorts of judgements that might be involved in making the decision concerning the morbidity of the 'mental symptom' will also have to draw on a wide range of mental activities. These will include a personal/individual interpretation of the subjective experience, which, in turn, is also likely to be based on a variety of factors (e.g. intensity of subjective experience, difference from 'normal' experience, context in which occurring, past experience, general understanding about mental illness, etc.).

Therefore, the judgements involved in making *sense* of an experience (whether this is demanded in terms of 'mental illness' or 'mental symptom') incorporate a range of heterogeneous judgements diverse in contents and type, and complexity. Thus, in contrast to the concept of awareness, the concept of insight, even in a narrow sense, in relation to psychiatric states, has an inherent *qualitative* aspect, which can be addressed in the elicitation of the clinical phenomenon. Patients are asked to judge in a wider sense what it is that they are experiencing in terms of what the experience means for *them* and how this might affect *them* in their ability to function and/or relate to others and possible implications for *them* (e.g. need for treatment) (Chapter 3). These judgements relate not just to the 'objective' characteristics of the problem or experience but to the personal *sense* the individuals make of these characteristics and, more directly, to the sense in which the experience is related to *themselves*. Consequently, such judgements are by their very nature qualitative in type, drawing on a wide range of experiences and knowledge held by the individual and related to the self. Here, in contrast to awareness, *it is the nature of insight in relation to the 'object' (mental illness/mental symptoms) that is being demanded of patients rather than insight in relation to the nature of the 'object' (mental illness)*. Insight, as a phenomenon, is thus assessed both quantitatively (patients can be said to have no insight, full insight or again a measure/score in between) and qualitatively (patients can be evaluated on the sorts of judgements they are expressing). This makes sense given the nature of the 'object' of insight assessment concerned, namely, its *positive* (presence of an abnormal/different experience) and its *subjective* (not accessible in a direct way by the external person) qualities. Hence, as far as insight is concerned, the focus has to be on the patient's understanding of the abnormal experience in terms of what sense the patient makes of his/her symptoms, how this links up with his/her knowledge and views, etc. These sorts of judgements are assessed by means of both quantitative (degree to which patient acknowledges problem) and qualitative (types of judgements expressed, e.g. acknowledgement of impact on different aspect of life, views on need for different treatments, views on cause of problems or experiences, etc.) measures. Qualitative aspects of insight are therefore inherent to the contents of judgements demanded. Thus, in contrast to the phenomenon of awareness in relation to impairments, the phenomenon of insight intrinsically linked to its 'object' of insight assessment will have its focus on qualitative features directed at the phenomenon itself rather than at the 'object' of insight.

8.1.2.3 Distinctions between awareness and insight

To illustrate the above described difference between 'awareness' and 'insight', it may be useful to look at specific instances. For example, the phenomenon of awareness into memory problems may be elicited by asking the individual to judge certain aspects of their memory, e.g. how frequently they experience memory difficulties or how severe these are considered to be, how they compare to memory of other people, etc. It is clear that generally such judgements tend to relate predominantly to features of memory function itself. The extent of the patient's awareness is based on the comparison between the patient's judgements and the clinician's/other's judgements of these memory function features. The phenomenon of insight into psychosis, on the other hand, may be elicited by asking the patient to judge his/her psychotic experiences. For example, the patient might be asked to decide what they represent, to determine whether they are abnormal or pathological, to think about whether they are related to a possible illness, to give a view whether treatment is needed, to give an opinion whether and/or in what way they affect functioning or have any impact on his/her life, etc. Such judgements, in contrast to the phenomenon of awareness into memory problems, relate less to 'objective' features of the abnormal experiences and more to a wider assimilation and interpretation of problems by the individual in relation to him/herself.

Bringing together some of the identified features helping to characterise and to distinguish between awareness and insight as distinct phenomena, it is evident that both reflect concepts which refer to some knowledge or understanding individuals have about themselves or about particular problems affecting them. Both have at some point been defined as *not* all-or-none concepts/phenomena and hence, could be described in quantitative terms. Individuals can have more or less insight and more or less awareness. We have seen that the concept of awareness, as used in the neurosciences, has referred predominantly to a perception or acknowledgement of some change happening to the self (i.e. loss of or impairment in some function or absence of a normal experience) as experienced by the individual. Judgements in this sense are simple in type because they refer to a *direct* appraisal of a specific impairment and can range from recognition of change (understanding there is a change and perhaps identifying the nature of the change, i.e. giving it a name) to evaluation of the severity/intensity of the change. Awareness is evaluated *quantitatively*. The qualitative aspects arising from awareness measures refer to the qualitative features imposed by the impairment itself. If the structure of the phenomenon of awareness is viewed as comprising of both the phenomenon of awareness together with its 'object' of awareness assessment in the bi-directional relationship as described earlier, then the focus of the qualitative aspects of awareness can be conceived as directed at the 'object'.

On the other hand, the concept of insight as used in general psychiatry has referred predominantly to a much wider concept of knowledge admitted by an individual. Judgements are complex in type because they refer to an *indirect* appraisal of a change to the self and depend on a range of subsidiary judgements relating to an individual's general knowledge, views, perceptions, past experiences, etc. Such judgements also range from recognition of change (understanding there is a change and perhaps identifying the nature of the change, i.e. giving it a name) to evaluation of the severity/intensity of the change, thus allowing for a quantitative assessment. However, in addition judgements are of a range and nature that enable a *qualitative* assessment. Here, the qualitative aspects of insight arising in relation to insight measures refer to the qualitative features imposed by the judgements themselves both in terms of the types of contents but also in terms of their self-directedness. Again, if the structure of the phenomenon of insight is viewed as comprising of both the phenomenon of insight together with its 'object' of insight assessment in the bi-directional relationship, then the focus of the qualitative aspects of insight in this case can be conceived as directed at the phenomenon rather than the 'object'.

Are there any other differences that can be identified between awareness as a narrow concept and insight as a wider concept? In fact, another interesting factor is raised when making a comparison between impaired awareness in patients and impaired insight in patients and that is one of *directionality*. This issue will be highlighted more clearly in the next section when an empirical study illustrating this will be examined. Here, however, in brief, one can consider the situation where a patient may complain of pain, which, to the external person or clinician, may appear to be out of proportion to the likely actual pain (as far as this can be evaluated). Alternatively, another situation might be one where patients are worried about some sort of minor deformity (e.g. blemish or scar on their face) to the extent that their beliefs and behaviours are adversely affected (e.g. they stop socialising with friends, use uncomfortable masking devices, believe they are ugly, etc.). In both these situations, one could argue that they seem to show *reduced insight* into their problems (i.e. it could be said that their judgements concerning the nature and effects of the 'objects' seem to be somewhat distorted or out of proportion to what is 'objectively' ascertainable). On the other hand, it could equally be argued that they seem to show *increased awareness* or apparent awareness of their problems (i.e. they are judging the 'object' of awareness to be of particularly high intensity).

In fact, because ultimately the patient's views are compared with those of the clinician, in these situations the problems would be formulated in terms of the patient's insight rather than the patient's awareness (even if termed interchangeably). This shows very obviously that reduced insight is not the same as reduced awareness.

The issue of directionality would seem to be of some importance in also distinguishing between the concepts of awareness and insight. Thus, awareness is generally conceived in terms of a *reduction* or absence of awareness in relation to a particular 'object' (e.g. in relation to memory impairment, to hemiplegia, etc.). When awareness is conceived or discussed in terms of an increase in awareness, this tends to be a relative increase from a level of poor awareness, rather than an increase from a 'normal' level of awareness (e.g. patients showing increased awareness of their difficulties/limitations following rehabilitation, etc.). Other situations when increased awareness may be conceived include the sorts of clinical experiences where qualitative aspects of awareness are also explored, e.g. some of the brain stimulation studies or various forms of epilepsy, but again here the focus is not on the understanding a patient is showing in relation to his/her experiences but on the nature of the experience itself.

Insight, on the other hand, tends to be more easily conceived as increasing as well as decreasing with respect to a 'normal' level. This difference between the two concepts is likely to be due to a number of factors. Firstly, the clinical backgrounds relating to these concepts are important. Awareness, in the neurosciences has tended to be modelled along neurological and neuropsychological frames in which 'awareness systems' (generalised or inherent to specific cognitive functions) are seen as structures or functions which can 'go wrong' in the same sort of way that other cognitive functions do. Thus, whilst it is conceivable that an awareness structure or function can become damaged by some brain lesion or disease, it is much more difficult to think of the same structure or function becoming enhanced in some way (without invoking the use of some specific stimulatory techniques akin to those used to enhance other aspects of cognitive function). The clinical background of insight in its broad conceptualisation is, as we have seen, very different and, in various ways, the psychiatric disciplines, psychoanalytic psychology and indeed Gestalt psychology all contribute to determining the potential for the concept of insight to increase as well as decrease from a 'normal' level. From the perspective of the psychiatric and psychoanalytic psychologies, this seems to relate to the issue of the complexity and of the judgements involved in constituting insight and the fact that, as was discussed earlier (Chapter 6), there is no clearly defined boundary to the different types and qualities of knowledge that can be held in relation to different 'objects'. Thus, there is always the possibility or potential for increasing insight, even from a 'normal' level. In the case of Gestalt psychology, we saw that insight was conceived very much in terms of newly acquired knowledge, and hence, involved an increase in capacity to solve particular problems.

Secondly, once again, the 'object' of insight/awareness assessment is also important in contributing to this difference in directionality. In the case of the neurosciences, the 'object' of awareness assessment is generally a loss or impairment of a normal function. 'Normal' or full awareness is simply linked to the presence of the function. Generally, there is not a case for exploring awareness into normal neurological or neuropsychological function and, in a sense, it is taken for granted that an individual can be aware of normal neurological or neuropsychological processes. Thus, an individual walks, talks and recalls things and, if asked at the relevant points, will be able to say that he is aware of walking, of talking and of recalling things, though will not necessarily be occupied with this awareness during such activities. As was seen earlier, researchers have sought to determine degrees of awareness in healthy subjects with respect to more complex neuropsychological functions, such as different types of memory capacities. This has been done mainly to establish the validity of tests designed to evaluate the awareness of patients with impairment in such functions (e.g. prediction of performance on specific memory tests, McGlynn & Kaszniak, 1991a, b). However, when the function becomes impaired or lost, then awareness of this impairment or loss can either be preserved or be likewise impaired but it makes little sense to conceive of awareness as increasing from a 'normal' level.

In the case of general psychiatry, the 'object' of insight assessment generally refers to the presence or appearance of an abnormal experience. Here the situation is different because the individual is being asked to make judgements about his/her new or additional experience rather than about a loss or impairment of a normal function. It is not the question of a 'normal' insight held into the new experience simply because it is a new experience. In other words, an abnormal experience is not linked to normal insight in the same way as a normal function is linked to normal awareness. Patients making sense of their new experiences can be conceived as developing more or less insight. Indeed, ultimately it is potentially possible that patients attain a greater level of insight than they held in their pre-morbid state because of the types of judgements they may be invoking (e.g. exploring their ideas and views about themselves as well as their experiences). In a similar sort of way, individuals embarking on psychoanalytic psychological treatment where the 'object' of insight assessment may relate not just to abnormal experiences but to behaviours and patterns of thinking, it is possible to conceive insight as increasing with respect to the types of judgements that individuals are exploring in themselves.

8.2 Empirical justification for distinguishing between awareness and insight

Having explored some of the theoretical reasons for making a distinction between awareness as a narrow concept and insight as a broad concept, let us consider an empirical study that may help illustrate some of the issues raised. The study is described in detail elsewhere (Marková *et al.*, 2004) and here only the salient aspects are presented and discussed. Essentially, the study was designed to explore insight into memory problems in a heterogeneous group of patients attending a memory clinic, i.e. in patients presenting with memory problems of various aetiologies. Crucially, such aetiologies spanned both 'organic' (e.g. neurological, mainly dementia) and 'non-organic' (e.g. depression, anxiety and others) factors. Hence, this study contrasted from previous studies which tended to focus on the exploration of insight in relation to either memory problems in dementias (e.g. Verhey *et al.*, 1993; Seltzer *et al.*, 1995a; Duke *et al.*, 2002; Chapter 5) or amnesic syndromes (e.g. Schacter, 1991; 1992; Chapter 4) but did not, generally, cut across the organic/non-organic categories.

The more specific aim of the Marková *et al.* (2004) study was to compare insight between patients with an organic basis (i.e. neurological pathology) and patients without an organic basis (i.e. no neurological pathology) to their memory problems. This perspective was taken in the light of some of the conceptual problems around insight raised earlier. Thus, in order to circumvent some of the identified preconceptions resulting from the conventional conceptualisations of insight in neurological/neuropsychological and the psychiatric disciplines, patients' insight was explored, in a sense, independently of the cause of the memory problem. All patients presented with memory complaints; and thus 'memory complaints' were chosen as the 'object' of insight assessment. By using the same instrument to assess insight across the diagnostic categories (i.e. loosely, 'organic' and 'non-organic'), and applying the same 'object' of insight assessment ('memory complaints'), the intention was to compare insight manifested between the patient groups and assess whether the phenomena of insight shared common patterns and hence could be 'explained' in terms of a single concept of insight or whether different patterns emerged and needed reference to more than one concept.

8.2.1 Methods and subjects

Insight into memory complaints was assessed by means of a simple 19-item questionnaire, the Memory Insight Questionnaire (MIQ), which asked patients to rate their problems in various memory-related areas (general functioning, memory itself, language and cognition). Scoring on the MIQ items was based on a 4-point scale: 1: improvement; 2: no change; 3: mildly worse and 4: much worse. A higher total score thus indicated a greater degree of perceived problem. In line with other studies in this area, insight was determined as the discrepancy in ratings between patients and carers (therefore assuming that carers gave the 'correct' appraisal) and so carers were asked to rate their assessments of patients' problems using the same questionnaire (but referring to the patient). The level of insight was calculated as the *difference* between ratings by patients and carers.

One hundred consecutive patients referred to the 'Memory Clinic' at Addenbrooke's Hospital, Cambridge, were given the MIQ as part of their overall assessment. Patients attending the clinic were examined in turn by the neurology, psychiatry and neuropsychology teams. Patients received a core neuropsychology battery which included: Verbal IQ (WAIS-R), NART IQ, digit span, vocabulary, arithmetic, similarities, block design, fragmented letters (VOSP), McKenna Naming Test, Warrington Recognition Memory Test for words and faces, Wechsler Memory Scale for passages and designs (immediate and delayed recall), verbal fluency, WCST and/or the Weigl (details and references of individual tests are in Lezak (1995). Patients and carers were interviewed separately and in addition to the psychiatric interview, patients completed a core of computerised psychiatric questionnaires: General Health Questionnaire 28 (Goldberg & Hillier, 1979), Cognitive Failures Questionnaire (Broadbent et al., 1982), Beck Depression Inventory (Beck et al., 1961), Signal Detection Memory Test (Miller & Berrios: Recognition memory by means of a word-based signal detection analysis, unpublished, based on Miller & Lewis, 1977), Irritability Scale (Snaith et al., 1978), Dissociation Questionnaire (Riley, 1988) and a Personality Inventory (Bedford & Foulds, 1978). Additional questionnaires relating to specific problems were given where appropriate, e.g. Maudsley Obsessional Compulsive Inventory (Rachman & Hodgson, 1980). Carers were asked to complete the TRIMS behavioural problem checklist (Niederehe, 1988).

On the basis of a unified diagnosis by the three clinical teams and for the purpose of analysis, patients were divided into those with 'neurological' memory dysfunction ($n = 56$), henceforth termed the 'neurological' group and those without 'neurological' memory dysfunction ($n = 44$), henceforth termed the 'psychiatric' group. In broad terms, the neurological group mainly included patients with Alzheimer's disease ($n = 32$) and a few patients with vascular dementia, traumatic brain damage, cerebrovascular incidents and encephalitis. The psychiatric group included patients with affective disorders classifiable under ICD-10 (World Health Organisation, 1992) and DSM-IV (American Psychiatric Association, 1994) as either depressive and/or anxiety disorder. Many however, could not be classified within the above systems but nevertheless showed patterns of affective/cognitive and behavioural symptoms, and personality traits which seemed to be related to some ongoing mental/personality disorder. They all had distressing and disabling memory complaints.

8.2.2 Results of study

8.2.2.1 Sociodemographic and clinical comparisons

Sociodemographic data are shown in Table 8.1. The 'neurological' sample was slightly older but there were no other differences in terms of sex ratio, duration of memory problems, education, alcohol dependency or smoking.

Table 8.1 Neurological and psychiatric patients compared on socio-demographic variables

Variable	Neurological group ($n = 56$)	Psychiatric group ($n = 44$)	Statistics
Mean age (S.D.)	63.02 (12.76)	52.16 (11.64)	$P < 0.001$[a]
Sex (males:females)	34:22	23:21	NS[b]
Mean duration of memory complaints in months (S.D.)	39.79 (35.89) ($n = 56$)	51.45 (38.18) ($n = 42$)	NS[a]
Alcohol (significant:non-significant intake)	3:53 ($n = 56$)	3:40 ($n = 43$)	NS[b]
Smoking (significant:non-significant)	11:37 ($n = 48$)	4:36 ($n = 40$)	NS[b]
Education (primary:secondary:higher)	19:26:10 ($n = 55$)	14:20:9 ($n = 43$)	NS[b]

[a] t-test for independent samples.
[b] Chi-squared.
S.D.: Standard Deviation.

Comparison of the two samples in terms of the computerised psychiatric questionnaires is shown in Table 8.2 and of neuropsychological performance in Table 8.3.

The 'neurological' sample scored significantly lower on the Beck Depression Inventory ($P < 0.0135$) and had significantly higher scores on the Cognitive Failures Questionnaire ($P < 0.0015$) and on the Signal Detection Memory Test (d' scores: $P < 0.0015$).

Unsurprisingly, the neurological patient group performed significantly worse on a number of neuropsychological measurements, particularly on the memory tests for recognition and recall but also on the McKenna Naming Test, fragmented letters and similarities. The neurological patients were also significantly worse on tests of frontal lobe dysfunction, i.e. the WCST and/or the Weigl ($\chi^2 = 9.57$, $P < 0.001$).

8.2.2.2 Comparison of MIQ scores between neurological and psychiatric groups

Total insight scores

For each of the 19 items on the MIQ, the patient's score was subtracted from the carer's score. The 19 discrepancy values fell into three groups:

1 discrepancy $= 0$ – indicating full agreement (i.e. good insight),
2 positive discrepancy values – indicating that the patient's memory problem was evaluated as more severe by the carer than the patient (i.e. poor insight),

Table 8.2 Neurological and psychiatric groups compared on main psychiatric measurements

| Psychiatric measure[a] | Median value (inter-quartile range) | | Mann–Whitney U | Significance[b] 2-tailed |
	Neurological group	Psychiatric group		
Beck Depression Inventory	6 (2.25–12) (n = 44)	10.5 (6–19) (n = 44)	570.0	P < 0.0135
Carers' Checklist (TRIMS-BPC)	47 (26–82) (n = 47)	73 (24.5–122.5) (n = 29)	579.5	NS
Cognitive Failures Questionnaire	93 (75–98) (n = 39)	73.5 (58–83) (n = 44)	422.5	P < 0.0015
Dissociation Questionnaire	7.5 (6–12) (n = 24)	10 (8–11) (n = 31)	329.0	NS
General Health Questionnaire 28	4 (1–8.75) (n = 48)	8.5 (2.25–14) (n = 44)	766.5	NS
Maudsley Obsessional Compulsive Inventory	6.5 (3.25–9.25) (n = 8)	7 (4–14) (n = 19)	67.0	NS
Personality Inventory dominance subscale	29 (27–30) (n = 31)	29 (26.75–31) (n = 34)	514.0	NS
Personality Inventory extrapunitive subscale	27 (25–29) (n = 31)	27.5 (25–30) (n = 34)	479.0	NS
Personality Inventory intropunitive subscale	32 (30–33) (n = 31)	30.5 (29–32.25) (n = 34)	394.5	NS
Signal Detection Memory – β value	1.31 (0.7–3.08) (n = 44)	3.66 (1.49–8.38) (n = 44)	572.5	P < 0.015
Signal Detection Memory – d' value	1.27 (0.63–1.67) (n = 44)	1.9 (1.54–2.28) (n = 44)	436.5	P < 0.0015
Snaith's Irritability Questionnaire – anxiety subscale	3 (2–5) (n = 34)	5 (3–9) (n = 35)	411.5	NS
Snaith's Irritability Questionnaire – depression subscale	3 (2.75–5) (n = 34)	5 (2–8) (n = 35)	478.0	NS
Snaith's Irritability Questionnaire – inward irritability	3 (1–4) (n = 34)	3 (1–4) (n = 35)	566.0	NS
Snaith's Irritability Questionnaire – outward irritability	3 (1–5) (n = 34)	4 (3–6) (n = 35)	457.5	NS

[a] References for psychiatric measures are in text.
[b] Bonferroni corrected.

3 negative discrepancy values – indicating that the patient's memory problem was evaluated as more severe by the patient than the carer (i.e. poor insight).

To obtain a quantitative assessment of insight in terms of the size by which evaluations were discrepant, the discrepancy values for all 19 items were added up for

Table 8.3 Neurological and psychiatric groups compared on main neuropsychological measurements

Neuropsychology measure[a]	Median value (inter-quartile range)		Mann–Whitney U	Significance[b] 2-tailed
	Neurological group	Psychiatric group		
Verbal IQ	96.5 (85.25–106.75) ($n = 44$)	103 (90–112) ($n = 31$)	518.5	NS
Arithmetic	9 (7–12) ($n = 46$)	11 (8–13) ($n = 31$)	565.5	NS
Block Design	9.5 (7–12.25) ($n = 50$)	12 (9–14) ($n = 31$)	525.5	NS
Digit Span	9 (7–11) ($n = 51$)	10 (7–11) ($n = 32$)	688.0	NS
Fragmented Letters (VOSP)	19 (18–19) ($n = 47$)	20 (19–20) ($n = 28$)	355.5	$P < 0.0075$
Similarities	8.5 (6–11) ($n = 50$)	11 (9–13) ($n = 32$)	479.0	$P < 0.03$
Vocabulary	9 (8–12) ($n = 50$)	11 (8–13) ($n = 32$)	612.5	NS
NART IQ	106 (96–116) ($n = 50$)	111.5 (97–117) ($n = 32$)	735.5	NS
McKenna Naming Test (raw score)	17 (9–21) ($n = 47$)	24 (19.75–26.25) ($n = 30$)	260.5	$P < 0.0015$
Verbal Fluency (using 'S')	12 (7–18.5) ($n = 41$)	16 (10.5–17) ($n = 29$)	431.5	NS
Wechsler Memory Scale: Passages – immediate recall[c]	16.5 (4–38.5) ($n = 32$)	63 (28–86) ($n = 27$)	185.5	$P < 0.003$
Wechsler Memory Scale: Passages – delayed recall[c]	8 (2–35) ($n = 29$)	51 (35.5–78.5) ($n = 25$)	110.5	$P < 0.0015$
Wechsler Memory Scale: Design – immediate recall[c]	31.5 (11.25–69.25) ($n = 26$)	94 (57–99) ($n = 19$)	85.5	$P < 0.003$
Warrington Recognition Memory Test: Words-50[c]	3 (3–9) ($n = 42$)	10 (6–12) ($n = 30$)	334.5	$P < 0.0135$
Warrington Recognition Memory Test: Faces-50[c]	5 (3–8) ($n = 32$)	8 (7–9) ($n = 28$)	223.0	$P < 0.009$

[a] References for the neuropsychological tests are in text.
[b] Bonferroni corrected.
[c] Raw scores have been age adjusted to give scale scores (Warrington) and percentiles (Wechsler).

each patient. Values were added up numerically, irrespective of direction (i.e. whether positive or negative) and the size of this global figure was interpreted as reflecting the patient's insight (thus, the greater the figure, the more discrepancies and therefore lower insight held by the patient).

Table 8.4 Comparison of total insight scores (as functions of discrepancy values on the MIQ) between neurological patients and psychiatric patients

| | Median value (inter-quartile range) | | | |
| | Neurological group | Psychiatric group | Mann– | Significance[a] |
Discrepancies on MIQ	($n = 56$)	($n = 44$)	Whitney U	2-tailed
Total discrepancy score	10.50 (7.00–15.00)	11.00 (7.25–16.00)	1143.5	NS
Total positive discrepancies	5.00 (2.25–11.75)	3.00 (1.25–5.00)	773.0	$P < 0.003$
Total negative discrepancies	3.00 (1.00–5.00)	7.00 (3.00–12.50)	662.5	$P < 0.0003$

[a] Bonferroni corrected.

To take account of the direction of the discrepancies, the sum of the positive and negative discrepancies were separately calculated for each patient. Results are shown in Table 8.4.

The results show that there is no significant difference in the total discrepancy scores between the patient groups. However, the neurological patients show significantly more positive discrepancies than the psychiatric patients and, conversely, the psychiatric patients show more negative discrepancies than the neurological patients. This indicates that the neurological patients evaluated their memory problems as less severe than their carers whereas, the psychiatric patients evaluated their memory problems as more severe than their carers.

Grouped insight scores

The 19 discrepancy values were parsed out in terms of the four areas of problems, i.e. with respect to general functioning, memory, language and cognition. The patient groups were compared on their insight into each area. The results are shown in Tables 8.5 and 8.6.

Table 8.5 shows a comparison of the *distribution* of discrepancies (positive, zero and negative) in relation to each area between the neurological and the psychiatric groups.

Table 8.6 shows a comparison of the *size* of insight held in relation to each area between the neurological and psychiatric groups.

Compared with the psychiatric group, the neurological group showed significantly more positive discrepancies but less negative discrepancies. This is consistent with reported results indicating that neurological patients evaluate their memory problems as less severe than their carers. The opposite was true for the psychiatric patients who, compared with their carers, evaluated their problems as more severe. Interestingly, both groups showed a higher relative frequency of negative discrepancies in the area of language, indicating that they both tended

Table 8.5 Distribution of insight responses compared between neurological and psychiatric patients in relation to the four areas on the MIQ: general, memory, language and cognitive

Clinical area	Neurological group ($n = 56$)	Psychiatric group ($n = 44$)	Chi-squared (D of F = 2)
General function	19/30/7*	10/25/9	8.75 ($P < 0.05$)
Memory	18/29/9	7/21/16	6.73 ($P < 0.05$)
Language	14/26/16	5/17/22	5.73 (NS)
Cognitive	17/29/10	5/23/16	7.28 ($P < 0.05$)

* (a/b/c): [a] distribution of positive discrepancies.
           [b] distribution of zero discrepancies (i.e. concordant responses).
           [c] distribution of negative discrepancies.

Table 8.6 Neurological and psychiatric patients compared on insight scores in relation to the four areas on the MIQ: general, memory, language and cognitive

Clinical area	Median value (inter-quartile range)		Mann–Whitney U	Significance 2-tailed
	Neurological group ($n = 56$)	Psychiatric group ($n = 44$)		
General function	1.00 (1.00–3.00)	1.00 (1.00–2.00)	1025.5	NS
Memory	3.00 (1.00–6.00)	3.00 (1.00–5.00)	1141.0	NS
Language	1.00 (0.25–2.00)	2.00 (1.00–3.00)	952.0	NS
				(Bonferroni correction: $P < 0.16$)
Cognitive	2.00 (1.00–2.00)	2.00 (1.00–5.00)	1154.5	NS

to evaluate their language function as more severely impaired than their carers did. In quantitative terms, both groups showed similar degrees of impaired insight (i.e. no significant difference in size of discrepancies) in each area.

8.2.3 Discussion of results

The most important finding from this study, from the perspective of this chapter, is the difference in the *type* of insight found between the two patient groups. Thus, whilst both the 'neurological' patient group and the 'psychiatric' patient group showed a similar range of total insight scores (Table 8.4) and a similar range of insight scores in the different clinical areas affected by memory problems (Table 8.6), they showed differences in the type of insight or phenomenon of insight manifested. The 'neurological' patients manifested a phenomenon of insight that was based on significantly more positive discrepancies and hence, indicated that patients seemed to show less awareness of memory difficulties, i.e. they were underestimating their memory problems. On the other hand, the 'psychiatric' patients manifested a phenomenon of insight that was based on significantly more negative discrepancies, indicating that these patients showed more apparent awareness of memory difficulties, i.e. they were overestimating their memory problems. As emphasised earlier, the issue here was not the detailed exploration of insight in patients with specific diagnoses. Instead, the issue was that, in a heterogeneous group of patients with a complaint cutting across diagnostic categories, *different aspects* (i.e. phenomena) of insight are elicited. In other words, the broad division of the patients into those with and those without a neurological basis to their memory problems yielded two types or phenomena of insight in regards to these two categories. If we examine these phenomena of insight in turn it can be seen that whilst each phenomenon can be understood within the rough disciplinary framework of the diagnostic category in which the phenomenon is elicited, it is more difficult to marry the phenomena within a unified framework.

Examining first the impaired insight in the patients with the neurological memory dysfunction, it is apparent, on the basis of the positive discrepancies obtained in this group, that these patients are underestimating their memory problems (in comparison with their carers' evaluations). Hence, given the 'objective' presence of such memory deficits (neuropsychology test results), they could be viewed as having *decreased awareness* of their difficulties. Thus, the impaired insight manifested in these patients, appears to be of a type that relates more to the *awareness* concept. Patients may not be perceiving (or rather, may not be perceiving the real extent of) the impairment that is affecting them. In response to questions about any problems with their memory, compared with others or compared with previous ability or in relation to general tasks and capacities, patients' lack of awareness (or only some awareness) into the basic impairment is then reflected in their judgements that they are functioning relatively well. In other words, if patients do not perceive or experience much wrong with their memory then they are unlikely to judge themselves as having difficulties with the memory related problems. Therefore, it would seem possible that the phenomenon elicited in these patients relates to awareness in its narrow sense as conceptualised in the neurosciences disciplines and as followed by the studies exploring insight in patients with organic memory impairment (e.g. Green *et al.*, 1993; Sevush & Leve, 1993; Starkstein *et al.*, 1997b, etc.). As we saw from such studies of awareness in dementia (Chapter 5), impaired awareness in these patients tended to be viewed either as inherent to the disease process (i.e. resulting from the mental disorganisation consequent to the brain degeneration) or to some form of motivated denial or indeed to a combination of these processes. Neuropsychological mechanisms postulated to underlie impaired awareness in this conceptualisation (excluding denial) have made reference to disturbance of some generalised awareness system or disturbance of a specific module-linked (in this case memory) awareness function (e.g. McGlynn & Schacter, 1989; Schacter, 1990).

Alternatively of course, the impaired insight manifested in these patients might be considered not as reduced awareness in the narrow sense but as reduced insight in the broader sense. In other words, irrespective of the degree to which patients may or may not experience the changes imposed by their memory deficits, it is at the level of their subsequent judgements that insight is impaired. However, this becomes over complicated. Here it makes sense to follow the other studies exploring awareness in such patients (as well as taking into account the contribution of the 'object' of insight assessment) and take a more parsimonious view of the phenomenon elicited and consider this as a problem of impaired awareness at its basic level (but see later for a caveat).

Let us examine in turn the impaired insight shown by the patients without the neurological memory dysfunction (i.e. the 'psychiatric' group). On the basis of the negative discrepancies obtained, it is apparent that these patients are overestimating their memory problems (in comparison with their carers' evaluations). Hence, they could be viewed as either having *increased awareness*, if we adhere to the same model as above, or *decreased insight* in the broader sense of the term, i.e. if impaired insight is viewed here as of the type relating to the concept of insight (rather than awareness). If we consider this latter option first, namely, conceive the type of insight shown by this patient group as belonging to the broader concept of *insight*, then, how is the elicited phenomenon to be interpreted? In response to questions about any problems with their memory as compared with others or as compared with previous ability or with respect to general tasks and capacities, patients' impaired insight can be viewed as resulting from poor or altered judgements concerning their experiences. For various reasons (e.g. mood disturbance, recent experiences, personality factors, etc.), patients may be experiencing changes (and drawing inferences about these changes) on the basis of more than direct perception. In other words, the *sense* patients make of their experiences may be affected by a range of different judgements which involve various aspects of general and personal knowledge.

On the other hand, if we conceive impaired insight in this group of patients as arising at the level of *awareness* (i.e. the direct perception of the impairment), then their overestimation of memory problems would have to be understood in terms of increased awareness of a deficit that had no 'objective' correlates (in terms of carers' evaluations or results on neuropsychological tests). Applying the neurosciences framework in this context would mean that one would have to consider such 'hyperawareness' as arising on the basis of some sort of stimulation of a generalised awareness system or a specific module-linked awareness function.

Therefore, the issue arising from this study is primarily concerned with the question of whether using a single concept or model will help to explain the different types of impaired insight seen in the patients or whether it makes more sense to view the impairment of insight in each patient group as reflecting, to some extent, different concepts. In fact, it is difficult to conceive of a unified model that could 'explain' in a plausible way both the 'reduced awareness' shown in one group of patients and the so-called 'increased awareness' shown in the other. I would contend that the two phenomena obtained in the different patient groups reflect the distinction, that has been argued for in this chapter, between *awareness* in the narrow sense and *insight* in the broad sense.

One further question that could be asked is, given that the same assessment instrument was used in both groups of patients and that the same 'object' of insight was being addressed, *why* should the two elicited phenomena of insight reflect two distinct concepts? Here, it is once again important to look properly at the 'object' of insight assessment. Although the 'object' of insight assessment in this study was ostensibly 'memory complaints', it is clear in fact that the actual 'object' of insight assessment was different in each patient group. In the 'neurological' group, the 'object' of insight assessment had to be 'memory dysfunction' (because comparisons were made with 'abnormal' results on psychometric testing). On the other hand, in the 'psychiatric' group, the 'object' of insight assessment was 'memory function' (because here comparisons were made with 'normal' results on psychometric testing). Hence, it makes sense that the different 'objects' played their part in determining the specific phenomenon of insight involved.

The study thus highlights that patients whose memory problems arise from different causes, manifest different types of impaired insight. This issue would not necessarily emerge if the patient groups were studied independently. In that situation, one study would show the 'neurological' patients as having poor insight (or awareness) and likewise another study would show 'psychiatric' patients as having poor insight (or awareness). The possibility of different 'types' of manifested impaired insight might not follow in the same way. However, our study design allowed for the emergence of these two distinct phenomena of impaired insight (underestimation and overestimation of problems) and consequently these needed explaining. The implications arising from this finding lie in questioning the assumption of equivalence between different insight phenomena. Clearly, the types of impaired insight shown by the patient groups are different and are likely to be underpinned by different mechanisms. It would make little sense to search for a common neurobiology (e.g. brain localisation of impaired insight) of poor insight in both cases. In crude terms, the phenomenon of aware-ness and the phenomenon of insight are likely to be organised differently in the brain.

At this point, it is important to stress another issue, in part arising from the results of this study but one that also may have been misconstrued from the analysis and justification for the distinction between awareness and insight made earlier in this chapter. Much of the argument presented for making this distinc-tion was based on highlighting some of the explicit differences in conceptual-isations of awareness/insight as explored in the neurosciences and those as explored in more general psychiatry and psychoanalytic psychology. Here, I want to emphasise that this was not intended to mean that exploration of awareness in the narrow sense was exclusive to the neurosciences disciplines and that explo-ration of insight in the broad sense was exclusive to clinical psychiatric disciplines. The differences in the way in which insight has been approached and explored in the different disciplines simply help to illustrate in a particularly overt way the dis-tinction that is argued for between the narrow and wide concepts of insight. However, it is a conceptual distinction, a differentiation that is made between two concepts on the basis of some identified specific differences in meaning. At the same time, whilst they are distinct, it is clear that they have features in common and that they interact in particular ways. I have touched upon this already and in the next chapter I shall examine the structural relationship between awareness and insight in some detail. In practical terms, it is clear that exploration of aware-ness/insight in patients is a mixed or combined enterprise in the sense that, gener-ally, clinicians may evaluate aspects of both awareness and insight in patients. Patients with various neurological/neuropsychological impairments, depending on the 'object' of insight assessment as well as on the degree of awareness held, may be asked about their views and judgements concerning the changes in a wider sense than those captured by 'awareness'. Hence, insight will be assessed as a com-bination of both awareness and insight. Similarly, in psychiatry, patients may be asked about signs (e.g. tardive dyskinesia) of which they may be 'unaware', i.e. they simply are not perceiving in a direct sense the 'object' that is observable to others. Hence, the phenomenon of insight elicited in relation to such 'objects' will in fact relate more closely to the narrow concept of awareness rather than to insight. Likewise, in the study described above, whilst both patient groups manifest impaired insight predominantly of the one type, the results show a mixture of both positive and negative discrepancies in both groups (see Table 8.5). In other words, both patient groups at some points overestimate their memory problems and at other points underestimate their difficulties. Whilst one has to consider here also the contribution to the 'insight score' from the carers in terms of the accuracy of their judgements of patients' problems, it is also likely that combinations of awareness and insight (i.e. wider judgements based on awareness) are elicited in both patient groups.

8.3 Conclusion

Amongst the many different perspectives on insight in different clinical specialities and within a single clinical area, the distinction between insight, as a narrow concept ('*awareness*') and insight, as a wide concept ('*insight*'), has emerged particularly prominently. *Awareness* refers to the simplest perception or direct appraisal of a particular state in an individual. This way of conceiving insight has been primarily employed in the exploration of insight in patients within the neurosciences disciplines and, consequently, the phenomenon of awareness has reflected this narrow approach. On the other hand, *insight* refers to more complex and diverse judgements made by an individual concerning the perceived state. This way of conceiving insight has been primarily employed in the exploration of insight within the disciplines of clinical psychiatry and in psychoanalytic psychology. Thus, similarly, the phenomenon of insight elicited in these clinical disciplines has reflected this wider approach.

The distinction between awareness and insight is apparent not only from the explicit descriptions of these concepts in the neurosciences and psychiatry but it also makes sense when we take into account the respective 'objects' of insight assessment in these clinical areas. Thus, in the neurosciences, 'objects' of insight assessment (e.g. hemiplegia, amnesia, dysphasia, etc.) tend to be *objective* in nature (i.e. directly accessible to an external person by observation or by test performance) and *negative* in type (i.e. referring to a loss or impairment of normal function). These features of the 'object' of insight assessment, as has been shown in the previous chapter, determine a phenomenon that is narrow and circumscribed, i.e. one which reflects the concept of *awareness*. In psychiatry, on the other hand, 'objects' of insight assessment (e.g. schizophrenia, depressive illness, hallucinations, delusions, etc.) tend to be *subjective* in nature (i.e. experiences which are not directly accessible to the external person), *positive* in type (i.e. referring to the presence of a new or abnormal experience) and/or referring to a more complex construct (e.g. 'mental disorder'). In turn, these features of the 'object' of insight assessment determine a phenomenon that is wider and based on a range of different judgements, i.e. one which reflects the concept of *insight*. The principal reason for this lies in the crucial role of the 'objects' of insight assessment in determining the clinical phenomena. In this case, these latter 'objects' simply demand judgements that are constituted by more than a direct appraisal of the 'object'. Thus, the phenomenon of insight elicited in relation to an 'object' such as 'mental illness' or 'hallucinations' depends on individuals, firstly, judging a change in their states (i.e. perceiving a change in the first place or, in other words, being aware of a change) but then making sense of this with respect to themselves and their experiences (hence the wider judgements involved). Since perceiving a change (i.e. awareness of some change in mental state) is inherent to the articulation of subjective complaints, then awareness, whilst a necessary component of insight in psychiatric disciplines, is not always a sufficient component of insight in these areas.

The clinical phenomena of awareness and insight share some characteristics but also have distinguishing features which help to determine in practical terms the division between awareness and insight. Both are phenomena that can be captured in quantitative terms, i.e. patients can show different degrees or extents of awareness and of insight. However, they differ in the source or focus of the qualitative features that are captured in clinical assessments. In the case of awareness, the focus of qualitative aspects determined by awareness measures is directed at the 'object' of awareness. In other words, patients are assessed in terms of *awareness in relation to the qualitative aspects of the 'object'* (e.g. the severity of an impairment, frequency with which the deficit interferes with function, etc.). In the case of insight, the focus of qualitative aspects determined by insight measures is directed at the phenomenon of insight itself. In other words, patients are assessed in terms of *qualitative aspects of insight* (i.e. different types of judgements held concerning, e.g. the nature of their experiences, whether these represent illness, in what way the experiences impact on their lives, etc.) *in relation to the 'object'*. In the previous chapter, the phenomenon of insight was proposed to be linked intrinsically with the 'object' of insight assessment, though, analysing the way in which the 'object' of insight assessment shaped the phenomenon of insight necessitated an artificial separation. The point however was that as far as the structure of the phenomenon of insight was concerned, the 'object' and the phenomenon were bound in a bi-directional relationship. Therefore, structurally the qualitative aspects of awareness are focused on the 'object' whereas the qualitative aspects of insight are focused on the phenomenon.

Another feature helping to differentiate the phenomenon of awareness from the phenomenon of insight is directionality. The quantitative assessment of awareness is generally described in terms of greater and lesser degrees but these degrees are all subsumed below an implicit 'normal' level of awareness. We can say that patients have reduced awareness of an impairment or they may show increased awareness following, e.g. rehabilitation, but there is not a situation where patients are expected to show greater levels of awareness than so-called 'normal' levels in relation to an impairment. In contrast, the phenomenon of insight has the potential for both a reduction below 'normal' and an increase above 'normal' levels.

The distinction highlighted between awareness and insight is crucially important because it provides a means of understanding the way in which different clinical phenomena relating to insight are obtained and, furthermore, helps to identify some of the specific ways in which such phenomena may be different. This carries implications for research on insight for it helps to clarify ways of determining equivalence between insight phenomena and thereby decide the limits of generalising between studies. In addition, as far as research on the neurobiology of insight is concerned, the distinction may help to select appropriate phenomena of insight for studies in this direction.

9

Towards a structure of insight: the relationship between awareness and insight

In Chapter 8 it was argued, on theoretical and empirical grounds, that there is an essential distinction between *awareness* as a narrow concept and *insight* as a wide concept. In consequence, the corresponding phenomena of awareness and insight could be differentiated on structural (nature of the constitutive judgements involved) and clinical (contents of individuals' utterances) grounds. The question addressed in this chapter concerns the nature of the relationship between awareness and insight. In other words, whilst a conceptual distinction can be made, it is equally evident that, given the interchangeableness of terms, overlap of, and generalisations between empirical studies, awareness and insight must share much in common. The question is how can their relationship be best understood? Is it possible to formulate an overall structure for insight that can help to clarify this relationship?

This chapter proposes a basic structure of insight in which the narrow and wider meanings can be integrated. The structure helps to understand the ways in which individual insight phenomena will be determined and delineated in relation to different 'objects' of insight. The clinical determinants and constituents of these insight phenomena will then be discussed in the light of the overall structure. Lastly, the implications carried by the model structure of insight for understanding insight in clinical terms and for directing future research on insight are explored.

9.1 The structure of insight

Throughout this work emphasis has been placed on the range of meanings of insight evident in the research and contributing to the variety of approaches taken to assess insight in patients with different clinical conditions. Within the range of meanings of insight a crucial distinction has been made between insight in its narrowest meaning as *awareness* i.e. the direct simplest perception of a particular stimulus/state affecting the individual and *insight* in its wider sense as self-knowledge, i.e. involving more complex judgements made by individuals concerning a particular state. Furthermore, it has been stressed that these latter judgements depend on, and relate to, an initial awareness of a particular state (though there are exceptions/qualifications but these will be discussed later). In other words, it is apparent that, in order to have insight of a clinical state in the wider sense, the individual has to first have an awareness of that state and subsequently, on the basis of that awareness, he/she can elaborate further judgements. At this stage, therefore, the relationship between awareness and insight can be tentatively formulated thus: *awareness provides the core element to insight as a whole.* For example, to have insight into his/her obsessive–compulsive disorder, the individual has to have some awareness of his/her thoughts and behaviours; in order to have insight into memory impairment, the individual has to have some awareness of difficulties with memory; in order to have insight into schizophrenia, the individual has to have some awareness of his/her abnormal experiences, and so on. Translated into a basic structure, insight must be constituted at its core by awareness. This can be represented schematically in a simple form as shown in Figure 9.1.

Figure 9.1 shows a simple representation of the structure of insight. The circumscribed core represents awareness and the arrows issuing outwards represent the various judgements that can be made in relation to awareness of a particular state. It has been argued already that insight is most usefully conceived as a mental

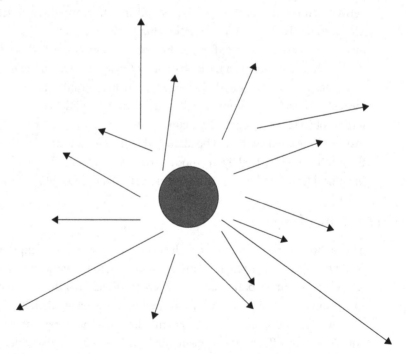

Figure 9.1   The structure of insight. A schematic representation of the structure for insight: *central sphere* represents core awareness and *arrows* represent judgements issuing from awareness of experience

state and as such there are no clearly defined limits to the numbers and types of judgements that can be invoked (see Chapter 6). Thus, as was seen in studies exploring insight in patients with psychoses, a wide variety of judgements demanded of patients concerning their experiences have been viewed as constitutive of insight. For example, researchers have included patients' views on the nature of their experiences, their judgements as to whether such experiences are pathological, their ideas on how the experiences affect their functioning or their relationship with others, their opinions on medication and other forms of treatment, etc. (refer to Chapter 3). In addition, apart from the range of types of judgements that can constitute insight, the level of knowledge required for 'complete' insight is far from clear and this again contributes to the lack of clear boundaries around the structure. What level of understanding should patients have of their illness or experiences? Do they need to know the details of the problems? To what degree do individuals need to judge the effects of their experiences on themselves and on the way they perceive and interact with their external environment? It can be seen that the sorts of judgements that can be made in relation to a particular clinical state (illness, symptoms, normal experiences, etc.) are infinite and ultimately for clinical/research purposes will have to be determined and limited by clinicians or researchers themselves.

In contrast, awareness is conceived as a more circumscribed concept. In clinical terms, patients are viewed as having or not having awareness or having various degrees of awareness of a particular state. Assessments of awareness are limited to capturing its quantitative aspects. Qualitative aspects of awareness are, as described in Chapter 8, directed at the 'object' of awareness and as such are constituted by the attributes of the particular object. This means that awareness itself in comparison to insight as a whole has more clearly defined boundaries.

It is important to emphasise at this point that the schematic representation of the basic structure of insight is intended to portray a *potential* basic structure. In other words, it is the *concept* of insight that is represented, i.e. insight as has been conceptualised within the clinical disciplines from the narrowest to the widest of theoretical conceptions. As is shown in Figure 1, the outward limits, in terms of the possible judgements that can constitute insight as a theoretical concept, cannot be properly demarcated. As a potential structure of insight, however, it provides a theoretical framework against which clinical *phenomena* of insight can be understood and positioned and delineated as described below.

If the basic structure of insight can be represented as constituted by core awareness underpinning a multiplex of judgements, where does the *phenomenon* of insight fit in? The phenomenon of insight has already been defined as referring to that aspect of insight that is manifested or elicited clinically. It has also been shown that it would be impractical to think that the phenomenon could capture everything that might be entailed by the concept of insight. As such, the phenomenon of insight might be thought of as a 'section' of the concept or structure of insight; i.e. incorporating only some of the chosen elements in terms of the types of judgements included. This could be represented in the same schematic diagram as simply a fraction of the structure, e.g. the area covered by the triangle outlined in Figure 9.2.

In other words, according to the choice made by clinicians/researchers, both in relation to a particular clinical state (or 'object' of insight assessment) and in relation to the types of judgements deemed to capture the concept of insight, the phenomenon of insight will encompass a particular fraction of the structure of insight. For example, the phenomenon of insight in relation to psychosis elicited using David's (1990) measure will incorporate some understanding of experienced psychotic symptoms as being pathological, judgements whether patients consider themselves as mentally ill and judgements as to whether medication is likely to be beneficial. On the other hand, the phenomenon of insight in relation to psychosis as assessed by the Amador *et al.* (1991) measure will have a different structure because the judgements demanded by the latter include ones of different contents

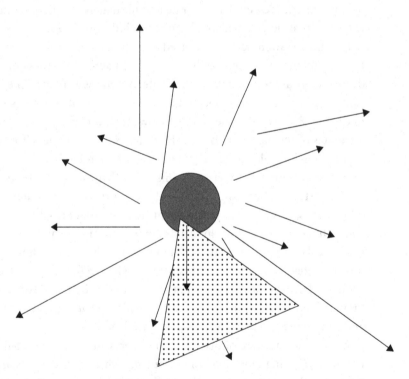

Figure 9.2   The basic phenomenon of insight (first level). A schematic representation of the structure for insight: *central sphere* represents core awareness; *arrows* represent judgements issuing from awareness of experience; and *stippled triangle* represents phenomenon of insight

such as the judgements concerning the social consequences of patients' experiences. Similarly the measures to capture insight employed by other researchers elicit phenomena of different structures depending on the types and number of judgements involved (e.g. Greenfeld *et al.*, 1989; Marková *et al.*, 2003).

It is important to emphasise again that such a *phenomenon* of insight simply captures the components of the insight structure *chosen* by the clinician or researcher. It does not mean that other aspects are not present or experienced by the patient. It means that, generally for practical reasons, there has to be a limit on the amount and type of understanding that is sought. Hence, as explained above, the structure of insight is to be conceived as a potential structure.

However, the structures of *phenomena* of insight are more complicated than simply involving sections of the concept of insight (see Chapter 6). It was argued that the *clinical* element, involved in the determination of insight, raises additional problems because of the issue of interpretation that is intrinsic to the elicitation of the phenomenon. Clinicians have to make a judgement of the patient's insight and this judgement will be based on *their* perception of what the patient says, how the patient behaves and/or how the patient manages certain tests. Depending on the measure chosen by the clinician, that judgement will include the interpretative elements constituted by the clinician/other factors (e.g. the clinician's particular perspective, knowledge, experience, biases, etc.). In other words, different approaches to assess the phenomenon of insight will influence the structure of the ensuing phenomenon by incorporating to varying extents the factors relating to the clinician judgement or the carer/family judgements or the factors relating to the interaction between patient and clinician in an interview situation, etc. (refer to Chapter 6). Thus, the structure of the phenomenon of insight might better be represented as shown in Figure 9.3.

Here, the additional bi-directional arrows facing the original phenomenon of insight represent the interacting influences of the type of approach used to elicit the phenomenon. The superimposed triangle represents the 'new' phenomenon of insight that ensues. This becomes a different or modified structure because it comprises not only of a selected fraction of the concept of insight as determined by the patient but includes also constituents determined by the individual judgements of the external assessor and/or the judgements developing within an interactive situation. For example, the phenomenon of insight in memory impairment will have a different structure when this is elicited within a clinician–patient interview situation than when this is elicited by means of a patient questionnaire, and it is different again when elicited using a discrepancy method.

Having outlined a very basic schematic representation of insight as a structure comprised of a core awareness around which a multitude of judgements arise and shown the different elements important in the determination of the structures of

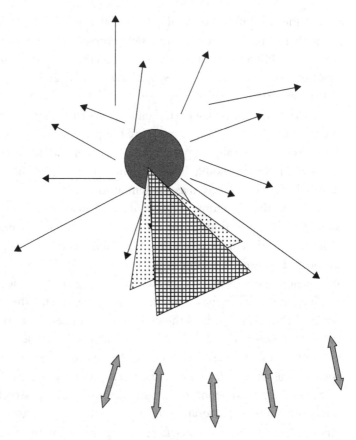

Figure 9.3   The phenomenon of insight (second level). A schematic representation of the structure for insight: *central sphere* represents core awareness; *arrows* represent judgements issuing from awareness of experience; *bi-directional arrows* represent interactional effects of clinician, type of 'insight' measure chosen, interview situation, other external individual, etc.; *stippled triangle* represents phenomenon of insight; and *superimposed triangle* represents 'new' phenomenon of insight incorporating changes as a result of the interactional effects

ensuing clinical phenomena, let us return to the relationship between awareness and insight. Although Figure 9.3 shows that phenomena of insight can vary depending on the types of judgements demanded of patients and depending on the type of measure used to elicit the phenomena, it could be questioned whether such differences are particularly important from a strictly structural point of view. In other words, the differences in the types of judgements demanded and/or the extent of knowledge elicited will give rise to different clinical phenomena of insight because of the consequent differences in *content* of such judgements. However, if such judgements, focused on making sense of personal experience, are assumed to share a similar *form*, then, it could be argued, that this might impose a common structure to these judgements irrespective of their specific contents. This would be much in the way that delusions are generally considered as sharing a basic structure irrespective of their contents and, likewise, obsessional thoughts, auditory hallucinations, etc. To briefly clarify, the structure of a symptom or mental phenomenon refers to its theoretical framework whilst the form and content have traditionally referred to the clinical representation of symptoms/mental phenomena (Marková & Berrios, 1995c). Thus, 'content' can be defined as the actual substance of the symptom whereas 'form' relates to the modality or medium in which the content is expressed, such as feeling, perception, thought, etc. (Jaspers, 1948). This is not the place to explore this issue in detail (and caveats would be needed in specific clinical areas, such as psychoanalytic psychology, where the structure of mental symptoms might be considered as dependent on symptom contents as much as their form). Certainly there are theoretical arguments against this view in that the judgements considered here are not unitary phenomena but a heterogeneous group which are constituted primarily from secondary judgements. Such secondary judgements are themselves complexes based on a range of other judgements, on various types of beliefs, on associated feelings, on past experiences, on general knowledge, attitudes and so on. Thus, although at a clinical level the judgements can be said to differ in content, this content in turn is dependent on a multitude of mental phenomena which themselves differ in form and content. In other words, there are theoretical grounds for suggesting that differences in phenomena of insight (in the broad sense) may be structurally meaningful. However, this issue, as well as that concerning the location of possible distinctions between judgements, to some extent remains to be determined empirically. It is highlighted here simply to illustrate that the nature of differences between phenomena of insight distinguished on the basis of judgements may be of a different order to the differences in phenomena which are distinguished on the basis of 'awareness' on the one hand and 'awareness and judgements' (insight in broader sense) on the other (see below).

As was argued in Chapter 8, the distinction between the phenomenon of awareness and the phenomenon of insight is based on a more striking structural difference between 'awareness' (as a direct perception of an 'object') and 'insight' (as 'awareness' together with the secondary judgements based on the awareness). It is important, therefore, to examine, in relation to the outlined insight structure, the determinants of phenomena of insight whose structures focus either on awareness or on insight in the wider sense. Understanding the ways in which awareness and insight are determined in this context may help to clarify their relationship in more detail. Following the argument developed in Chapter 7 concerning the crucial role of the 'object' of insight assessment in determining the clinical phenomenon of insight, the structure of the phenomenon of insight will be examined in relation to different types of 'objects' of insight assessment. For the purposes here, this will be limited to three types of 'objects' of insight assessment, namely, (i) subjective mental states, (ii) loss or impairment of function, and (iii) specific diagnostic constructs (e.g. mental illness).

9.1.1 Insight phenomena determined by 'subjective mental states'

The term 'subjective mental state' refers here to any mental experience, 'normal' or pathological, that an individual is able to identify in some way as relating to him/herself; e.g. feelings of happiness, sadness, anger, perplexity, hearing 'voices', 'seeing' things not visible to others, worrying thoughts, beliefs of special powers, beliefs of being persecuted, etc. Whether offered spontaneously or elicited on questioning such descriptions represent the individual's interpretation of his/her particular mental state. Thus, as was pointed out earlier (see Chapter 7), awareness of the mental experience is a prerequisite for such interpretation. Individuals will say they are hearing voices on the basis of awareness of some new or change in mental experience that is then interpreted and judged in that particular way. Similarly, individuals may describe themselves as feeling happy or angry and, in turn, such a judgement is based on interpretation of a particular mental state about which they are aware. Awareness of a mental experience is therefore inherent to the formation of a subjective mental state.

What does this mean in terms of understanding the structure of the phenomenon of insight that is elicited in relation to (and determined by) subjective mental states? It follows that when the phenomenon of insight is assessed in relation to a subjective mental state, it is not sufficient to elicit awareness (i.e. insight in its narrow sense) of the mental state since that would mean, in effect, to elicit only the subjective mental state itself. Awareness is inherent to the subjective mental state and cannot be accessed independently of the mental state. Instead, the phenomenon of insight determined by a subjective mental state has to relate to the *sense* the individual makes regarding the subjective mental state. Figure 9.4 illustrates this schematically using the original representation.

Ignoring, for simplicity's sake, the influence of interpretative factors on the phenomenon of insight, Figure 9.4 indicates the area under the triangle as representing the structure of the phenomenon of insight when determined by subjective mental states. The area represented by the pale triangle relates to the core awareness whereas the area within the stippled area relates to various judgements made in relation to the subjective mental state. Since, however, awareness is necessary and intrinsic to subjective mental states, it is not possible to separate the two and, hence, in practical or clinical terms, the phenomenon of insight will be elicited *solely* in terms of the wider judgements concerning the individual's views on the nature and effects of the mental state. For example, an individual recognising

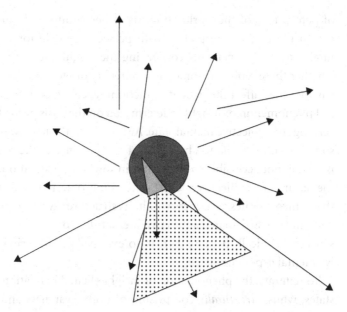

Figure 9.4   The phenomenon of insight in relation to 'subjective mental states'. A schematic representation of the structure for insight; *central sphere* represents core awareness; *arrows* represent judgements issuing from awareness of experience; *stippled triangle* represents phenomenon of insight; and *pale triangle* within the stippled triangle represents the awareness that is intrinsic to, and hence inseparable from, the subjective state itself

him/herself as feeling happy may describe this as feeling good and bright. In this sense, he/she is interpreting an awareness of a particular mental state and giving it a specific name, i.e. happiness. At this stage, the individual would be described as reporting a subjective mental state but it is unlikely this would be termed insight. Similarly, a patient complaining of people plotting against him and being unable to accept evidence to the contrary would be described as reporting a subjective fear/worry that was not amenable to reasoning (and the clinician might then describe this as a delusional belief). However, the reporting of the worry on the part of the patient would not, in itself, be viewed as insightful even though the patient is reporting this on the basis of an awareness of some change in his/her mental state. In other words, in both these cases, the reporting of subjective states whilst, by definition, are indicative of awareness of particular changes in mental state, is not sufficient for determining insight. The phenomenon of insight would demand, in both these examples, further judgements concerning the nature and effects of the articulated subjective state. In the case of the individual reporting feeling happy, elicitation of insight into the happiness might, for example, involve judgements concerning how the happiness affects him/her in terms of general feelings, in terms of perceptions of the world, in terms of behaviours and interaction with others, etc. In the case of the patient with persecutory delusions, elicitation of insight might include judgements concerning the origin and nature of his/her worries, whether these represent some form of reality or whether they might reflect illness, whether they affect the patient's functioning, etc. In both these examples, the clinical phenomenon of insight is determined on the basis of further judgements concerning the subjective mental state. Awareness in the narrow sense of perception of some stimulus or change, by virtue of its inherence to the subjective mental state, is simply not accessible to elicitation in the clinical situation. Or, in other words, the nature of a subjective mental state as the 'object' of insight assessment is such that it incorporates awareness within its structure. Awareness of the mental experience and the articulated subjective mental state on which this is based cannot be separated clinically because there is no 'external' way of verifying the actual subjective mental experience itself.

To reiterate, the phenomenon of insight elicited in relation to subjective mental states, whilst *structurally* comprising of both awareness and insight in its wider sense, *clinically* will only be accessible in terms of the wider sense, i.e. in terms of the secondary judgements made in relation to the subjective mental state (Figure 9.4). Concerning such judgements and indeed those that come into the interpretation of awareness of a particular mental state in the first place, this is an area of particular complexity for various reasons.

Firstly, there is little known about how such judgements develop nor what sort of factors may determine them. The range of insight that can be found in regards to both 'normal' mental states/behaviours and pathological mental states, suggests that probably a multitude of factors are likely to be important. Some empirical research has suggested that the type of background general knowledge held by an individual is likely to influence the sorts of judgements individuals make (e.g. Lam et al., 1996; Chung et al., 1997); social and cultural factors have also been considered important in determining judgements not only concerning the sense the individual makes of his subjective mental state but also in interpreting the original mental state experience on which he/she determines its name though there has been little in the way of empirical work exploring this (Johnson & Orrell, 1995; Clare, 2004). Other factors, more speculative, may include the individual's past experiences of similar mental states (Thompson et al., 2001), individual personality factors (Weinstein et al., 1994; Lysaker et al., 1999; 2002), level of intelligence, tendency to introspect, family/peer influences, etc. (see Chapter 3).

Secondly, in regards to mental illness, there is as yet no coherent model developed in regards to symptom (including subjective mental states) formation. Some preliminary suggestions have been proposed in general terms (e.g. Berrios et al., 1995; Marková & Berrios, 1995b, c) and various models from specialised perspectives have been put forward in relation to specific individual symptoms (e.g. Garety & Hemsley, 1994). However, from the perspective of making sense of psychopathology as a whole, in terms of understanding the ways in which symptoms/signs may develop, the factors affecting these, the assumptions that need to be taken into account and the extents and limits to which different types of approaches help acquire such knowledge, much research remains to be done. It is in this context that further understanding concerning the sort of factors and likely mechanisms underlying impairment of insight in relation to pathological mental states might be developed.

Thirdly, and relating to this, there is little knowledge so far concerning the effects of mental illness as a whole on the judgements made relating to insight. In other words, in spite of the numerous empirical studies exploring the relationship between levels of insight and illness/disease variables (refer to Chapters 3–5), the contribution of the illness itself on different types of judgements has not been clarified. The situation is different as regards awareness, or insight in its narrow sense (see below), where research has, with greater validity, indicated some association between impaired *awareness* and neurological and/or neurocognitive dysfunction (e.g. Prigatano, 1991; Derouesné *et al.*, 1999). However, in terms of insight in its wider sense, i.e. in terms of the relationship between specific judgements relating to insight and the mental illness itself, then at present little is known. For example, does having schizophrenia or bipolar affective disorder or a delusional disorder affect the way in which individuals think about themselves, does it affect perceptions concerning themselves and their functioning, are perhaps only some types of judgements affected or is there a pervasive influence on reasoning? Thus, the original question as posed by the early alienists and echoed by subsequent researchers, as to whether and/or to what extent a 'disordered' mind can judge its own problems has not yet been answered.

9.1.2 Insight phenomena determined by 'loss/impairment of function' ('objective' dysfunction)

The term 'loss or impairment of function' refers here to a loss or reduction of a 'normal' function or ability such as mobility, memory, speech and resulting in, e.g. hemiplegia, amnesia, dysphasia, etc. This loss or impairment can occur either acutely as might happen following a cerebrovascular accident or progressively as in the case of a neurodegenerative disorder such as Alzheimer's disease. The most striking difference between this type of 'object' of insight assessment and the sort of 'object' exemplified by a 'subjective mental state' is that in contrast to the latter, the loss or impairment in function is something that is in some specific way externally evident and verifiable. As was discussed in Chapters 7 and 8, this carries important consequences for the phenomenon of insight that is determined by such an 'object'.

Precisely because the loss/impairment of function can be verified or determined by an external individual or test, the phenomenon of insight in its narrow sense, i.e. awareness, can be accessed directly. In contrast to the situation with subjective mental states, a direct comparison between the patient's perception and the clinician's perception (or test result) of the dysfunction is possible. Therefore, the patient's awareness of the dysfunction can be elicited directly. Again, a schematic representation of the phenomenon in this case is illustrated in Figure 9.5.

The white triangle within the core awareness aspect of the insight structure represents the phenomenon of awareness in relation to loss or impairment of function. The phenomenon of insight is focused in this case on *awareness* of the problem/dysfunction. In relation to the dysfunction, the patient's awareness is either present or reduced or absent. Qualitative aspects of awareness are limited to judgements made concerning the characteristics of the dysfunction itself rather than the wider judgements demanded in relation to subjective mental states. For example, eliciting insight into memory problems in a patient with dementia might depend on a comparison between the patient's perceptions of his/her memory difficulties and the clinician's assessment of problems on the basis of psychometric tests. Or, in a patient with hemiplegia following a stroke, eliciting insight might depend on a

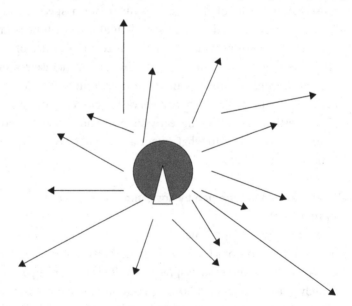

Figure 9.5   The phenomenon of insight in relation to 'objective dysfunction'. A schematic representation of the structure for insight; *central sphere* represents core awareness; *arrows* represent judgements issuing from awareness of experience; and *white triangle* within the core awareness represents the phenomenon of insight in relation to the dysfunction. Clinically represented therefore only by awareness. Further judgements focused on the features of the dysfunction itself (see text)

comparison between the patient's perception of his/her ability to move and direct observation of the patient's movements. Depending on the degree of awareness held by the patients in relation to such dysfunction, further judgements can be demanded, generally relating to observable or measurable features of the dysfunction itself, such as severity of the problem, the frequency with which it causes difficulties, etc. Clearly, where patients lack complete awareness of the dysfunction, further judgements cannot be determined.

The phenomenon of insight determined by 'objects' of insight assessment relating to 'objective dysfunction' (i.e. loss/impairment of function), therefore, whilst comprising both *structurally* and *clinically* of awareness and insight in its wider sense, is focused predominantly on awareness, i.e. on insight in its narrow sense. This results in a more circumscribed phenomenon whose boundaries are fixed by the limits imposed by quantitative assessment. Patients will have either awareness of say, a hemiplegia or dyskinesia, or reduced or absent awareness of the same. The concept of increased awareness, i.e. beyond 'normal' awareness does not apply because the external verification of the dysfunction is carried out quantitatively and has a finite limit. And, awareness is judged on the basis of a comparison with this external verification. Thus, a patient who is unable to move a leg can state that he/she cannot move a leg thus displaying awareness of this problem. Alternatively, the patient may say that he/she has some difficulty in moving a leg, indicating reduced awareness of the problem and finally, the patient could say that he/she is able to move the leg normally, suggesting absent awareness (anosognosia). However, the patient would not be described as having increased awareness of the problem. Qualitative assessment of awareness, from the point of view of eliciting patients' understanding of a dysfunction, is not 'measurable' simply because there is no external concomitant. Thus, to reinforce the argument from Chapter 8, qualitative descriptions around the phenomenon of awareness in relation to dysfunctions are constrained to characterising the dysfunctions themselves. These features characterising the phenomenon of awareness together with the relative lack of judgements elaborated in the wider sense suggest that the structure of this phenomenon in relation to verifiable dysfunction might lend itself more easily to research seeking to explore the neurobiology of awareness.

9.1.3 Insight phenomena determined by 'diagnostic constructs'

A 'diagnostic construct' such as 'mental illness' or 'schizophrenia' or 'dementia' refers here to a different category of 'objects' of insight assessment, namely, one which incorporates not only the identified signs and symptoms of the particular psychopathology but, in addition, all the elements (social, cultural, historical, political, etc.) that might contribute to the 'meaning' of the term (see Chapter 7). This makes this category of 'objects' very different from the previous types of 'objects' of insight assessment. In other words, and again, as was argued earlier, because of these 'extra' elements contained within 'diagnostic constructs', then in contrast to the previous 'objects' of insight assessment, there is not the same one-to-one relationship between the 'diagnostic construct' and its determinable manifestation. Eliciting insight into persecutory delusions relates to judgements patients are making about a particular mental state they are experiencing. Similarly, eliciting insight into memory dysfunction relates to judgements patients make about an 'overt' or 'objectively determined' problem. Eliciting insight into schizophrenia, however, may require judgements not only of particular mental experiences and/or problems the patient may be having but also judgements made in relation to a concept that, through its social, cultural and political elements, may be quite distant to a personal experience. In fact, different sorts of insight phenomena may be determined by such a construct.

One sort of phenomenon may be elicited where the focus is on the judgements made by patients based on the sum of individual abnormal mental experiences thought to be the symptoms and signs of illness. For example, some approaches to assessing insight in patients with schizophrenia include questions concerning whether the 'abnormal' experiences they are having are the result of mental illness (e.g. Amador *et al.*, 1991). This can again be represented schematically as in Figure 9.6.

Figure 9.6 shows three triangles extending from the core awareness and incorporating wider judgements. These represent the same sorts of phenomena of insight that are obtained in relation to subjective mental states (i.e. comprising of both awareness of a particular mental state, as inherent to the subjective mental state, and judgements based on this awareness) (Figure 9.4). In addition, these phenomena reach out to a larger stippled triangle which represents judgements that are based on other information (i.e. not on awareness itself) in terms of general knowledge, personal views and biases, individual experiences, etc. relating to the wider elements of the construct. In other words, the composite phenomenon of insight in relation to schizophrenia in this case becomes constituted of both personal and more general judgements. As was the case in relation to the phenomenon of insight determined by subjective mental states, *structurally* this composite phenomenon is constituted of both awareness and insight in the wider sense and, *clinically*, the phenomenon is composed of a multitude of judgements ranging in complexity. In contrast, however, to the phenomenon of insight determined by subjective mental states, this phenomenon also includes judgements which are not purely based on awareness of a particular mental state but are based, in addition, on the individual's general knowledge and opinions about the 'object' in question. It could be argued that these latter judgements are likewise important in the formation of the insight phenomenon in relation to subjective mental states. Indeed, these sorts of factors were raised earlier as likely to influence the sorts of judgements

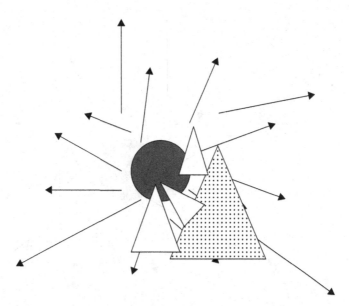

Figure 9.6   The phenomenon of insight in relation to 'diagnostic constructs'. A schematic
representation of the structure for insight: *central sphere* represents core awareness;
arrows represent judgements issuing from awareness of experience; *white triangles*
represent phenomena of insight in relation to individual subjective mental states; and
stippled triangle represents phenomenon of insight in relation to diagnostic construct as
a composite of: (1) insight in relation to subjective states, and (2) judgements based on
other knowledge/perspectives, e.g. cultural contexts, general views, past experiences

held by patients concerning the nature and effects of subjective mental states.
However, the difference in this case is that, whilst it is likely the factors will interact, there is in addition the added element that perhaps more of the wider judgements which are elicited will be unrelated to the patient's actual experience. This
can be illustrated further by examining another sort of phenomenon of insight
that might be determined by a construct such as 'mental illness'.

For example, other approaches to assessing insight in patients with schizophrenia include questions which ask the patients directly whether they think they are
suffering from a mental illness (e.g. David, 1990). This could result in a somewhat
different phenomenon of insight as illustrated in Figure 9.7.

Figure 9.7 shows a phenomenon of insight, represented by the stippled triangle,
that is composed entirely of different sorts of judgements in relation to the construct but there is no relationship to any sort of awareness of a mental state or
experienced problem. In other words, and in qualification to what has been said
earlier, in some situations, the phenomenon of insight in the wider sense may not
be dependent on awareness of a particular state. For example, it is possible that a

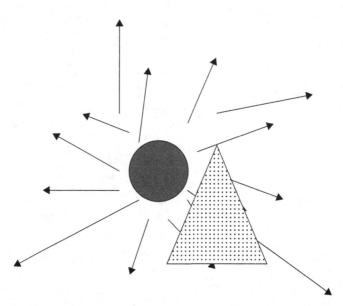

Figure 9.7   An alternative phenomenon of insight in relation to 'diagnostic constructs'. A schematic
representation of the structure for insight: *central sphere* represents core awareness;
arrows represent judgements issuing from awareness of experience; and *stippled triangle*
represents phenomenon of insight in relation to diagnostic construct not based on current
subjective experiences. Therefore, clinically composed of judgements based on other
types of knowledge only, e.g. general views, cultural contexts, personal biases, past
experiences, etc. (i.e. insight without awareness).

patient with schizophrenia may not 'feel' ill in any way or may not perceive that
he/she has particular problems and, yet, the patient may judge on the basis of
information given to him/her by others that he/she is suffering from schizophrenia. This could be considered similar to the situation where patients with, for
example, silent or asymptomatic cancer are diagnosed with the condition (and
given information about it including management and prognosis), and acknowledge that they have the disease, understand the effects this may have on their life
and the implications for treatment again without necessarily feeling ill in any way.

The phenomena of insight determined by 'objects' of insight assessment relating
to diagnostic constructs can therefore be of different kinds. Some will be similar to
the phenomena of insight elicited in relation to subjective mental states and thus
comprise *structurally* of awareness and insight in its wider sense though *clinically*
only in insight in its wider sense. Others will comprise both *structurally* and *clinically* only of insight in its wider sense and, because of this, *clinically* the judgements
formed in relation to the construct will not be based on awareness of a particular

state (i.e. relating to experience of components of the construct) but will be based on other sources of information.

9.2 Clinical and research implications

Having presented a possible structure underlying insight, various questions naturally arise. Most practical perhaps are the questions of how does the proposed structure help to understand the clinical phenomenon of insight? And, what implications does the structure carry for future research on insight in psychiatry? This section addresses these questions by examining in more detail some specific points highlighted by the structure. Most importantly, however, the proposed structure represents, in a relatively straightforward schematic form, the conceptualisation of insight in the light of the theoretical analyses of insight based on the historical and clinical approaches to the study of insight reviewed in this book. In other words, the conceptual analysis undertaken here has detailed in a specific way some of the complexities inherent to the study of insight and argued for distinctions that can help to address the complexities. This has entailed the examination of a number of individual problems at various levels and involved, inevitably, some repetitious arguments. The structure that has culminated from this work, however, can summarise in a simple manner the complex issues that are relevant for both the clinical understanding of insight and for research purposes.

9.2.1 Awareness and insight: clinical and research implications

One of the main points illustrated by the structure of insight is the relationship between awareness and insight. The structure of insight highlights two issues in this regard. First, it shows awareness and insight to be separate though related structures. Secondly, it shows that the relationship between awareness and insight changes according to the 'object' of insight assessment and, hence, according to clinical context. What does this imply for the general or clinical understanding of insight?

In the first place, it means that awareness and insight should not be considered as synonymous. This is important from a professional (as opposed to lay) perspective, particularly given the confusion around the interchangeableness of terms. Individuals evidently can have awareness without insight and insight without awareness. Or, patients can have *good awareness together with poor insight* (as in the case of patients complaining of hearing voices and attributing these to some alien intervention) and *poor awareness but good insight* (as in the case of patients understanding they are affected by a condition on the basis of information given to them by others but without any concomitant subjective experiences). In other words, it makes clinical sense to distinguish between awareness as the primary appraisal of a particular perception/experience and insight as constituted by the more complex judgements pertaining to a specific experience. The structure of insight makes it clear that this distinction can be understood at both the *clinical* level (i.e. manifesting itself in the differences between patients' utterances) and at the *structural* level (i.e. implying different underlying processes or mechanisms).

In the second place, the structure of insight shows how the relationship between awareness and insight is determined to some extent by different 'objects' of insight assessment. Thus, in clinical terms, the phenomenon of insight elicited in relation to subjective mental states such as depressed mood, anxiety or auditory hallucinations, will mainly reflect the secondary judgements of insight rather than the primary appraisal or awareness of the subjective experience itself. Insight determined by subjective mental states has to relate to the sense patients make of their experiences. On the other hand, the phenomenon of insight elicited in relation to 'objective' dysfunction such as dyskinesia, amnesia or psychomotor retardation, will predominantly reflect the extent of patients' awareness or primary appraisal of the problem. The relative importance of awareness and insight in the constitution of the clinical phenomena elicited thus varies according to the clinical context in which the phenomenon of insight is elicited. Once again this illustrates that not only will patients be expressing different types of experiences in relation to the clinical context (or 'object' of insight assessment) but that the processes or mechanisms underlying such expressions are likely to be different.

The structure of insight also makes clear that there is little evidence that awareness and insight (together with denial and anosognosia) represent different points of severity on a continuum as has been suggested by some authors (e.g. Ghaemi, 2003). Indeed this is already apparent from the fact that, as was demonstrated earlier in this book, the concepts of awareness, insight, anosognosia, denial, etc. have different historical origins and have been approached in different ways in relation to different clinical populations. However, the structure of insight helps to shows this more clearly by delineating, first of all, a clear division between awareness and insight as independent though interrelated structures. Thus, as described above, the difference between awareness and insight is dependent on different underlying processes or mechanisms, i.e. a difference in *kind* rather than a difference in *grade*. Secondly, the structure of insight shows that further divisions can be postulated between insight phenomena depending on the various judgements involved. The differences between such subsequent insight phenomena therefore would be dependent on the contents of judgements rather than on a different degree of severity or intensity of one particular judgement.

The structure of insight thus helps to clarify understanding of insight in terms of the distinctions between awareness and insight and their interrelationship in different clinical contexts. In addition, this understanding also carries implications for research on insight. Most importantly, as far as research into brain representation of insight is concerned, the distinction between awareness and insight may help to direct such research in particular areas. For example, the structural differences between awareness and insight highlighted by the schematic representation of insight suggest more than that the processes underlying awareness and insight are different. Instead, the implication is also drawn that whilst awareness can be represented by a relatively circumscribed and contained structure, by contrast, insight is conceived as a structure whose boundaries are undefined and whose content encompasses limitless judgements. The arguments supporting this structural distinction were expounded earlier when the characteristics of the respective phenomena were delineated, for example, in terms of qualitative and quantitative aspects, directionality, etc. (refer to Chapter 8). The proposed insight structure however shows this difference in an explicit albeit simplistic way. From this, though, it follows that research aiming to explore possible brain representation or neurobiology of insight might more usefully focus on awareness rather than on insight in its wider sense. In other words, it would seem to be a more legitimate enterprise to be exploring associations between brain function and a structure that, because of its circumscribed nature, is not only more reliably accessed but is also likely to be underpinned by a common and consistent mechanism.

Secondly, again from the perspective of research into brain representation, and following from the above, it makes sense to concentrate on eliciting phenomena which are constituted primarily by 'awareness' as opposed to 'insight'. To this end, the dependency of insight phenomena on their 'object' of insight assessment indicates that exploring insight in relation to, for example, 'objective' dysfunction will determine a phenomenon that will more meaningfully lend itself to such correlational research. On the other hand, exploring insight in relation to 'subjective mental states' or to 'diagnostic constructs' will determine phenomena that are constituted mainly by the wider judgements pertaining to insight and, as such, are unlikely to associate consistently with a specific neuronal system.

Apart from research into the neurobiology of insight, the structure of insight carries implications for research on insight in psychiatry in other directions. In particular, it is evident that much research is needed to develop further understanding around the nature of phenomena of insight in the wider sense. Here, as indicated earlier, many questions need exploring both from a theoretical perspective but also by empirical means. For example, it seems plausible, though needs empirical testing, that some insight phenomena, based on particular types of judgements, might be of more predictive value, in terms of prognosis or quality of life, than other insight phenomena. Similarly, it might be that phenomena of insight based on different judgements may be clinically important or useful in different ways. Again this would need addressing empirically. Other questions alluded to earlier concern the possibility of further distinguishing between different insight phenomena. In other words, might there be some validity in making further distinctions between insight phenomena based on the types and contents of judgements involved? In a different vein, but crucially, research into insight might usefully concentrate on exploring the factors that might be important in the formation of the judgements that constitute insight. For example, one important focus here might concern distinguishing between 'illness' factors (e.g. current mood, past experience of similar states, cognitive problems) and non-illness factors (e.g. cultural, social and environmental influences). In addition, and as mentioned earlier, research may need to address the question of 'symptom' formation, i.e. look at developing models for the ways in which mental symptoms may arise and be expressed.

9.2.2 Determinants of the phenomenon of insight: clinical and research implications

The other main point illustrated by the structure of insight is the location and structure of the phenomenon of insight both within the concept of insight as a whole, and within the external context in which it is elicited. There are several aspects of this that are highlighted by the schematic representation of insight and which are important for the clinical understanding of insight and which also carry implications for future research.

First, the structure of insight shows clearly the distinction between the clinical phenomenon of insight and the theoretical construct. This helps to understand that the phenomenon of insight, that is that aspect of insight which is elicited clinically, is not to be considered as equivalent to insight as this is viewed in its theoretical totality. The phenomenon of insight can only represent an aspect of insight. In other words, it would be impractical to attempt to determine insight clinically in terms of all its possible potential constituents.

Second, the schematic representation of insight shows the phenomenon of insight to be a product not only of the theoretical construct of insight but also of external influences. In terms of the latter, two such influences are clearly identified. Thus, firstly, as already described in the previous section, the 'object' of insight determines significantly the relative contribution of awareness and insight to the structure of the insight phenomenon elicited. Assessing insight into memory dysfunction or dyskinesia, for example, elicits a phenomenon whose structure is focused mainly on awareness. On the other hand, assessing insight into schizophrenia or into psychotic experiences elicits a phenomenon whose structure is focused mainly on the judgements that constitute insight in the wider sense. Secondly, in addition, the phenomenon of insight is also seen to be influenced by the specific method employed to assess insight. Figure 9.3 represents this influence simply by the presence of the external arrows causing a change in the resultant phenomenon which becomes reconstituted through the effects of such influence. Thus, the individual judgements, experiences and interactive factors of an external assessor will contribute to the final insight phenomenon elicited. Similarly, tests based on various discrepancies will contribute to the resultant structure of the elicited insight phenomenon. Once again the grounds for this have been put forward previously (Chapter 6) but the schematic representation of insight helps to bring this out in a more explicit way. In turn, this helps to understand the factors likely to influence the assessment of insight and expression of insight in a clinical setting.

Third, the schematic representation of insight and the phenomenon of insight situated against this framework highlight the *descriptive* nature of this model. In other words, the structure of insight, both as a concept and phenomenon, is depicted in terms of its possible and potential constituents and their likely interrelationships. On the other hand, mechanisms postulated to underlie changes in insight, such as denial in its psychodynamic sense or specific neuronal dysfunction or others, have to be addressed separately. The essential point, however, is that exploration of such mechanisms are necessarily dependent on an understanding of the insight phenomenon at its descriptive level.

Knowledge concerning the determinants of insight phenomena also carries implications for further research. Thus, understanding about the way in which different 'objects' of insight assessment can determine a particular phenomenon of insight allows for a clearer appreciation of the structure of the phenomenon that is elicited. In turn, from a research perspective, this allows for more valid comparisons between phenomena of insight elicited in studies within and between clinical areas. Furthermore, it also enables researchers to choose and devise measures which, on theoretical grounds, can most usefully assess the particular phenomenon under study. Likewise, understanding about the contribution of judgements made by clinicians, instruments and the interactive situation towards the formation of the clinical phenomenon of insight allows for a clearer appreciation of the structure of the insight phenomenon elicited. Again this is important from a research perspective as such factors may be important to take into account when exploring insight in patients and when making comparisons between different insight phenomena. In addition, this is an area where empirical work would be useful in order to help determine the levels and types of influence possessed by different insight measures. Such knowledge, in turn, would be important once again for choosing a particular method of assessing patients' insight in different clinical situations.

9.3 Conclusion

Clinical exploration of insight is hampered, amongst other things, by complexities inherent in the concept of insight itself. Based on identification and individuation of some specific problems contributing to the complexities, a basic structure for insight has been proposed and schematically represented. The structure revolves around the distinction made between awareness and insight and proposes that, in relation to any self-experience, awareness forms the core around which insight, in terms of more complex and elaborate judgements, is constructed. Although judgements forming the wider structure of insight are shown as independent entities issuing from the core awareness, it is understood that this is an oversimplification and that relevant judgements are elaborated not only on the basis of awareness but on the basis of and interaction with other judgements. For the purposes here, the crucial issue is the fundamental distinction between awareness and insight. Whether subsequent distinctions between different levels of judgements are possible is a matter for further theoretical and empirical research.

The structure provides a framework against which clinical phenomena of insight can be defined and delineated. Different 'objects' of insight assessment determine phenomena of insight that differ structurally and clinically mainly on account of the relative proportion of awareness and further judgements in their constitution. The structure provides the space to show the added contribution of external factors (i.e. in terms of clinician/measure contribution) to the determination of the insight phenomenon. The focus on the 'object' of insight assessment allows the external factors contributing to the phenomenon of insight to be considered more specifically in relation to the nature of the 'object' itself. In these ways, the structure of insight helps to organise understanding about clinical phenomena of insight explored in different clinical situations. In addition, it helps to identify areas where research may usefully focus.

The relationship between awareness and insight is evidently not straightforward and it has been argued here that the terms are not synonymous. Individuals are able to have at the same time poor awareness and good insight and conversely good awareness together with poor insight. The structural distinction between awareness and insight suggests that research aimed at exploring the nature and correlates of insight needs to make a like distinction since different approaches to such study may be required in each case.

References

Abramowitz, S.I. & Abramowitz, C.Z. (1974) Psychological-mindedness and benefit from insight-oriented group therapy. *Archives of General Psychiatry*, 30, 610–615.

Abrams, S. (1981) Insight. The Teiresian gift. In *The Psychoanalytic Study of the Child*, Eds. A.J. Solnit, R.S. Eissler, A. Freud, M. Kris & P.B. Neubauer, vol. 36. New Haven: Yale University Press, pp. 289–305.

Ackerknecht, E.H. (1967) *Medicine at the Paris Hospital 1794–1848*. Baltimore: Johns Hopkins Press.

Adelung, T. (1811) *Grammatisch-Kritisches Wörterbuch der hohdeutschen Mundart*. Vienna: Bauer.

Agnew, S.K. & Morris, R.G. (1998) The heterogeneity of anosognosia for memory impairment in Alzheimer's disease: a review of the literature and a proposed model. *Aging & Mental Health*, 2, 7–19.

Alexander, F. & French, T.M. (1946) *Psychoanalytic Therapy: Principles and Applications*. New York: Ronald Press.

Allen, C.C. & Ruff, R.M. (1990) Self-rating versus neuropsychological performance of moderate versus severe head-injured patients. *Brain Injury*, 4, 7–17.

Almeida, O.P., Levy, R., Howard, R.J. & David, A.S. (1996) Insight and paranoid disorders in late life (late paraphrenia). *International Journal of Geriatric Psychiatry*, 11, 653–658.

Amador, X.F. & David, A.S. (Eds) (1998) *Insight and Psychosis*. Oxford: Oxford University Press.

Amador, X. & David, A. (Eds) (2004) *Insight and Psychosis. Awareness of Illness in Schizophrenia and Related Disorders*, 2nd edn. Oxford: Oxford University Press.

Amador, X.F. & Gorman, J.M. (1998) Psychopathological domains and insight in schizophrenia. *The Psychiatry Clinics of North America*, 21, 27–42.

Amador, X.F. & Kronengold, H. (1998) The description and meaning of insight in psychosis. In *Insight and Psychosis*, Eds. X.F. Amador & A.S. David, 1st edn. Oxford: Oxford University Press, pp. 15–32.

Amador, X.F. & Strauss, D.H. (1993) Poor insight in schizophrenia. *Psychiatric Quarterly*, 64, 305–318.

Amador, X.F., Strauss, D.H., Yale, S.A. & Gorman, J.M. (1991) Awareness of illness in schizophrenia. *Schizophrenia Bulletin*, 17, 113–132.

Amador, X.F., Strauss, D.H., Yale, S.A., Flaum, M.M., Endicott, J. & Gorman, J.M. (1993) Assessment of insight in psychosis. *American Journal of Psychiatry*, 150, 873–879.

Amador, X.F., Flaum, M., Andreason, N.C., Strauss, D.H., Yale, S.A., Clark, S.C. & Gorman, J.M. (1994) Awareness of illness in schizophrenia and schizoaffective and mood disorders. *Archives of General Psychiatry*, 51, 826–836.

Amador, X.F., Friedman, J.H., Kasapis, C., Yale, S.A., Flaum, M. & Gorman, J.M. (1996) Suicidal behavior in schizophrenia and its relationship to awareness of illness. *American Journal of Psychiatry*, 153, 1185–1188.

American Psychiatric Association (1987) *Diagnostic and Statistical Manual of Mental Disorders*, 3rd edn. revised (DSM-III-R). Washington, DC: APA.

American Psychiatric Association (1994) *Diagnostic and Statistical Manual of Mental Disorders*, 4th edn. (DSM-IV). Washington, DC: APA.

Aminoff, M.J., Marshall, J., Smith, E.M. & Wyke, M.A. (1975) Pattern of intellectual impairment in Huntington's chorea. *Psychological Medicine*, 5, 169–172.

Anderson, S.W. & Tranel, D. (1989) Awareness of disease states following cerebral infarction, dementia and head trauma: standardized assessment. *The Clinical Neuropsychologist*, 3, 327–339.

Ansburg, P.I. (2000) Individual differences in problem solving via insight. *Current Psychology: Developmental, Learning, Personality, Social*, 19, 143–146.

Anton, G. (1899) Ueber die Selbstwahrnehmung der Herderkrankungen des Gehirns durch den Kranken bei Rindenblindheit und Rindentaubheit. *Archiv für Psychiatrie und Nervenkrankheiten*, 32, 86–127.

Apel, K-O. (1987) Dilthey's distinction between 'explanation' and 'understanding' and the possibility of its 'mediation'. *Journal of the History of Philosophy*, 25, 131–149.

Appelbaum, P.S., Mirkin, S.A. & Bateman, A.L. (1981) Empirical assessment of competency to consent to psychiatric hospitalization. *American Journal of Psychiatry*, 138, 1170–1176.

Appelros, P., Karlsson, G.M., Seiger, Å. & Nydevik, I. (2002) Neglect and anosognosia after first-ever stroke: incidence and relationship to disability. *Journal of Rehabilitation Medicine*, 34, 215–220.

Arango, C., Adami, H., Sherr, J.D., Thaker, G.K. & Carpenter, W.T. (1999) Relationship of awareness of dyskinesia in schizophrenia to insight into mental illness. *American Journal of Psychiatry*, 156, 1097–1099.

Arduini, L., Kalyvoka, A., Stratta, P., Rinaldi, O., Daneluzzo, E. & Rossi, A. (2003) Insight and neuropsychological function in patients with schizophrenia and bipolar disorder with psychotic features. *Canadian Journal of Psychiatry*, 48, 338–341.

Arndt, E. (1905) Zur Analyse des Krankheitsbewusstseins bei Psychosen. *Centralblatt für Nervenheilkunde und Psychiatrie*, 16, 773–797.

Aschaffenburg, G. (1915) Allgemeine Symptomatologie der Psychosen. Krankheitsgefühl und Krankheitseinsicht. In *Handbuch der Psychiatrie*, Ed. G. Aschaffenburg. Leipzig: Franz Deuticke, pp. 367–371.

Auchus, A.P., Goldstein, F.C., Green, J. & Green, R.C. (1994) Unawareness of cognitive impairments in Alzheimer's disease. *Neuropsychiatry Neuropsychology, and Behavioral Neurology*, 7, 25–29.

Azam, É.E. (1892) Double consciousness. In *A Dictionary of Psychological Medicine*, Vol. 1, Ed. D. Hack Tuke. London: J. & A. Churchill, pp. 401–406.

Babinski, M.J. (1914) Contribution à l'étude des troubles mentaux dans l'hémiplégie organique cérébrale (anosognosie). *Revue Neurologique*, 27, 845–848.

Baddeley, A. (1987) *Working Memory*. Oxford: Oxford University Press.

Baier, M., DeShay, E., Owens, K., Robinson, M., Lasar, K., Peterson, K. & Bland, R.S. (2000) The relationship between insight and clinical factors for persons with schizophrenia. *Archives of Psychiatric Nursing*, 14, 259–265.

Baillarger, J.G.F. (1853) Essai sur une classification des différents genres de folie. *Annales Médico-Psychologiques*, 5, 545–566.

Ballard, C.G., Chithiramohan, R.N., Handy, S., Bannister, C., Davis, R. & Todd, N.B. (1991) Information reliability in dementia sufferers. *International Journal of Geriatric Psychiatry*, 6, 313–316.

Baron-Cohen, S. (1995) *Mindblindness*. Cambridge, MA: MIT Press.

Barrett, A.M., Eslinger, P.J., Ballentine, N.H. & Heilman, K.M. (2005) Unawareness of cognitive deficits (cognitive anosognosia) in probably AD and control subjects. *Neurology*, 64, 693–699.

Bartkó, G., Herczeg, I. & Zádor, G. (1988) Clinical symptomatology and drug compliance in schizophrenic patients. *Acta Psychiatrica Scandinavica*, 77, 74–76.

Bauer, R.M. (1984) Autonomic recognition of names and faces in prosopagnosia: a neuropsychological application of the guilty knowledge test. *Neuropsychologia*, 22, 457–469.

Bauer, R.M. (1993) Agnosia. In *Clinical Neuropsychology*, Eds. K.M. Heilman & E. Valenstein, 3rd edn. Oxford: Oxford University Press, pp. 215–278.

Bauer, R.M., Tobias, B. & Valenstein, E. (1993) Amnesic disorders. In *Clinical Neuropsychology*, Eds. K.M. Heilman & E. Valenstein, 3rd edn. Oxford: Oxford University Press, pp. 523–602.

Bear, D.M. (1983) Hemispheric specialization and the neurology of emotion. *Archives of Neurology*, 40, 195–202.

Beaumont, J.G., Kenealy, P.M. & Rogers, M.J.C. (Eds) (1999) *The Blackwell Dictionary of Neuropsychology*. Oxford: Blackwell Publishers Ltd.

Beck, A.T., Ward, C.H., Mendelson, M., Mock, J. & Erbaugh, J. (1961) An inventory for measuring depression. *Archives of General Psychiatry*, 4, 561–571.

Bedford, A. & Foulds, G. (1978) *Personality Deviance Scale (Manual)*. Windsor, Berkshire: NFER Publishing Company.

Benton, A. & Tranel, D. (1993) Visuoperceptual, visuospatial, and visuoconstructive disorders. In *Clinical Neuropsychology*, Eds. K.M. Heilman & E. Valenstein, 3rd edn. Oxford: Oxford University Press, pp. 165–213.

Berrios, G.E. (1992) Phenomenology, psychopathology and Jaspers: a conceptual history. *History of Psychiatry*, 3, 303–327.

Berrios, G.E. (1993) European views on personality disorders: a conceptual history. *Comprehensive Psychiatry*, 34, 14–30.

Berrios, G.E. (1994a) Historiography of mental symptoms and diseases. *History of Psychiatry*, 5, 175–190.

Berrios, G.E. (1994b) Delusions: selected historical and clinical aspects. In *The Neurological Boundaries of Reality*, Ed. E.M.R. Critchley. London, UK: Farrand, pp. 251–267.

Berrios, G.E. (1996) *The History of Mental Symptoms*. Cambridge, UK: Cambridge University Press.

Berrios, G.E. (2000) The history of psychiatric concepts. In *Contemporary Psychiatry: Foundations of Psychiatry*, Vol. 1, Eds. F. Henn, N. Sartorius, H. Helmchen & H. Lauter. Heidelberg: Springer, pp. 1–30.

Berrios, G.E. & Marková, I.S. (2001) Psychiatric disorders mimicking dementia. In *Early-Onset Dementia. A Multidisciplinary Approach*, Ed. J.R. Hodges. Oxford: Oxford University Press, pp. 104–123.

Berrios, G.E. & Marková, I.S. (2002) Conceptual issues. In *Biological Psychiatry*, Eds. H. D'haenen, J.A. den Boer & P. Willner. Chichester, UK: John Wiley & Sons, Ltd., pp. 3–24.

Berrios, G.E. & Marková, I.S. (2003) The self and psychiatry: a conceptual history. In *The Self in Neuroscience and Psychiatry*, Eds. T. Kircher & A. David. Cambridge, UK: Cambridge University Press, pp. 9–39.

Berrios, G.E. & Porter, R. (Eds) (1995) *A History of Clinical Psychiatry. The Origin and History of Psychiatric Disorders*. London, UK: Athlone Press.

Berrios, G.E., Marková, I.S. & Olivares, J.M. (1995) Retorno a los síntomas mentales: hacia una nueva metateoría. *Psiquitría Biológica*, 2, 13–24.

Berti, A. & Rizzolatti, G. (1992) Visual processing without awareness: evidence from unilateral neglect. *Journal of Cognitive Neuroscience*, 4, 345–351.

Berti, A., Làdavas, E., Stracciari, A., Giannarelli, C. & Ossola, A. (1998) Anosognosia for motor impairment and dissociations with patients' evaluation of the disorder: theoretical considerations. *Cognitive Neuropsychiatry*, 3, 21–44.

Bibring, E. (1954) Psychoanalysis and the dynamic psychotherapies. *Journal of the American Psychoanalytic Association*, 2, 745–770.

Billod, E. (1870) Discussion sur les aliénés avec conscience. *Annales Médico-Psychologiques*, 3, 264–281.

Billod, E. (1882) Des aliénés avec conscience de leur état. In *Des Maladies Mentales et Nerveuses*. Paris: Masson, pp. 492–512.

Birchwood, M., Smith, J., Drury, V., Healy, J., Macmillan, F. & Slade, M.A. (1994) A self-report insight scale for psychosis: reliability, validity and sensitivity to change. *Acta Psychiatrica Scandinavica*, 89, 62–67.

Bisiach, E. & Geminiani, G. (1991) Anosognosia related to hemiplegia and hemianopia. In *Awareness of Deficit After Brain Injury*, Eds. G.P. Prigatano & D.L. Schacter. Oxford: Oxford University Press, pp. 17–39.

Bisiach, E., Vallar, G., Perani, D., Papagno, C. & Berti, A. (1986) Unawareness of disease following lesions of the right hemisphere: anosognosia for hemiplegia and anosognosia for hemianopia. *Neuropsychologia*, 24, 471–482.

Blonder, L.X. & Ranseen, J.D. (1994) Awareness of deficit following right hemisphere stroke. *Neuropsychiatry, Neuropsychology, and Behavioral Neurology*, 7, 260–266.

Blum, H.P. (1979) The curative and creative aspects of insight. *Journal of the American Psychoanalytic Association*, 27, 41–69.

Blum, H.P. (1992) Psychic change: the analytic relationship(s) and agents of change. *International Journal of Psycho-Analysis*, 73, 255–265.

Bogetto, F. & Ladu, M.A. (1989) Evaluation of the change in psychotherapy: an experimental study. *European Journal of Psychiatry*, 3, 171–177.

Bologna, S.M. & Camp, C.J. (1997) Covert versus overt self-recognition in late stage Alzheimer's disease. *Journal of the International Neuropsychological Society*, 3, 195–198.

Boring, E.G. (1953) A history of introspection. *Psychological Bulletin*, 50, 169–189.

Bourgeois, M., Swendsen, J., Young, F., Amador, X., Pini, S., Cassano, G.B., Lindenmayer, J-P., Hsu, C., Alphs, L., Meltzer, H.Y. & The InterSePT Study Group (2004) Awareness of disorder and suicide risk in the treatment of schizophrenia: results of the International Suicide Prevention Trial. *American Journal of Psychiatry*, 161, 1494–1496.

Boutroux, E. (1908) De l'influence de la philosophie Écossaise sur la philosophie Française. In *Études d'Histoire de la philosophie*. Paris: Felix Alcan.

Brain, R. (1958) The physiological basis of consciousness. *Brain*, 81, 426–455.

Brentano, F. (1874/1973) *Psychology from an Empirical Standpoint*, Trans. A.C. Rancurello, D.B. Terrell & L.L. McAlister. London: Routledge and Kegan Paul.

Brierre de Boismont, A. (1853) De l'état des facultés dans les délires partiels ou monomanies. *Annales Médico-Psychologiques*, 5, 567–591.

Broadbent, D.E., Cooper, P.F., FitzGerald, P. & Parkes, K.R. (1982) The cognitive failures questionnaire (CFQ) and its correlates. *British Journal of Clinical Psychology*, 21, 1–16.

Brooks, G.P. (1976) The faculty psychology of Thomas Reid. *Journal of the History of the Behavioral Sciences*, 12, 65–67.

Buchanan, A. (1992) A two-year prospective study of treatment compliance in patients with schizophrenia. *Psychological Medicine*, 22, 787–797.

Buchtel, H.A., Henry, T.R. & Aboukhalil, B. (1992) Memory for neurological deficits during the intracarotid amytal procedure: a hemispheric difference. *Journal of Clinical and Experimental Neuropsychology*, 14, 96–97.

Buckley, P.F., Hasan, S., Friedman, L. & Cerny, C. (2001) Insight and schizophrenia. *Comprehensive Psychiatry*, 42, 39–41.

Bucknill, J. & Tuke, D.H. (1858) *A Manual of Psychological Medicine*. London: John Churchill.

Bulbrook, M.E. (1932) An experimental inquiry into the existence and nature of 'insight'. *The American Journal of Psychology*, 44, 409–453.

Burke, J., Knight, R.G. & Partridge, F.M. (1994) Priming deficits in patients with dementia of the Alzheimer type. *Psychological Medicine*, 24, 987–993.

Burke, W.J., Roccaforte, W.H., Wengel, S.P., McArthur-Miller, D., Folks, D.G. & Potter, J.F. (1998) Disagreement in the reporting of depressive symptoms between patients with dementia of the Alzheimer type and their collateral sources. *American Journal of Geriatric Psychiatry*, 6, 308–319.

Burns, A., Jacoby, R. & Levy, R. (1990) Psychiatric phenomena in Alzheimer's disease. III: disorders of mood. *British Journal of Psychiatry*, 157, 81–86.

Butler, S. (1880/1920) *Unconscious Memory*, 3rd edn. London: A.C. Fifield.

Butters, N., Heindel, W.C. & Salmon, D.P. (1990) Dissociation of implicit memory in dementia: neurological implications. *Bulletin of the Psychonomic Society*, 28, 359–366.

Caine, E.D. & Shoulson, I. (1983) Psychiatric syndromes in Huntington's disease. *American Journal of Psychiatry*, 140, 728–733.

Caine, E.D., Hunt, R.D., Weingartner, H. & Ebert, M.H. (1978) Huntington's dementia, clinical and neuropsychological features. *Archives of General Psychiatry*, 35, 377–384.

Cappa, S., Sterzi, R., Vallar, G. & Bisiach, E. (1987) Remission of hemineglect and anosognosia during vestibular stimulation. *Neuropsychologia*, 25, 775–782.

Caracci, G., Mukherjee, S., Roth, S.D. & Decina, P. (1990) Subjective awareness of abnormal involuntary movements in chronic schizophrenia. *American Journal of Psychiatry*, 147, 295–298.

Carroll, A., Fattah, S., Clyde, Z., Coffey, I., Owens, D.G.C. & Johnstone, E.C. (1999) Correlates of insight and insight change in schizophrenia. *Schizophrenia Research*, 35, 247–253.

Carsky, M., Selzer, M.A., Terkelsen, K. & Hurt, S.W. (1992) The PEH: a questionnaire to assess acknowledgement of psychiatric illness. *Journal of Nervous and Mental Disease*, 180, 458–464.

Carveth, D.L. (1998) Is there a future in disillusion? Insight psychotherapy in the new millennium. *Journal of the Melanie Klein and Object Relations*, 16, 555–587.

Cassidy, F., McEvoy, J.P., Yang, Y.K. & Wilson, W.H. (2001) Insight is greater in mixed than in pure manic episodes of bipolar I disorder. *Journal of Nervous and Mental Disease*, 189, 398–399.

Cautela, J.H. (1965) Desensitization and insight. *Behavior Research and Therapy*, 3, 59–64.

Cermak, L.S., Talbot, N., Chandler, K. & Wolbarst, L.R. (1985) The perceptual priming phenomena in amnesia. *Neuropsychologia*, 23, 615–622.

Chen, E.Y.H., Kwok, C.L., Chen, R.Y.L. & Kwong, P.P.K. (2001) Insight changes in acute psychotic episodes. A prospective study of Hong Kong Chinese patients. *Journal of Nervous and Mental Disease*, 189, 24–30.

Chung, K.F., Chen, E.Y.H., Lam, L.C.W., Chen, R.Y.L. & Chan, C.K.Y. (1997) How are psychotic symptoms perceived? A comparison between patients, relatives and the general public. *Australia & New Zealand Journal of Psychiatry*, 31, 756–761.

Clare, L. (2003) Managing threats to self: awareness in early stage Alzheimer's disease. *Social Science & Medicine*, 57, 1017–1029.

Clare, L. (2004) The construction of awareness in early-stage Alzheimer's disease: a review of concepts and models. *British Journal of Clinical Psychology*, 43, 155–175.

Clare, L., Wilson, B.A., Carter, G., Roth, I. & Hodges, J.R. (2002) Assessing awareness in early-stage Alzheimer's disease: development and piloting of the Memory Awareness Rating Scale. *Neuropsychological Rehabilitation*, 12, 341–362.

Clare, L., Marková, I.S., Verhey, F. & Kenny, G. (2005) Awareness in dementia: a review of assessment methods and measures. *Aging & Mental Health*, 9, 394–413.

Collins, A.A., Remington, G.J., Coulter, K. & Birkett, K. (1997) Insight, neurocognitive function and symptom clusters in chronic schizophrenia. *Schizophrenia Research*, 27, 37–44.

Condillac, E.B., Abbé de (1746/1924) *Essai sur l'Origine des Connaissances Humaines. Publié avec notice biographique et bibliographique par R. Lenoir*. Paris: Librairie Armand Colin.

Conrad, K. (1958) *Die Beginnende Schizophrenie*. Stuttgart: Georg Thieme Verlag.

Coons, W.H. (1957) Interaction and insight in group psychotherapy. *Canadian Journal of Psychology*, 11, 1–8.

Cooper, R. (2004) What is wrong with the DSM? *History of Psychiatry*, 15, 5–25.

Cooter, R.J. (1979) Phrenology and British alienists c1825–1845, part I & part II. *Medical History*, 20, 1–21, 135–151.

Correa, D.D., Graves, R.E. & Costa, L. (1996) Awareness of memory deficit in Alzheimer's disease patients and memory-impaired older adults. *Aging, Neuropsychology and Cognition*, 3, 215–228.

Cotrell, V. & Wild, K. (1999) Longitudinal study of self-imposed driving restrictions and deficit awareness in patients with Alzheimer's disease. *Alzheimer Disease and Associated Disorders*, 13, 151–156.

Critchley, M. (1953) *The Parietal Lobes*. London: Arnold.

Crits-Christoph, P., Barber, J.P., Miller, N.E. & Beebe, K. (1993) Evaluating insight. In *Psychodynamic Treatment Research*, Eds. N.E. Miller, L. Luborsky, J.P. Barber & J.P. Docherty. New York: BasicBooks, Harper Collins, pp. 407–422.

Crosson, B., Barco, P.P., Velozo, C.A., Bolesta, M.M., Cooper, P.V., Werts, D. & Brobeck, T.C. (1989) Awareness and compensation in postacute head injury rehabilitation. *Journal of Head Trauma Rehabilitation*, 4, 46–54.

Csikszentmihalyi, M. & Sawyer, K. (1995) Creative insight: the social dimension of a solitary moment. In *The Nature of Insight*, Eds. R.J. Sternberg & J.E. Davidson. Cambridge, Massachusetts: MIT Press, pp. 329–363.

Cuesta, M.J. & Peralta, V. (1994) Lack of insight in schizophrenia. *Schizophrenic Bulletin*, 20, 359–366.

Cuesta, M.J., Peralta, V., Caro, F. & de Leon, J. (1995) Is poor insight in psychotic disorders associated with poor performance on the Wisconsin card sorting test? *American Journal of Psychiatry*, 152, 1380–1382.

Cuesta, M.J., Peralta, V. & Zarzuela, A. (1998) Psychopathological dimensions and lack of insight in schizophrenia. *Psychological Reports*, 83, 895–898.

Cuesta, M.J., Peralta, V. & Zarzuela, A. (2000) Reappraising insight in psychosis. Multi-scale longitudinal study. *British Journal of Psychiatry*, 177, 233–240.

Cuffel, B.J., Alford, J., Fischer, E.P. & Owen, R.R. (1996) Awareness of illness in schizophrenia and outpatient treatment adherence. *Journal of Nervous and Mental Disease*, 184, 653–659.

Cummings, J.L., Ross, W., Absher, J., Gornbein, J. & Hadjiaghai, L. (1995) Depressive symptoms in Alzheimer disease: assessment and determinants. *Alzheimer Disease and Associated Disorders*, 9, 87–93.

Currin, J. (2000) What are the essential characteristics of the analytic attitude? Insight, the use of enactments and relationship. *Journal of Clinical Psychoanalysis*, 9, 75–91.

Cutting, J. (1978) Study of anosognosia. *Journal of Neurology, Neurosurgery and Psychiatry*, 41, 548–555.

Dagonet, M.H. (1881) Conscience et aliénation mentale. *Annales Médico-Psychologiques*, 5, 368–397, 6, 19–32.

Dalla Barba, G., Parlato, V., Iavarone, A. & Boller, F. (1995) Anosognosia, intrusions and 'frontal' functions in Alzheimer's disease and depression. *Neuropsychologia*, 33, 247–259.

Danielczyk, W. (1983) Various mental behavioral disorders in Parkinson's disease, primary degenerative senile dementia, and multiple infarction dementia. *Journal of Neural Transmission*, 56, 161–176.

David, A.S. (1990) Insight and psychosis. *British Journal of Psychiatry*, 156, 798–808.

David, A. & Kemp, R. (1997) Five perspectives on the phenomenon of insight in psychosis. *Psychiatric Annals*, 27, 791–797.

David, A.S. & Cutting, J.C. (Eds) (1994) *The Neuropsychology of Schizophrenia*. Hove, UK: Lawrence Erlbaum Associates.

David, A.S., Buchanan, A., Reed, A. & Almeida, O. (1992) The assessment of insight in psychosis. *British Journal of Psychiatry*, 161, 599–602.

David, A.S., van Os, J., Jones, P., Harvey, I., Foerster, A. & Fahy, T. (1995) Insight and psychotic illness – cross-sectional and longitudinal associations. *British Journal of Psychiatry*, 167, 621–628.

Davidoff, S.A., Forester, B.P., Ghaemi, S.N. & Bodkin, J.A. (1998) Effect of video self-observation on development of insight in psychotic disorders. *Journal of Nervous and Mental Disease*, 186, 697–700.

Davidson, J.E. (1995) The suddenness of insight. In *The Nature of Insight*, Eds. R.J. Sternberg & J.E. Davidson. Cambridge, Massachusetts: MIT Press, pp. 125–155.

Davidson, J.E. & Sternberg, R.J. (1986) What is insight? *Educational Horizon*, 64, 177–179.

Davies, W.G. (1873) Consciousness and 'unconscious cerebration'. *Journal of Mental Science*, 19, 202–217.

De Bettignies, B.H., Mahurin, R.K. & Pirozzolo, F.J. (1990) Insight for impairment in independent living skills in Alzheimer's disease and multi-infarct dementia. *Journal of Clinical and Experimental Neuropsychology*, 12, 355–363.

Debowska, G., Grzywa, A. & Kucharska-Pietura, K. (1998) Insight in paranoid schizophrenia – its relationship to psychopathology and premorbid adjustment. *Comprehensive Psychiatry*, 39, 255–260.

Deckel, A.W. & Morrison, D. (1996) Evidence of a neurologically based 'denial of illness' in patients with Huntington's disease. *Archives of Clinical Neuropsychology*, 11, 295–302.

De Jonghe, F., Rijnierse, P. & Janssen, R. (1992) The role of support in psychoanalysis. *Journal of the American Psychoanalytic Association*, 40, 475–499.

Delasiauve, L.J.F. (1853) De la monomanie au point de vue psychologique et légal. *Annales Médico-Psychologiques*, 5, 353–371.

Delasiauve, L.J.F. (1861) Des diverses formes mentales. *Journal de Médecine Mentale*, 1, 4–14.

Delasiauve, L.J.F. (1863) Délire partiel diffus ou pseudo-monomanie. *Journal de Médecine Mentale*, 3, 80–106.

Delasiauve, L.J.F. (1865) Des diverses formes mentales, folies partielles. *Journal de Médecine Mentale*, 5, 11–20.

Delasiauve, L.J.F. (1866) Discussion sur la folie raisonnante. *Annales Médico-Psychologiques*, 7, 426–431.

Delasiauve, L.J.F. (1870) Discussion sur les aliénés avec consciences. *Annales Médico-Psychologiques*, 3, 103–109, 126–130, 290–291, 307–309.

Dening, T.R. & Berrios, G.E. (1992) The Hachinski ischaemic score: a reevaluation. *International Journal of Geriatric Psychiatry*, 7, 585–589.

Derouesné, C., Thibault, S., Lagha-Pierucci, S., Baudouin-Madec, V., Ancri, D. & Lacomblez, L. (1999) Decreased awareness of cognitive deficit in patients with mild dementia of the Alzheimer's type. *International Journal of Geriatric Psychiatry*, 14, 1019–1030.

Descartes, R. (1648/1991) Conversation with Burman, 16th April 1648. In *The Philosophical Writings of Descartes*, Vol. III, Trans. J. Cottingham, R. Stoothoff, D. Murdoch & A. Kenny. The Correspondence. Cambridge, UK: Cambridge University Press.

Despine, P. (1875) *De la Folie au point de vue Philosophique ou plus spécialement psychologique*. Paris: Savy.

Dickerson, F.B., Boronow, J.J., Ringel, N. & Parente, F. (1997) Lack of insight among outpatients with schizophrenia. *Psychiatric Services*, 48, 195–199.

Dilthey, W. (1976) *Selected Writings*. Cambridge, UK: Cambridge University Press.

Dittman, J. & Schüttler, R. (1990) Disease consciousness and coping strategies of patients with schizophrenic psychosis. *Acta Psychiatrica Scandinavica*, 82, 318–322.

Dixon, M., King, S. & Steiger, H. (1998) The contribution of depression and denial towards understanding the unawareness of symptoms in schizophrenic outpatients. *British Journal of Medical Psychology*, 71, 85–97.

Dominowski, R.L. & Dallob, P. (1995) Insight and problem solving. In *The Nature of Insight*, Eds. R.J. Sternberg & J.E. Davidson. Cambridge, Massachusetts: MIT Press, pp. 33–62.

Doyle, M., Flanagan, S., Browne, S., Clarke, M., Lydon, D., Larkin, E. & O'Callaghan, C. (1999) Subjective and external assessments of quality of life in schizophrenia: relationship to insight. *Acta Psychiatrica Scandinavica*, 99, 466–472.

Drake, R.J. & Lewis, S.W. (2003) Insight and neurocognition in schizophrenia. *Schizophrenia Research*, 62, 165–173.

Drake, R.J., Pickles, A., Bentall, R.P., Kinderman, P., Haddock, G., Tarrier, N. & Lewis, S.W. (2004) The evolution of insight, paranoia and depression during early schizophrenia. *Psychological Medicine*, 34, 285–292.

Duke, L., Seltzer, B., Seltzer, J.E. & Vasterling, J.J. (2002) Cognitive components of deficit awareness in Alzheimer's disease. *Neuropsychology*, 16, 359–369.

Dunbar, K. (1995) How scientists really reason: scientific reasoning in real-world laboratories. In *The Nature of Insight*, Eds. R.J. Sternberg & J.E. Davidson. Cambridge, MA: MIT Press, pp. 365–395.

Duncker, K. (1945) On problem-solving, Trans. L.S. Lees. *Psychological Monographs*, 58, whole no. 270.

Dymond, R.F. (1948) A preliminary investigation of the relation of insight and empathy. *Journal of Consulting Psychology*, 12, 228–233.

Dywan, C.A., McGlone, J. & Fox, A. (1995) Do intracarotid barbiturate injections offer a way to investigate hemispheric models of anosognosia? *Journal of Clinical and Experimental Neuropsychology*, 17, 431–438.

Edelman, G.M. (2003) Naturalizing consciousness: a theoretical framework. *Proceedings of the National Academic Sciences*, 100, 5520–5524.

Ehrenfels, C. von (1890) Ueber 'Gestaltqualitäten'. *Vierteljahrsschrift für wissenschaftliche Philosophie*, 14, 242–292.

Eisen, J.L., Phillips, K.A., Baer, L., Beer, D.A., Atala, K.D. & Rasmussen, S.A. (1998) The Brown assessment of beliefs scale: reliability and validity. *American Journal of Psychiatry*, 155, 102–108.

Eisen, J.L., Rasmussen, S.A., Phillips, K.A., Price, L.H., Davidson, J., Lydiard, R.B., Ninan, P. & Piggott, T. (2001) Insight and treatment outcome in obsessive-compulsive disorder. *Comprehensive Psychiatry*, 42, 494–497.

Eisen, J.L., Phillips, K.A., Coles, M.E. & Rasmussen, S.A. (2004) Insight in obsessive compulsive disorder and body dysmorphic disorder. *Comprehensive Psychiatry*, 45, 10–15.

Ellen, P. & Pate, J.L. (1986) Is insight merely response chaining?: a reply to Epstein. *The Psychological Record*, 36, 155–160.

Elliott, R., Shapiro, D.A., Firth-Cozens, J., Stiles, W.B., Hardy, G.E., Llewelyn, S.P. & Margison, F.R. (1994) Comprehensive process analysis of insight events in cognitive-behavioral and psychodynamic-interpersonal psychotherapies. *Journal of Counselling Psychology*, 41, 449–463.

Endicott, J., Spitzer, R.L., Fleiss, J.L. & Cohen, J. (1976) The global assessment scale. *Archives of General Psychiatry*, 33, 766–771.

Eskey, A. (1958) Insight and prognosis. *Journal of Clinical Psychology*, 14, 426–429.

Esquirol, E. (1819) Monomanie. In *Dictionnaire Des Sciences Médicales*, Vol. 34, Eds. Adelon, Alibert, Barbier *et al.* Paris: Panckoucke, pp. 114–125.

Esquirol, E. (1838) *Des Maladies Mentales Considérés Sous Les Rapports Médical, Hygiénique Et Médico-Légal*, 2 volumes. Paris: Baillière.

Etchegoyen, R.H. (1993) Psychoanalytic technique today: a personal view. *Journal of Clinical Psychoanalysis*, 2, 529–540.

Exner, J.E. & Murillo, L. (1975) Early prediction of post-hospitalization relapse. *Journal of Psychiatric Research*, 12, 231–237.

Fabre Dr. (Ed) (1840) *Dictionnaire des Dictionnaires de Medicine Français et Etrangers*. Paris: Béthune et Plon.

Falret, J.P. (1866) Discussion sur la folie raisonnante. *Annales Médico-Psychologiques*, 7, 382–426.

Falret, J.P. (1870) Discussion sur les aliénés avec conscience. *Annales Médico-Psychologiques*, 3, 120–121, 126.

Feher, E.P., Mahurin, R.K., Inbody, S.B., Crook, T.H. & Pirozzolo, F.J. (1991) Anosognosia in Alzheimer's disease. *Neuropsychiatry, Neuropsychology and Behavioral Neurology*, 4, 136–146.

Feher, E.P., Larrabee, G.J. & Crook, T.H. (1992) Factors attenuating the validity of the Geriatric Depression Scale in a dementia population. *Journal of the American Geriatrics Society*, 40, 906–909.

Feher, E.P., Larrabee, G.J., Sudilovsky, A. & Crook, T.H. (1994) Memory self-report in Alzheimer's disease and in age-associated memory impairment. *Journal of Geriatrics, Psychiatry and Neurology*, 7, 58–65.

Feldman, M.J. & Bullock, D.H. (1955) Some factors related to insight. *Psychological Reports*, 1, 143–152.

Fenichel, O. (1945) *The Psychoanalytic Theory of Neurosis*. New York: W.W. Norton & Company, Inc.

Fennig, S., Everett, E., Bromet, E.J., Jandorf, L., Fennig, S.R., Tanenberg-Karant, M. & Craig, T.J. (1996) Insight in first-admission psychotic patients. *Schizophrenia Research*, 22, 257–263.

Ferris, S.H., Hofeldt, G.T., Carbone, G., Masciandaro, P., Troetel, W.M. & Imbimbo, B.P. (1999) Suicide in two patients with a diagnosis of probable Alzheimer disease. *Alzheimer Disease and Associated Disorders*, 13, 88–90.

Fingarette, H. (1969) *Self-deception*. London: Routledge & Kegan Paul.

Finke, R.A. (1995) Creative insight and preinventive forms. In *The Nature of Insight*, Eds. R.J. Sternberg & J.E. Davidson. Cambridge, MA: MIT Press, pp. 255–280.

Fiore, S.M. & Schooler, J.W. (1998) Right hemisphere contributions to creative problem solving: converging evidence for divergent thinking. In *Right Hemisphere Language Comprehension. Perspectives from Cognitive Neuroscience*, Eds. M. Beeman & C. Chiarello. Mahwah, NJ: Lawrence Erlbaum Associates, pp. 349–371.

Fisher, S. & Greenberg, R.P. (1977) *The Scientific Credibility of Freud's Theories and Therapy*. New York: Harvester Press.

Flashman, L.A., McAllister, T.W., Andreasen, N.C. & Saykin, A.J. (2000) Smaller brain size associated with unawareness of illness in patients with schizophrenia. *American Journal of Psychiatry*, 157, 1167–1169.

Flashman, L.A., McAllister, T.W., Johnson, S.C., Rick, J.H., Green, R.L. & Saykin, A.J. (2001) Specific frontal lobe subregions correlated with unawareness of illness in schizophrenia: a preliminary study. *Journal of Neuropsychiatry and Clinical Neurosciences*, 13, 255–257.

Foa, E.B. (1979) Failure in treating obsessive-compulsives. *Behaviour Research and Therapy*, 17, 169–176.

Foa, E.B. & Kozak, M.J. (1995) DSM-IV field trial: obsessive-compulsive disorder. *American Journal of Psychiatry*, 152, 90–96.

Foa, E.B., Abramowitz, J.S., Franklin, M.E. & Kozak, M.J. (1999) Feared consequences, fixity of belief and treatment outcome in patients with obsessive-compulsive disorder. *Behavior Therapy*, 30, 717–724.

Folstein, M.F., Folstein, S.E. & McHugh, P.R. (1975) 'Mini-mental state': a practical method for grading the cognitive state of patients for the clinician. *Journal of Psychiatric Research*, 12, 189–198.

Foucault, M. (1971) *Madness and Civilization*, Trans. R. Howard. London: Routledge.

Fournet, (no initials) (1870) Discussion sur les aliénés avec conscience. *Annales Médico-Psychologiques*, 3, 121–125.

Francis, J.L. & Penn, D.L. (2001) The relationship between insight and social skill in persons with severe mental illness. *Journal of Nervous and Mental Disease*, 189, 822–829.

Frank, K.A. (1993) Actions, insight and working through. Outline of an integrative approach. *Psychoanalytic Dialogues*, 3, 535–577.

Freud, A. (1981) Insight. Its presence and absence as a factor in normal development. In *The Psychoanalytic Study of the Child*, Vol. 36, Eds. A.J. Solnit, R.S. Eissler, A. Freud, M. Kris & P.B Neubauer. New Haven: Yale University Press, pp. 241–249.

Freud, S. (1900) Preface to the 3rd (revised) English edition to the interpretation of dreams. In *The Standard Edition of the Complete Psychological Works of Sigmund Freud*, Vol. IV. Ed. J. Strachey, 1954. London: Hogarth Press.

Freud, S. (1973a) *Introductory Lectures on Psychoanalysis*, Trans. J. Strachey, 1963, Harmondsworth: Penguin Books Ltd.

Freud, S. (1973b) *New Introductory Lectures on Psychoanalysis*, Trans. J. Strachey, 1964, Harmondsworth: Penguin Books Ltd.

Freudenreich, O., Deckersbach, T. & Goff, D.C. (2004) Insight into current symptoms of schizophrenia. Association with frontal cortical function and affect. *Acta Psychiatrica Scandinavica*, 110, 14–20.

Friedman, R.S. & Förster, J. (2000) The effects of approach and avoidance motor actions on the elements of creative insight. *Journal of Personality and Social Psychology*, 79, 477–492.

Garety, P.A. & Hemsley, D.R. (1994) *Delusions. Investigations into the Psychology of Delusional Reasoning*. Oxford: Oxford University Press.

Gasquoine, P. (1992) Affective state and awareness of sensory and cognitive effects after closed head injury. *Neuropsychology*, 6, 187–196.

Gasquoine, P.G. & Gibbons, T.A. (1994) Lack of awareness of impairment in institutionalized, severely, and chronically disabled survivors of traumatic brain injury: a preliminary investigation. *Journal of Head Trauma Rehabilitation*, 9, 16–24.

Gedo, P.M. & Schaffer, N.D. (1989) An empirical approach to studying psychoanalytic process. *Psychoanalytic Psychology*, 6, 277–291.

Gelder, M., Gath, D., Mayou, R. & Cowen, P. (1996) *Oxford Textbook of Psychiatry*, 3rd edn. Oxford: Oxford University Press.

Gelso, C.J., Hill, C.E. & Kivlighan, D.M. (1991) Transference, insight and the counselor's intentions during a counselling hour. *Journal of Counseling and Development*, 69, 428–433.

Gelso, C.J., Kivlighan, D.M., Wine, B., Jones, A. & Friedman, S.C. (1997) Transference, insight and the course of time-limited therapy. *Journal of Counseling Psychology*, 44, 209–217.

Georget, E. (1820) *De la Folie. Considérations sur cette maladie.* Paris: Crevot.

Geschwind, N. (1965) Disconnexion syndromes in animals and man. *Brain*, 88, 237–294, 585–644.

Ghaemi, S.N. (2003) *The Concepts of Psychiatry. A Pluralistic Approach to the Mind and Mental Illness.* Baltimore and London: John Hopkins Press.

Ghaemi, S.N., Stoll, A.L. & Pope, H.G. (1995) Lack of insight in bipolar disorder. *Journal of Nervous and Mental Disease*, 183, 464–467.

Ghaemi, S.N., Hebben, N., Stoll, A.L. & Pope, H.G. (1996) Neuropsychological aspects of lack of insight in bipolar disorder: a preliminary report. *Psychiatry Research*, 65, 113–120.

Ghaemi, S.N., Sachs, G.S., Baldassano, C.F. & Truman, C.J. (1997) Insight in seasonal affective disorder. *Comprehensive Psychiatry*, 38, 345–348.

Gialanella, B. & Mattioli, F. (1992) Anosognosia and extrapersonal neglect as predictors of functional recovery following right hemisphere stroke. *Neuropsychological Rehabilitation*, 2, 169–178.

Gick, M.L. & Holyoak, K.J. (1980) Analogical problem solving. *Cognitive Psychology*, 12, 306–355.

Gick, M.L. & Holyoak, K.J. (1983) Schema induction and analogical transfer. *Cognitive Psychology*, 15, 1–38.

Gick, M.L. & Lockhart, R.S. (1995) Cognitive and affective components of insight. In *The Nature of Insight*, Eds. R.J. Sternberg & J.E. Davidson. Cambridge, MA: MIT Press, pp. 197–228.

Gil, R., Arroyo-Anllo, E.M., Ingrand, P., Gil, M., Neau, J.P., Ornon, C. & Bonnaud, V. (2001) Self-consciousness and Alzheimer's disease. *Acta Neurologica Scandinavica*, 104, 296–300.

Gillett, G. (1994) Insight, delusion, and belief. *Philosophy, Psychiatry and Psychology*, 1, 227–236.

Gilmore, R.L., Heilman, K.M., Schmidt, R.P., Fennell, E.M. & Quisling, R. (1992) Anosognosia during Wada testing. *Neurology*, 42, 925–927.

Giovannetti, T., Libon, D.J. & Hart, T. (2002) Awareness of naturalistic action errors in dementia. *Journal of the International Neuropsychological Society*, 8, 633–644.

Girard de Gailleux (1870) Discussion sur les aliénés avec conscience de leur état. *Annales Médico-Psychologiques*, 3, 466–471.

Glisky, E.L., Schacter, D.L. & Tulving, E. (1986) Computer learning by memory-impaired patients: acquisition and retention of complex knowledge. *Neuropsychologia*, 24, 313–328.

Gloor, P., Olivier, A., Quesney, L.F., Andermann, F. & Horowitz, S. (1982) The role of the limbic system in experiential phenomena of temporal lobe epilepsy. *Annals of Neurology*, 12, 129–144.

Glucksman, M.L. (1993) Insight, empathy, and internalization: elements of clinical change. *Journal of the American Academy of Psychoanalysis*, 21, 163–181.

Godfrey, G.P.D., Partridge, F.M., Knight, R.G. & Bishara, S. (1993) Course of insight disorder and emotional dysfunction following closed head injury: a controlled cross-sectional follow-up study. *Journal of Clinical and Experimental Neuropsychology*, 15, 503–515.

Goldberg, D.P. & Hillier, V.F. (1979) A scaled version of the General Health Questionnaire. *Psychological Medicine*, 9, 139–145.

Goldberg, E. & Barr, W.B. (1991) Three possible mechanisms of unawareness of deficit. In *Awareness of Deficit After Brain Injury*, Eds. G.P. Prigatano & D.L. Schacter. Oxford: Oxford University Press, pp. 152–175.

Goldberg, R.W., Green-Paden, L.D., Lehman, A.F. & Gold, J.M. (2001) Correlates of insight in serious mental illness. *Journal of Nervous and Mental Disease*, 189, 137–145.

Goldstein, J. (1987) *Console and Classify. The French Psychiatric Profession in the Nineteenth Century*. Cambridge, UK: Cambridge University Press.

Gordon, J. (1815) The doctrines of Gall and Spurzheim. *Edinburgh Review*, 25, 227–268.

Graf, P. & Schacter, D.L. (1985) Implicit and explicit memory for new associations in normal and amnesic subjects. *Journal of Experimental Psychology: Learning, Memory and Cognition*, 11, 501–518.

Green, J., Goldstein, F.C., Sirockman, B.E. & Green, R.C. (1993) Variable awareness of deficits in Alzheimer's disease. *Neuropsychiatry, Neuropsychology and Behavioral Neurology*, 6, 159–165.

Greenfeld, D., Strauss, J.S., Bowers, M.B. & Mandelkern, M. (1989) Insight and interpretation of illness in recovery from psychosis. *Schizophrenia Bulletin*, 15, 245–252.

Greenfeld, D.G., Anyon, W.R., Hobart, M., Quinlan, D. & Plantes, M. (1991) Insight into illness and outcome in anorexia nervosa. *International Journal of Eating Disorders*, 10, 101–109.

Grenyer, B.F.S. & Luborsky, L. (1996) Dynamic change in psychotherapy: mastery of interpersonal conflicts. *Journal of Consulting and Clinical Psychology*, 64, 411–416.

Grimm, J. & Grimm, W. (1862) *Deutsches Wörterbuch*, Vol. 12. Leipzig: S. Hirzel.

Gruber, H.E. (1995) Insight and affect in the history of science. In *The Nature of Insight*, Eds. R.J. Sternberg & J.E. Davidson. Cambridge, MA: MIT Press, pp. 397–431.

Grut, M., Jorm, A.F., Fratiglioni, L., Forsell, Y., Viitanen, M. & Winblad, B. (1993) Memory complaints of elderly people in a population survey: variation according to dementia stage and depression. *Journal of the American Geriatrics Society*, 41, 1295–1300.

Guislain, J. (1852) *Leçons Orales sur les Phrénopathies, ou Traité Théorique et Pratique des Maladies Mentales*. Gand: Hebbelynck.

Gustafson, L. & Nilsson, L. (1982) Differential diagnosis of presenile dementia on clinical grounds. *Acta Psychiatrica Scandinavica*, 65, 194–209.

Guy, W. & Ban, T.A. (1982) *The AMDP-System. Manual for the Assessment and Documentation of Psychopathology*. Berlin: Springer-Verlag.

Hachinski, V.C., Iliff, L.D., Zilhka, E., Du Boulay, G.H., McAllister, V.L., Marshall, J., Russell, R.W.R. & Symon, L. (1975) Cerebral blood flow in dementia. *Archives of Neurology*, 32, 632–637.

Haight, M.R. (1980) *A Study of Self-deception*. Brighton: Harvester Press.

Hameroff, S.R., Kaszniak, A.W. & Scott, A.C. (Eds) (1996) *Toward a Science of Consciousness*. Cambridge, MA: MIT Press.

Hamilton, M. (1967) Development of a rating scale for primary depressive illness. *British Journal of Social and Clinical Psychology*, 6, 278–296.

Hamlyn, D.W. (1977) Self-knowledge. In *The Self: Psychological and Philosophical Issues*, Ed. T. Mischel. Oxford: Blackwell.

Hankoff, L.D., Engelhardt, D.M., Freedman, N., Mann, N. & Margolis, R. (1960a) Denial of illness in schizophrenic outpatients: the effects of psychopharmacological treatment. *Archives of General Psychiatry*, 3, 657–664.

Hankoff, L.D., Engelhardt, D.M. & Freedman, N. (1960b) Placebo response in schizophrenic out-patients. *Archives of General Psychiatry*, 2, 33–42.

Hart, T., Sherer, M., Whyte, J., Polansky, M. & Novack, T.A. (2004) Awareness of behavioral, cognitive, and physical deficits in acute traumatic brain injury. *Archives of Physical Medicine and Rehabilitation*, 85, 1450–1456.

Hartlage, L.C. (1970) Subprofessional therapists' use of reinforcement versus traditional psychotherapeutic techniques with schizophrenics. *Journal of Consulting and Clinical Psychology*, 34, 181–183.

Hartmann, G.W. (1931) The concept and criteria of insight. *Psychological Review*, 38, 242–253.

Hartmann, G.W. (1932) Insight and the context of Gestalt theory. *American Journal of Psychology*, 44, 576–578.

Harwood, D.G. & Sultzer, D.L. (2002) Life is not worth living: hopelessness in Alzheimer's disease. *Journal of Geriatrics Psychiatry and Neurology*, 15, 38–43.

Harwood, D.G., Sultzer, D.L. & Wheatley, M.V. (2000) Impaired insight in Alzheimer's disease: association with cognitive deficits, psychiatric symptoms and behavioural disturbances. *Neuropsychiatry, Neuropsychology and Behavioral Neurology*, 13, 83–88.

Hatcher, R.L. (1973) Insight and self-observation. *Journal of the American Psychoanalytic Association*, 21, 377–398.

Healton, E.B., Navarro, C., Bressman, S. & Brust, J.C.M. (1982) Subcortical neglect. *Neurology*, 32, 776–778.

Heilman, K.M. (1991) Anosognosia: possible neuropsychological mechanisms. In *Awareness of Deficit After Brain Injury*, Eds. G.P. Prigatano & D.L. Schacter. Oxford: Oxford University Press, pp. 53–62.

Heilman, K.M., Watson, R.T. & Valenstein, E. (1993) Neglect and related disorders. In *Clinical Neuropsychology*, Eds. K.M. Heilman & E. Valenstein, 3rd edn. Oxford: Oxford University Press, pp. 279–336.

Heindel, W.C., Salmon, D.P., Shults, C.W., Walicke, P.A. & Butters, N. (1989) Neuropsychological evidence for multiple implicit memory systems: a comparison of Alzheimer's, Huntington's and Parkinson's disease patients. *Journal of Neuroscience*, 9, 582–587.

Heinrichs, E.L., Cohen, B.P. & Carpenter, W.T. (1985) Early insight and the management of schizophrenic decompensation. *Journal of Nervous and Mental Disease*, 173, 133–138.

Henley, R. (1999) Distinguishing insight from intuition. *Journal of Consciousness Studies*, 6, 287–290.

Hering, E. (1870/1920) On memory as a universal function of organised matter. Lecture translated in S. Butler *Unconscious Memory* (1880/1920). London: A.C. Fifield, pp. 63–86.

Hermann, D.J. (1982) Know the memory: the use of questionnaires to assess and study memory. *Psychological Bulletin*, 92, 434–452.

Hier, D.B., Mondlock, J. & Caplan, L.R. (1983a) Behavioral abnormalities after right hemisphere stroke. *Neurology*, 33, 337–344.

Hier, D.B., Mondlock, J. & Caplan, L.R. (1983b) Recovery of behavioral abnormalities after right hemisphere stroke. *Neurology*, 33, 345–350.

Hodges, J.R. (1994) *Cognitive Assessment for Clinicians*. Oxford: Oxford University Press.

Hoffbauer, J.C. (1808/1827) *Médecine Légale relative aux Aliénés et aux Sourds-muets*, Trans A.M. Chambeyron, Notes E. Esquirol & J.M.G. Itard, 3rd edn. Paris: JB. Baillière.

Horton, P.C. (1976) Personality disorder and parietal lobe dysfunction. *American Journal of Psychiatry*, 133, 782–785.

Howorth, P. & Saper, J. (2003) The dimensions of insight in people with dementia. *Aging and Mental Health*, 7, 113–122.

Hutchinson, E.D. (1941) The nature of insight. *Psychiatry Journal for the Study of Interpersonal Processes*, 4, 31–43.

Insel, T.R. & Akiskal, H.S. (1986) Obsessive-compulsive disorder with psychotic features: a phenomenologic analysis. *American Journal of Psychiatry*, 143, 1527–1533.

Ippolito, M.F. & Tweney, R.D. (1995) The inception of insight. In *The Nature of Insight*, Eds. R.J. Sternberg & J.E. Davidson. Cambridge, MA: MIT Press, pp. 433–462.

Iqbal, Z., Birchwood, M., Chadwick, P. & Trower, P. (2000) Cognitive approach to depression and suicidal thinking in psychosis. 2. Testing the validity of a social ranking model. *British Journal of Psychiatry*, 177, 522–528.

Ireland, W.W. (1875) Can unconscious cerebration be proved? *Journal of Mental Science*, 21, 366–387.

Isaak, M.I. & Just, M.A. (1995) Constraints on thinking in insight and invention. In *The Nature of Insight*, Eds. R.J. Sternberg & J.E. Davidson. Cambridge, MA: MIT Press, pp. 281–325.

Jacoby, L.L. & Kelley, C. (1992) Unconscious influences of memory: dissociations and automaticity. In *The Neuropsychology of Consciousness*, Eds. A.D. Milner & M.D. Rugg. London: Academic Press, pp. 201–233.

Jacoby, L.L. & Witherspoon, D. (1982) Remembering without awareness. *Canadian Journal of Psychology*, 36, 300–324.

Janet, P. (1904) L'amnésie et la dissociation des souvenirs par l'émotion. *Journal de Psychologie*, 5, 417–453.

Jaspers, K. (1913) *Allgemeine Psychopathologie*, 1st edn. Berlin: Springer.

Jaspers, K. (1948) *Allgemeine Psychopathologie*, 5th edn. Berlin: Springer.

Jehkonen, M., Ahonen, J-P., Dastidar, P., Laippala, P. & Vilkki, J. (2000) Unawareness of deficits after right hemispheric stroke: double-dissociations of anosognosias. *Acta Neurologica Scandinavica*, 102, 378–384.

Johnson, S. & Orrell, M. (1995) Insight and psychosis: a social perspective. *Psychological Medicine*, 25, 515–520.

Johnson, S. & Orrell, M. (1996) Insight, psychosis and ethnicity: a case-note study. *Psychological Medicine*, 26, 1081–1084.

Jørgensen, P. (1995) Recovery and insight in schizophrenia. *Acta Psychiatrica Scandinavica*, 92, 436–440.

Jorm, A.F., Christensen, H., Henderson, A.S., Korten, A.E., Mackinnon, A.J. & Scott, R. (1994) Complaints of cognitive decline in the elderly: a comparison of reports by subjects and informants in a community survey. *Psychological Medicine*, 24, 365–374.

Joyce, A. & Stoker, J. (2000) Insight and the nature of therapeutic action in the psychoanalysis of 4- and 5-year-old children. *International Journal of Psychoanalysis*, 81, 1139–1154.

Kageyama, J. (1984) Sur l'histoire de la monomanie. *L'Evolution Psychiatrique*, 49, 155–162.

Kahn, R.L. & Fink, M. (1959) Personality factors in behavioral response to electroshock therapy. *Journal of Neuropsychiatry*, 1, 45–49.

Kaplan, C.A. & Simon, H.A. (1990) In search of insight. *Cognitive Psychology*, 22, 374–419.

Kaplan, R.F., Meadows, M.E., Cohen, R.A., Bromfield, E.B. & Ehrenberg, B.L. (1993) Awareness of deficit after the sodium amobarbital (Wada) test. *Journal of Clinical and Experimental Neuropsychology*, 15 (Abstract), 383.

Kaszniak, A.W. & Christenson, G.D. (1996) Self-awareness of deficit in patients with Alzheimer's disease. In *Toward a Science of Consciousness. The First Tucson Discussions and Debates*, Eds. S.R. Hameroff, A.W. Kaszniak & A.C. Scott. Cambridge, MA: MIT Press, pp. 227–242.

Kay, S.R., Fiszbein, A. & Opler, L.A. (1987) The positive and negative syndrome scale (PANSS) for schizophrenia. *Schizophrenia Bulletin*, 13, 261–276.

Keane, M. (1989) Modelling problem solving in Gestalt 'insight' problems. *The Irish Journal of Psychology*, 10, 201–215.

Keane, M.M., Gabrieli, J.D.E., Fennema, A.C., Growden, J.H. & Corkin, S. (1991) Evidence for a dissociation between perceptual and conceptual priming in Alzheimer's disease. *Behavioral Neurosciences*, 105, 326–342.

Kellogg, W.N. (1938) An eclectic view of some theories of learning. *Psychological Review*, 45, 165–184.

Kemp, R. & David, A. (1996) Psychological predictors of insight and compliance in psychotic patients. *British Journal of Psychiatry*, 169, 444–450.

Kemp, R.A. & Lambert, T.J.R. (1995) Insight in schizophrenia and its relationship to psychopathology. *Schizophrenia Research*, 18, 21–28.

Kennedy, H. (1979) The role of insight in child analysis: a developmental viewpoint. *Journal of the American Psychoanalytic Association*, 27, 9–28.

Keshavan, M.S., Rabinowitz, J., DeSmedt, G., Harvey, P.D. & Schooler, N. (2004) Correlates of insight in first episode psychosis. *Schizophrenia Research*, 70, 187–194.

Kim, Y., Sakamoto, K., Kamo, T., Sakamura, Y. & Miyaoka (1997) Insight and clinical correlates in schizophrenia. *Comprehensive Psychiatry*, 38, 117–123.

Kivlighan, D.M., Multon, K.D. & Patton, M.J. (2000) Insight and symptom reduction in time-limited psychoanalytic counseling. *Journal of Counseling Psychology*, 47, 50–58.

Kiyak, H.A., Teri, L. & Borson, S. (1994) Physical and functional health assessment in normal aging and in Alzheimer's disease: self-reports vs family reports. *The Gerontologist*, 34, 324–330.

Koffka, K. (1925/1980) *The Growth of the Mind*, 2nd edn. New Brunswick, NJ: Transaction Books.

Koffka, K. (1935/1963) *Principles of Gestalt Psychology*. New York: Harcourt, Brace & World Inc.

Köhler, W. (1924/1957) *The Mentality of Apes*, Trans. E. Winter, 1925, 2nd edn. Harmondsworth, Middlesex: Penguin Books Ltd.

Kohut, H. (1977) *The Restoration of the Self*. New York: International Universities Press.

Koltai, D.C., Welsh-Bohmer, K.A. & Schmeckel, D.E. (2001) Influence of anosognosia on treatment outcome among dementia patients. *Neuropsychological Rehabilitation*, 11, 455–475.

Korsakoff, S.S. (1889) Étude médico-psychologique sur une forme des maladies de la mémoire. *Revue Philosophique*, 28, 501–530.

Koss, E., Patterson, M.B., Ownby, R., Stuckey, J.C. & Whitehouse, P.J. (1993) Memory evaluation in Alzheimer's disease, caregivers' appraisals and objective testing. *Archives of Neurology*, 50, 92–97.

Kotler-Cope, S. & Camp, C.J. (1995) Anosognosia in Alzheimer's disease. *Alzheimer Disease and Associated Disorders*, 9, 52–56.

Kraepelin, E. (1913/1919) *Dementia Praecox and Paraphrenia*, Trans. R.M. Barclay. Edinburgh: E. & S. Livingstone.

Krafft-Ebing, R. (1893) *Lehrbuch der Psychiatrie*, 5th edn. Stuttgart: F. Enke.

Kris, E. (1956) On some vicissitudes of insight in psychoanalysis. *International Journal of Psycho-Analysis*, 37, 445–455.

Kuriansky, J.B., Gurland, B.J. & Fleiss, J.L. (1976) The assessment of self-care capacity in geriatric psychiatric patients by objective and subjective methods. *Journal of Clinical Psychology*, 32, 95–102.

Lam, D. & Wong, G. (1997) Prodromes, coping strategies, insight and social functioning in bipolar affective disorders. *Psychological Medicine*, 27, 1091–1100.

Lam, L.C., Chan, C.K. & Chen, E.Y. (1996) Insight and general public attitude on psychotic experiences in Hong Kong. *International Journal of Social Psychiatry*, 42, 10–17.

Lamar, M., Lasarev, M.R. & Libon, D.J. (2002) Determining levels of unawareness in dementia research. *Journal of Neuropsychiatry and Clinical Neurosciences*, 14, 430–437.

Lange, K. (1906) *Über Apperzeption*. Leipzig: R. Voigtländers Verlag.

Langer, K.G. & Padrone, F.J. (1992) Psychotherapeutic treatment of awareness in acute rehabilitation of traumatic brain injury. *Neuropsychological Rehabilitation*, 2, 59–70.

Larøi, F., Fannemel, M., Rønneberg, U., Flekkøy, K., Opjordsmoen, S., Dullerud, R. & Haakonsen, M. (2000) Unawareness of illness in chronic schizophrenia and its relationship to structural brain measures and neuropsychological tests. *Psychiatry Research*, 100, 49–58.

Larrabee, G.J., West, R.L. & Crook, T.H. (1991) The association of memory complaint with computer-simulated everyday memory performance. *Journal of Clinical and Experimental Neuropsychology*, 13, 466–478.

Legrand du Saulle, H. (1864) *La Folie devant les Tribunaux*. Paris: Savy.

Lehmkuhl, U. (1989) Wie läßt sich Einsicht vermitteln? Zur Methode und zur Wirkung von Deutungen. *Zeitschrift für Individualpsychologie*, 14, 227–233.

Lelliott, P.T., Noshirvani, H.F., Baþoðlu, M., Marks, I.M. & Monteiro, W.O. (1988) Obsessive-compulsive beliefs and treatment outcome. *Psychological Medicine*, 18, 697–702.

Lélut, F. (1837) *Qu'est-ce que la Phrenologie?* Bruxelles: Établissement Encyclographique.

Lélut, F. (1843) *Rejet de l'organologie phrénologique de Gall, et de ses successeurs*. Paris: Masson.

Levenson, E. (1998) Awareness, insight and learning. *Contemporary Psychoanalysis*, 34, 239–249.

Levin, H.S., High, W.M., Goethe, K.E., Sisson, R.A., Overall, J.E., Rhoades, H.M., Eisenberg, H.M., Kalisky, Z. & Gary, H.E. (1987) The neurobehavioural rating scale: assessment of the behavioural sequelae of head injury by the clinician. *Journal of Neurology, Neurosurgery and Psychiatry*, 50, 183–193.

Levine, H.B. (1994) The analyst's participation in the analytic process. *International Journal of Psycho-Analysis*, 75, 665–676.

Levine, D.N., Calvanio, R. & Rinn, W.E. (1991) The pathogenesis of anosognosia for hemiplegia. *Neurology*, 41, 1770–1781.

Lewis, A. (1934) The psychopathology of insight. *Journal of Medical Psychology*, 14, 332–348.

Lewis, L. (1991) Role of psychological factors in disordered awareness. In *Awareness of Deficit After Brain Injury*, Eds. G.P. Prigatano & D.L. Schacter. Oxford: Oxford University Press, pp. 223–239.

Lezak, M.D. (1995) *Neuropsychological Assessment*, 3rd edn. Oxford: Oxford University Press.

Lin, I.F., Spiga, R. & Fortsch, W. (1979) Insight and adherence to medication in chronic schizophrenics. *Journal of Clinical Psychiatry*, 40, 430–432.

Lindén, J. (1984) Insight and its classification. *Psychoanalysis and Contemporary Thought*, 7, 99–114.

Lindén, J. (1985) Insight through metaphor in psychotherapy and creativity. *Psychoanalysis and Contemporary Thought*, 8, 375–406.

Linn, E.L. (1965) Relevance of psychotic patients' 'insight' to their prognosis. *Archives of General Psychiatry*, 13, 424–428.

Lishman, W.A. (1998) *Organic Psychiatry*, 3rd edn. Oxford: Blackwell.

Locke, J. (1700/1979) *An Essay Concerning Human Understanding*, 4th edn. Oxford: Clarendon Press.

Loebel, J.P., Dager, S.R., Berg, G. & Hyde, T.S. (1990) Fluency of speech and self-awareness of memory deficit in Alzheimer's disease. *International Journal of Geriatric Psychiatry*, 5, 41–45.

Loewald, H.W. (1960) On the therapeutic action of psychoanalysis. *International Journal of Psycho-Analysis*, 41, 16–33.

Loewenstein, R.M. (1956) Some remarks on the role of speech in psycho-analytic technique. *International Journal of Psychoanalysis*, 37, 460–468.

Logsdon, R.G. & Teri, L. (1995) Depression in Alzheimer's disease patients: caregivers as surrogate reporters. *Journal of the American Geriatric Society*, 43, 150–155.

Lopez, O.L., Becker, J.T., Somsak, D., Dew, M.A. & DeKosky, S.T. (1994) Awareness of cognitive deficits and anosognosia in probable Alzheimer's disease. *European Neurology*, 34, 277–282.

Luborsky, L., Diguer, L., Luborsky, E., Singer, B., Dickter, D. & Schmidt, K.A. (1993) The efficacy of dynamic psychotherapies: is it true that 'everyone has won and all must have prizes'? In *Psychodynamic Treatment Research*, Eds. N.E. Miller, L. Luborsky, J.P. Barber & J.P. Docherty. New York: BasicBooks, Harper Collins, pp. 497–516.

Luria, A.R. (1976) *The Neuropsychology of Memory*. New York: Wiley.

Lysaker, P. & Bell, M. (1994) Insight and cognitive impairment. *Journal of Nervous and Mental Disease*, 182, 656–660.

Lysaker, P. & Bell, M. (1995) Work rehabilitation and improvements in insight in schizophrenia. *Journal of Nervous and Mental Disease*, 183, 103–106.

Lysaker, P., Bell, M., Milstein, R., Bryson, G. & Beam-Goulet, J. (1994) Insight and psychosocial treatment compliance in schizophrenia. *Psychiatry*, 57, 307–315.

Lysaker, P.H., Bell, M.D., Bryson, G. & Kaplan, E. (1998a) Neurocognitive function and insight in schizophrenia: support for an association with impairments in executive function but not with impairments in global function. *Acta Psychiatrica Scandinavica*, 97, 297–301.

Lysaker, P.H., Bell, M.D., Bryson, G.J. & Kaplan, E. (1998b) Insight and interpersonal function in schizophrenia. *Journal of Nervous and Mental Disease*, 186, 432–436.

Lysaker, P.H., Bell, M.D., Bryson, G.J. & Kaplan, E. (1999) Personality as a predictor of the variability of insight in schizophrenia. *Journal of Nervous and Mental Disease*, 187, 119–122.

Lysaker, P.H., Bryson, G.J., Lancaster, R.S., Evans, J.D. & Bell, M.D. (2002) Insight in schizophrenia: associations with executive function and coping style. *Schizophrenia Research*, 59, 41–47.

Lysaker, P.H., Lancaster, R.S., Davis, L.W. & Clements, C.A. (2003) Patterns of neurocognitive deficits and unawareness of illness in schizophrenia. *Journal of Nervous and Mental Disease*, 191, 38–44.

MacKenzie, T.B., Robiner, W.N. & Knopman, D.S. (1989) Differences between patient and family assessments of depression in Alzheimer's disease. *American Journal of Psychiatry*, 146, 1174–1178.

MacPherson, R. & Collis, R. (1992) Tardive dyskinesia. Patients' lack of awareness of movement disorder. *British Journal of Psychiatry*, 160, 110–112.

MacPherson, R., Jerrom, B. & Hughes, A. (1996) Relationship between insight, educational background and cognition in schizophrenia. *British Journal of Psychiatry*, 168, 718–722.

McAndrews, M.P., Glisky, E.L. & Schacter, D.L. (1987) When priming persists: long-lasting implicit memory for a single episode in amnesic patients. *Neuropsychologia*, 25, 497–506.

McCabe, R., Quayle, E., Beirne, A. & Duane, M.A. (2000) Is there a role for compliance in the assessment of insight in chronic schizophrenia? *Psychology, Health and Medicine*, 5, 173–178.

McCabe, R., Quayle, E., Beirne, A. & Duane, M.M.A. (2002) Insight, global neuropsychological functioning and symptomatology in chronic schizophrenia. *Journal of Nervous and Mental Disease*, 190, 519–525.

McDaniel, K.D., Edland, S.D., Heyman, A. & the CERAD Clinical Investigators (1995) Relationship between level of insight and severity of dementia in Alzheimer disease. *Alzheimer Disease and Associated Disorders*, 9, 101–104.

McEvoy, J.P. (1998) The relationship between insight in psychosis and compliance with medications. In *Insight and Psychosis*, Eds. X.F. Amador & A.S. David, 1st edn. Oxford: Oxford University Press, pp. 289–306.

McEvoy, J.P., Freter, S., Everett, G., Geller, J.L., Appelbaum, P., Apperson, L.J. & Roth, L. (1989a) Insight and the clinical outcome of schizophrenic patients. *Journal of Nervous and Mental Disease*, 177, 48–51.

McEvoy, J.P., Apperson, L.J., Appelbaum, P.S., Ortlip, P., Brecosky, J., Hammill, K., Geller, J.L. & Roth, L. (1989b) Insight in schizophrenia. Its relationship to acute psychopathology. *Journal of Nervous and Mental Disease*, 177, 43–47.

McEvoy, J.P., Appelbaum, P.S., Apperson, L.J., Geller, J.L. & Freter, S. (1989c) Why must some schizophrenic patients be involuntarily committed? The role of insight. *Comprehensive Psychiatry*, 30, 13–17.

McEvoy, J.P., Freter, S., Merritt, M. & Apperson, L.J. (1993a) Insight about psychosis among outpatients with schizophrenia. *Hospital and Community Psychiatry*, 44, 883–884.

McEvoy, J.P., Schooler, N.R., Friedman, E., Steingard, S. & Allen, M. (1993b) Use of psychopathology vignettes by patients with schizophrenia or schizoaffective disorder and by mental health professionals to judge patients' insight. *American Journal of Psychiatry*, 150, 1649–1653.

McEvoy, J.P., Hartman, M., Gottlieb, D., Goodwin, S., Apperson, L.J. & Wilson, W. (1996) Common sense, insight and neuropsychological test performance in schizophrenia patients. *Schizophrenia Bulletin*, 22, 635–641.

McGlashan, T.H. & Carpenter, W.T. (1981) Does attitude toward psychosis relate to outcome? *American Journal of Psychiatry*, 138, 797–801.

McGlashan, T.H. & Miller, G.H. (1982) The goals of psychoanalysis and psychoanalytic psychotherapy. *Archives of General Psychiatry*, 39, 377–388.

McGlone, J., Gupta, S., Humphrey, D. & Oppenheimer, T. (1990) Screening for early dementia using memory complaints from patients and relatives. *Archives of Neurology*, 47, 1189–1193.

McGlynn, S.M. & Kaszniak, A.W. (1991a) When metacognition fails: impaired awareness of deficit in Alzheimer's disease. *Journal of Cognitive Neuroscience*, 3, 183–189.

McGlynn, S.M. & Kaszniak, A.W. (1991b) Unawareness of deficits in dementia and schizophrenia. In *Awareness of Deficit After Brain Injury*, Eds. G.P. Prigatano & D.L. Schacter. Oxford: Oxford University Press, pp. 84–110.

McGlynn, S.M. & Schacter, D.L. (1989) Unawareness of deficits in neuropsychological syndromes. *Journal of Clinical and Experimental Neuropsychology*, 11, 143–205.

McGorry, P. & McConville, S.B. (1999) Insight in psychosis: an elusive target. *Comprehensive Psychiatry*, 40, 131–142.

McKenna, P.J. (1994) *Schizophrenia and Related Syndromes*. Oxford: Oxford University Press.

McKhann, G., Drachman, D., Folstein, M., Katzman, R., Price, D. & Stadlan, E.M. (1984) Clinical diagnosis of Alzheimer's disease: report of the NINCDS-ADRDA work group under the auspices of the Department of Health and Human Services Task Force on Alzheimer's disease. *Neurology*, 34, 939–944.

McLoughlin, D.M., Cooney, C., Holmes, C. & Levy, R. (1996) Carer informants for dementia sufferers: carer awareness of cognitive impairment in an elderly community-resident sample. *Age and Ageing*, 25, 367–371.

Makkreel, R.A. (1992) *Dilthey*. Princeton: Princeton University Press.

Mangham, C.A. (1981) Insight. Pleasurable affects associated with insight and their origins in infancy. In *The Psychoanalytic Study of the Child*, Vol. 36. Eds. A.J. Solnit, R.S. Eissler, A. Freud, M. Kris & P.B. Neubauer. New Haven: Yale University Press, pp. 271–277.

Mangone, C.A., Hier, D.B., Gorelick, P.B., Ganellen, R.J., Langenberg, P., Boarman, R. & Dollear, W.C. (1991) Impaired insight in Alzheimer's disease. *Journal of Geriatric Psychiatry and Neurology*, 4, 189–193.

Mann, J.H. & Mann, C.H. (1959) Insight as a measure of adjustment in three kinds of group experience. *Journal of Consulting Psychology*, 23, 91.

Marcel, A.J. & Bisiach, E. (Eds) (1988) *Consciousness in Contemporary Science*. Oxford: Oxford University Press.

Marder, S.R., Mebane, A., Chien, C., Winslade, W.J., Swann, E. & Van Putten, T. (1983) A comparison of patients who refuse and consent to neuroleptic treatment. *American Journal of Psychiatry*, 140, 470–472.

Marková, I.S. & Berrios, G.E. (1992a) The meaning of insight in clinical psychiatry. *British Journal of Psychiatry*, 160, 850–860.

Marková, I.S. & Berrios, G.E. (1992b) The assessment of insight in clinical psychiatry: a new scale. *Acta Psychiatrica Scandinavica*, 86, 159–164.

Marková, I.S. & Berrios, G.E. (1995a) Insight in clinical psychiatry revisited. *Comprehensive Psychiatry*, 36, 367–376.

Marková, I.S. & Berrios, G.E. (1995b) Insight in clinical psychiatry: a new model. *Journal of Nervous and Mental Disease*, 183, 743–751.

Marková, I.S. & Berrios, G.E. (1995c) Mental symptoms: are they similar phenomena? The problem of symptom heterogeneity. *Psychopathology*, 28, 147–157.

Marková, I.S. & Berrios, G.E. (2000) Insight into memory deficits. In *Memory Disorders in Psychiatric Practice*, Eds. G.E. Berrios & J.R. Hodges. Cambridge, UK: Cambridge University Press.

Marková, I.S. & Berrios, G.E. (2001) The 'object' of insight assessment: relationship to insight 'structure'. *Psychopathology*, 34, 245–252.

Marková, I.S., Roberts, K.H., Gallagher, C., Boos, H., McKenna, P.J. & Berrios, G.E. (2003) Assessment of insight in psychosis: a re-standardization of a new scale. *Psychiatry Research*, 119(1–2), 81–88.

Marková, I.S., Berrios, G.E. & Hodges, J.R. (2004) Insight into memory function. *Neurology, Psychiatry and Brain Research*, 11, 115–126.

Marks, K.A., Fastenau, P.S., Lysaker, P.H. & Bond, G.R. (2000) Self-appraisal of illness questionnaire (SAIQ): relationship to researcher-rated insight and neuropsychological function in schizophrenia. *Schizophrenia Research*, 45, 203–211.

Martin, A.R. (1952) The dynamics of insight. *American Journal of Psychoanalysis*, 12, 24–38.

Maudsley, H. (1885) *Responsibility in Mental Disease*. London: Kegan Paul & Trench.

Maudsley, H. (1895) *The Pathology of Mind*. London: Macmillan & Co.

Maudsley, H. (1916) *Organic to Human Psychological and Sociological*. London: Macmillan & Co.

Maury, A.L.F (1870) Discussion sur les aliénés avec consciences. *Annales Médico-Psychologiques*, 3, 119–120.

Mayer, R.E. (1995) The search for insight: grappling with Gestalt psychology's unanswered questions. In *The Nature of Insight*, Eds. R.J. Sternberg & J.E. Davidson. Cambridge, MA: MIT Press, pp. 3–32.

Mead, G.H. (1934) *Mind, Self and Society*. Chicago and London: University of Chicago Press.

Mead, G.H. (1936) *Movements of Thought in the Nineteenth Century*. Chicago and London: University of Chicago Press.

Mercier, C.A. (1892) Consciousness. In *A Dictionary of Psychological Medicine*, Vol. 1, Ed. D. Hack Tuke. London: J. & A. Churchill, pp. 249–262.

Mesulam, M-M. (1986) Frontal cortex and behavior. *Annals of Neurology*, 19, 320–325.

Metcalfe, J. (1986a) Feeling of knowing in memory and problem solving. *Journal of Experimental Psychology: Learning, Memory, and Cognition*, 12, 288–294.

Metcalfe, J. (1986b) Premonitions of insight predict impending error. *Journal of Experimental Psychology: Learning, Memory, and Cognition*, 12, 623–634.

Metcalfe, J. (1998) Insight and metacognition. In *Metacognition and Cognitive Neuropsychology*, Eds. G. Mazzoni & T.O. Nelson. Mahwah, NJ: Lawrence Erlbaum Associates, pp. 181–197.

Metcalfe, J. & Shimamura, A.P. (1994) *Metacognition. Knowing about Knowing*. Cambridge: MIT Press.

Metcalfe, J. & Wiebe, D. (1987) Intuition in insight and noninsight problem solving. *Memory & Cognition*, 15, 238–246.

Michalakeas, A., Skoutas, C., Charatambous, A., Peristeris, A., Marinos, V., Keramari, E. & Theologou, A. (1994) Insight in schizophrenia and mood disorders and its relation to psychopathology. *Acta Psychiatrica Scandinavica*, 90, 46–49.

Michon, A., Deweer, B., Pillon, B., Agid, Y. & Dubois, B. (1992) Anosognosia and frontal dysfunction in SDAT. *Neurology* (Suppl. 3), 42, 221.

Michon, A., Deweer, B., Pillon, B., Agid, Y. & Dubois, B. (1994) Relation of anosognosia to frontal lobe dysfunction in Alzheimer's disease. *Journal of Neurology, Neurosurgery and Psychiatry*, 57, 805–809.

Migliorelli, R., Tesón, A., Sabe, L., Petracca, G., Petracchi, M., Leiguarda, R. & Starkstein, S.E. (1995) Anosognosia in Alzheimer's disease: a study of associated factors. *Journal of Neuropsychiatry and Clinical Sciences*, 7, 338–344.

Miller, E. & Lewis, P. (1977) Recognition memory in elderly patients with depression and dementia: a signal detection analysis. *Journal of Abnormal Psychology*, 86, 84–86.

Milner, A.D. & Rugg, M.D (Eds) (1992) *The Neuropsychology of Consciousness*. London: Academic Press Ltd.

Mintz, A.R., Dobson, K.S. & Romney, D.M. (2003) Insight in schizophrenia: a meta-analysis. *Schizophrenia Research*, 61, 75–88.

Mintz, A.R., Addington, J. & Addington, D. (2004) Insight in early psychosis: a 1-year follow-up. *Schizophrenia Research*, 67, 213–217.

Mohamed, S., Fleming, S., Penn, D.L. & Spaulding, W. (1999) Insight in schizophrenia: its relationship to measures of executive functions. *Journal of Nervous and Mental Disease*, 187, 525–531.

Moore, O., Cassidy, E., Carr, A. & O'Callaghan, E. (1999) Unawareness of illness and its relationship with depression and self-deception in schizophrenia. *European Psychiatry*, 14, 264–269.

Morgan, R., Luborsky, L., Crits-Christoph, P., Curtis, H. & Solomon, J. (1982) Predicting the outcomes of psychotherapy by the Penn Helping Alliance rating method. *Archives of General Psychiatry*, 39, 397–402.

Morel, B.A. (1870) Discussion sur les aliénés avec conscience. *Annales Médico-Psychologiques*, 3, 110–119.

Morris, L. (1972) *The Discovery of the Individual, 1050–1200*. New York: Harper and Row.

Moulin, C.J.A., Perfect, T.J. & Jones, R.W. (2000) Global predictions of memory in Alzheimer's disease: evidence for preserved metamemory monitoring. *Aging, Neuropsychology and Cognition*, 7, 230–244.

Mullen, R., Howard, R., David, A. & Levy, R. (1996) Insight in Alzheimer's disease. *International Journal of Geriatric Psychiatry*, 11, 645–651.

Mutsatsa, S.H., Joyce, E.M., Hutton, S.B., Webb, E., Gibbins, H., Paul, S. & Barnes, T.R.E. (2003) Clinical correlates of early medication adherence: West London first episode schizophrenia study. *Acta Psychiatrica Scandinavica*, 108, 439–446.

Myerson, P.G. (1960) Awareness and stress: post-psycho-analytic utilization of insight. *International Journal of Psycho-Analysis*, 41, 147–156.

Myerson, P.G. (1965) Modes of insight. *Journal of the American Psychoanalytic Association*, 13, 771–792.

Myslobodsky, M.S. (1986) Anosognosia in tardive dyskinesia: 'tardive dysmentia' or 'tardive dementia'? *Schizophrenia Bulletin*, 12, 1–6.

Neary, D., Snowden, J.S., Bowen, D.M., Sims, N.R., Mann, D.M.A., Benton, J.S., Northen, B. Yates, P.O. & Davison, A.N. (1986) Neuropsychological syndromes in presenile dementia due to cerebral atrophy. *Journal of Neurology, Neurosurgery and Psychiatry*, 49, 163–174.

Neubauer, P.B. (1979) The role of insight in psychoanalysis. *Journal of the American Psychoanalytic Association*, 27, 29–40.

Neundorfer, M.M. (1997) Awareness of variability in awareness. *Alzheimer Disease and Associated Disorders*, 11, 121–122.

Niederehe, G. (1988) TRIMS behavioral problem checklist (BPC). *Psychopharmacology Bulletin*, 24, 771–773.

Nisbett, R.E. & Wilson, T.D. (1977) Telling more than we can know: verbal reports on mental processes. *Psychological Review*, 84, 231–259.

O'Connor, R. & Herrman, H. (1993) Assessment of contributions to disability in people with schizophrenia during rehabilitation. *Australia and New Zealand Journal of Psychiatry*, 27, 595–600.

O'Connor, L.E., Edelstein, S., Berry, J.W. & Weiss, J. (1994) Changes in the patient's level of insight in brief psychotherapy: two pilot studies. *Psychotherapy*, 31, 533–544.

O'Mahoney, P.D. (1982) Psychiatric patient denial of mental illness as a normal process. *British Journal of Medical Psychology*, 55, 109–118.

Oddy, M., Coughlan, T., Tyerman, A. & Jenkins, D. (1985) Social adjustment after closed head injury: a further follow-up seven years after injury. *Journal of Neurology, Neurosurgery and Psychiatry*, 48, 564–568.

Ogden, R.M. (1932) Insight. *American Journal of Psychology*, 44, 350–356.

Ohlsson, S. (1984a) Restructuring revisited. I. Summary and critique of the Gestalt theory of problems solving. *Scandinavian Journal of Psychology*, 25, 65–78.

Ohlsson, S. (1984b) Restructuring revisited. II. An information processing theory of restructuring and insight. *Scandinavian Journal of Psychology*, 25, 117–129.

Olmos-de-Paz, T. (1990) Working-through and insight in child psychoanalysis. *Melanie Klein and Object Relations*, 8, 99–112.

Orange, W. (1892) Criminal responsibility. In *A Dictionary of Psychological Medicine*, Vol. 1, Ed. D. Hack Tuke. London: J. & A. Churchill, pp. 294–320.

Orrell, M.W. & Sahakian, B.J. (1991) Dementia of frontal lobe type. *Psychological Medicine*, 21, 553–556.

Osgood, C.E. (1964) *Method and Theory in Experimental Psychology*. New York: Oxford University Press.

Ott, B.R. & Fogel, B.S. (1992) Measurement of depression in dementia: self vs clinician rating. *International Journal of Geriatric Psychiatry*, 7, 899–904.

Ott, B.R., Lafleche, G., Whelihan, W.M., Buongiorno, G.W., Albert, M.S. & Fogel, B.S. (1996a) Impaired awareness of deficits in Alzheimer disease. *Alzheimer Disease and Associated Disorders*, 10, 67–76.

Ott, B.R., Noto, R.B. & Fogel, B.S. (1996b) Apathy and loss of insight in Alzheimer's disease: A SPECT imaging study. *Journal of Neuropsychiatry and Clinical Neurosciences*, 8, 41–46.

Paillard, J., Michel, F. & Stelmack, G. (1983) Localization without content. A tactile analogue of 'blind sight'. *Archives of Neurology*, 40, 548–551.

Pallanti, S., Quercioli, L., Pazzagli, A., Rossi, A., Dell'Osso, L., Pini, S. & Cassano, G.B. (1999) Awareness of illness and subjective experience of cognitive complaints in patients with bipolar I and bipolar II disorder. *American Journal of Psychiatry*, 156, 1094–1096.

Parant,V. (1888) *La Raison dans la Folie*. Paris: Doin.

Paul, G.L. (1967) Insight versus desensitization in psychotherapy two years after termination. *Journal of Consulting Psychology*, 31, 333–348.

Pauleikhoff, B. & Mester, H. (1973) Einsicht. In *Lexikon der Psychiatrie*, Ed. C. Müller. Heidelberg: Springer, pp. 150–151.

Pedersen, P.M., Jörgensen, H.S., Nakayama, H., Raaschou, H.O. & Olsen, T.S. (1996) Frequency, determinants and consequences of anosognosia in acute stroke. *Journal of Neurological Rehabilitation*, 10, 243–250.

Penfield, W. (1975) *The Mystery of the Mind. A Critical Study of Consciousness and the Human Brain*. Princeton: Princeton University Press.

Peralta, V. & Cuesta, M.J. (1994) Lack of insight: its status within schizophrenic psychopathology. *Biological Psychiatry*, 36, 559–561.

Peralta, V. & Cuesta, M.J. (1998) Lack of insight in mood disorders. *Journal of Affective Disorders*, 46, 55–58.

Perenin, M.T. & Jeannerod, M. (1975) Residual vision in cortically blind hemifields. *Neuropsychologia*, 13, 1–7.

Perenin, M.T. & Jeannerod, M. (1978) Visual function within the hemianopic field following early cerebral hemidecortication in man, parts I & II. *Neuropsychologia*, 16, 1–13, 697–708.

Perenin, M.T., Ruel, J. & Hécaen, H. (1980) Residual visual capacities in a case of cortical blindness. *Cortex*, 16, 605–612.

Perkins, D.N. (1981) *The Mind's Best Work*. Cambridge, MA: Harvard University Press.

Perkins, D.N. (1995) Insight in minds and genes. In *The Nature of Insight*, Eds. R.J. Sternberg & J.E. Davidson. Cambridge, MA: MIT Press, pp. 495–533.

Perkins, J.A. (1969) *The Concept of the Self in the French Enlightenment*. Geneva: Libraire Droz.

Persson, G. & Alström, J.E. (1983) A scale for rating suitability for insight-oriented psychotherapy. *Acta Psychiatrica Scandinavica*, 68, 117–125.

Persson, G. & Alström, J.E. (1984) Suitability for insight-oriented psychotherapy as a prognostic factor in treatment of phobic women. *Acta Psychiatrica Scandinavica*, 69, 318–326.

Phinney, A. (2002) Fluctuating awareness and the breakdown of the illness narrative in dementia. *Dementia*, 1, 329–344.

Pick, A. (1882) Ueber Krankheitsbewusstsein in psychischen Krankheiten. *Archiv für Psychiatrie und Nervenkrankheiten*, 13, 518–581.

Pico della Mirandola, G. *On the Dignity of Man*, Trans. C.G. Wallis (1965). Indianapolis and New York: Bobbs-Merrill.

Picton, T.W. & Stuss, D.T. (1994) Neurobiology of conscious experience. *Current Opinion in Neurobiology*, 4, 256–265.

Pierce, B.H. (1999) An evolutionary perspective on insight. In *Evolution of the Psyche*, Eds. D.H. Rosen & M.C. Luebbert. Westport, Connecticut: Praeger Publishers, pp. 106–122.

Pinel, Ph. (1801) *Traité Médico-philosophique sur l'Aliénation Mentale, ou la Manie*. Paris: Richard, Caille et Ravier.

Pinel, Ph. (1809) *Traité médico-philosophique sur l'aliénation mentale*, 2nd edn. Paris: Brosson.

Pini, S., Cassano, G.B., Dell'Osso, L. & Amador, X.F. (2001) Insight into illness in schizophrenia, schizoaffective disorder and mood disorder with psychotic features. *American Journal of Psychiatry*, 158, 122–125.

Plato (1892) Alcibiades, I. In *The Dialogues of Plato*, vol. II, Ed. & Trans. B. Jowett. Oxford: Clarendon Press.

Plato (1987) Charmides. In *Plato, Early Socratic Dialogues*, Trans. D. Watt. Harmondsworth: Penguin Press.

Poland, W.S. (1988) Insight and the analytic dyad. *Psychoanalytic Quarterly*, 57, 341–369.

Pollock, G.H. (1981) Reminiscences and insight. In *The Psychoanalytic Study of the Child*, Vol. 36, Eds. A.J. Solnit, R.S. Eissler, A. Freud, M. Kris & P.B. Neubauer. New Haven: Yale University Press, pp. 289–305.

Porter, R. (1987) *A Social History of Madness*. London: Phoenix Giant, Orion Books Ltd.

Porter, R. (1990) *Mind-Forg'd Manacles*. Harmondsworth: Penguin Books Ltd.

Price, B.H. & Mesulam, M. (1985) Psychiatric manifestation of right hemisphere infarctions. *Journal of Nervous and Mental Disease*, 173, 610–614.

Prichard, J.C. (1835) *A Treatise on Insanity and other Disorders Affecting the Mind*. London: Sherwood, Gilbert and Piper.

Prigatano, G.P. (1991) Disturbances of self-awareness of deficit after traumatic brain injury. In *Awareness of Deficit After Brain Injury*, Eds. G.P. Prigatano & D.L. Schacter. Oxford: Oxford University Press, pp. 111–126.

Prigatano, G.P. (1996) Behavioral limitations TBI patients tend to underestimate: a replication and extension to patients with lateralized cerebral dysfunction. *Clinical Neuropsychologist*, 10, 191–201.

Prigatano, G.P. & Altman, I.M. (1990) Impaired awareness of behavioral limitations after traumatic brain injury. *Archives of Physical Medicine and Rehabilitation*, 71, 1058–1064.

Prigatano, G.P. & Schacter, D.L. (Eds) (1991) *Awareness of Deficit After Brain Injury*. Oxford: Oxford University Press.

Prigatano, G.P., Fordyce, D.J., Zeiner, H.K., Roueche, J.R., Pepping, M. & Wood, B.C. (1986) *Neuropsychological Rehabilitation After Brain Injury*. Baltimore: Johns Hopkins University Press.

Prigatano, G.P., Ogano, M. & Amakusa, B. (1997) A cross-cultural study on impaired self-awareness in Japanese patients with brain dysfunction. *Neuropsychiatry, Neuropsychology and Behavioral Neurology*, 10, 135–143.

Pulver, S.E. (1992) Psychic change: insight or relationship. *International Journal of Psychoanalysis*, 73, 199–206.

Pyne, J.M., Bean, D. & Sullivan, G. (2001) Characteristics of patients with schizophrenia who do not believe they are mentally ill. *Journal of Nervous and Mental Disease*, 189, 146–153.

Rachman, S.J. & Hodgson, R.J. (1980) *Obsessions and Compulsions*. New Jersey: Prentice-Hall, Inc.

Reber, A.S. (1993) *Implicit Learning and Tacit Knowledge. An Essay on the Cognitive Unconscious*. Oxford: Oxford University Press.

Reder, L.M. (1996) *Implicit Memory and Metacognition*. New Jersey: Lawrence Erlbaum.

Redlich, F.C. & Dorsey, J.F. (1945) Denial of blindness by patients with cerebral disease. *Archives of Neurology and Psychiatry*, 53, 407–417.

Reed, B.R., Jagust, W.J. & Coulter, L. (1993) Anosognosia in Alzheimer's disease: relationships to depression, cognitive function, and cerebral perfusion. *Journal of Clinical and Experimental Neuropsychology*, 15, 231–244.

Reid, T. (1785/1994) *The Works of Thomas Reid*, Ed. W. Hamilton (1863). Bristol: Thoemmes Press.

Reid, J.R. & Finesinger, J.E. (1952) The role of insight in psychotherapy. *American Journal of Psychiatry*, 108, 726–734.

Reifler, B.V., Larson, E. & Hanley, R. (1982) Coexistence of cognitive impairment and depression in geriatric outpatients. *American Journal of Psychiatry*, 139, 623–626.

Reisberg, B., Ferris, S.H., de Leon, M.J. & Crook, T. (1982) The global deterioration scale for assessment of primary degenerative dementia. *American Journal of Psychiatry*, 139, 1136–1139.

Reisberg, B., Gordon, B., McCarthy, M., Ferris, S.H. & deLeon, M.J. (1985) Insight and denial accompanying progressive cognitive decline in normal aging and Alzheimer's disease. In *Geriatric Psychiatry: Ethical and Legal Issues*, Ed. B. Stanley. Washington, DC: American Psychiatric Press, pp. 38–79.

Rhee, D. (1990) The Tao, psychoanalysis and existential thought. *Psychotherapy and Psychosomatics*, 53, 21–27.

Richfield, J. (1954) An analysis of the concept of insight. *Psychoanalytic Quarterly*, 23, 390–408.

Riley, K.C. (1988) Measurement of dissociation. *Journal of Nervous and Mental Disease*, 176, 449–450.

Ritter, J. (1972) *Historisches Wörterbuch der Philosophie*. Darmstadt: Wissenschaftliche Buchgesellschaft.

Ritti, A. (1879) Folie avec conscience. In *Dictionnaire Encyclopédique des Sciences Médicales*, Vol. 39, Ed. A. Dechambre. Paris: Masson, pp. 307–320.

Roback, H.B. (1971) The comparative influence of insight and non-insight psychotherapies on therapeutic outcome: a review of the experimental literature. *Psychotherapy: Theory, Research and Practice*, 8, 23–25.

Roback, H.B. (1972) Experimental comparison of outcomes in insight- and non-insight-oriented therapy groups. *Journal of Consulting and Clinical Psychology*, 38, 411–417.

Roback, H.B. (1974) Insight: a bridging of the theoretical and research literatures. *The Canadian Psychologist*, 15, 61–88.

Roback, H.B. & Abramowitz, S.I. (1979) Insight and hospital adjustment. *Canadian Journal of Psychiatry*, 24, 233–236.

Robert, P.H., Clairet, S., Benoit, M., Koutaich, J., Bertogliati, C., Tible, O., Caci, H., Borg, M., Brocker, P. & Bedoucha, P. (2002) The apathy inventory: assessment of apathy and awareness in Alzheimer's disease, Parkinson's disease and mild cognitive impairment. *International Journal of Geriatric Psychiatry*, 17, 1099–1105.

Rohde, K., Peskind, E.R. & Raskind, M.A. (1995) Suicide in two patients with Alzheimer's disease. *Journal of the American Geriatrics Society*, 43, 187–189.

Rose, G. (1878) *Neues Wörterbuch der Französischen und Deutschen Sprache*. Berlin: Schreiter.

Rossell, S-L., Coakes, J., Shapleske, J., Woodruff, P.W. & David, A.S. (2003) Insight: its relationship with cognitive function, brain volume and symptoms in schizophrenia. *Psychological Medicine*, 33, 111–119.

Roth, M. (1949) Disorders of the body image caused by lesions of the right parietal lobe. *Brain*, 72, 89–111.

Roth, N. (1944) Unusual types of anosognosia and their relation to the body image. *Journal of Nervous and Mental Disease*, 100, 35–43.

Rubens, A.B. & Garrett, M.F. (1991) Anosognosia of linguistic deficits in patients with neurological deficits. In *Awareness of Deficit After Brain Injury*, Eds. G.P. Prigatano & D.L. Schacter. Oxford: Oxford University Press, pp. 40–52.

Rubenstein, L.Z., Schairer, C., Wieland, G.D. & Kane, R. (1984) Systematic biases in functional status assessment of elderly adults: effects of different data sources. *Journal of Gerontology*, 39, 686–691.

Rubinštejn, S.L. (1960) *O Myslení A Spôsobech Jeho Vyskumu*. Bratislava: Slovenske Pedagogické Nakladatelstvo.

Rugg, M.D. (1995) Memory and consciousness: a selective review of issues and data. *Neuropsychologia*, 33, 1131–1141.

Rullier (1815) Faculté. In *Dictionnaire Des Sciences Médicales*, Vol. 14, Eds. Adelon, Alard, Alibert *et al*. Paris: Panckoucke, pp. 389–420.

Russo, R. & Spinnler, H. (1994) Implicit verbal memory in Alzheimer's disease. *Cortex*, 30, 359–375.

Ryle, G. (1949/1990) *The Concept of Mind*. Harmondsworth: Penguin Books.

Rymer, S., Salloway, S., Norton, L., Malloy, P., Correia, S. & Monast, D. (2002) Impaired awareness, behaviour disturbance and caregiver burden in Alzheimer disease. *Alzheimer Disease and Associated Disorders*, 16, 248–253.

Samoilov, A., Goldfried, M.R. & Shapiro, D.A. (2000) Coding system for therapeutic focus on action and insight. *Journal of Consulting and Clinical Psychology*, 68, 513–514.

Sampson, H. (1991) Experience and insight in the resolution of transferences. *Contemporary Psychoanalysis*, 27, 200–207.

Sanz, M., Constable, G., Lopez-Ibor, I., Kemp, R. & David, A.S. (1998) A comparative study of insight scales and their relationship to psychopathological and clinical variables. *Psychological Medicine*, 28, 437–446.

Sargent, H.D. (1953) *The Insight Test*. New York: Grune & Stratton.

Sayer, N.A., Sackeim, H.A., Moeller, J.R., Prudic, J., Devanand, D.P., Coleman, E.A. & Kiersky, J.E. (1993) The relations between observer-rating and self-report of depressive symptomatology. *Psychological Assessment*, 5, 350–360.

Schacter, D.L. (1987) Implicit memory: history and current status. *Journal of Experimental Psychology: Learning, Memory and Cognition*, 13, 501–518.

Schacter, D.L. (1990) Toward a cognitive neuropsychology of awareness: implicit knowledge and anosognosia. *Journal of Clinical and Experimental Neuropsychology*, 12, 155–178.

Schacter, D.L. (1991) Unawareness of deficit and unawareness of knowledge in patients with memory disorders. In *Awareness of Deficit After Brain Injury*, Eds. G.P. Prigatano & D.L. Schacter. Oxford: Oxford University Press, pp. 127–151.

Schacter, D.L. (1992) Consciousness and awareness in memory and amnesia: critical issues. In *The Neuropsychology of Consciousness*, Eds. A.D. Milner & M.D. Rugg. London: Academic Press, pp. 179–200.

Schacter, D.L. (1995) Implicit memory: a new frontier for cognitive neuroscience. In *The Cognitive Neurosciences*, Ed. M.S. Gazzaniga. Cambridge, MA: MIT Press, pp. 815–824.

Schacter, D.L. (1999) Implicit vs explicit memory. In *The MIT Encyclopedia of the Cognitive Sciences*, Eds. R.A. Wilson & F.C. Keil. Cambridge, MA: MIT Press, pp. 394–395.

Schacter, D.L., Chiu, C.-Y.P. & Ochsner, K.N. (1993) Implicit memory: a selective review. *Annual Review of Neuroscience*, 16, 159–182.

Schmukler, A.G. (1999) Use of insight in child analysis. *Psychoanalytic Study of the Child*, 54, 339–355.

Schneck, M.K., Reisberg, B. & Ferris, S.H. (1982) An overview of current concepts in Alzheimer's disease. *American Journal of Psychiatry*, 139, 165–173.

Schooler, J.W., Ohlsson, S. & Brooks, K. (1993) Thoughts beyond words: when language overshadows insight. *Journal of Experimental Psychology: General*, 122, 166–183.

Schooler, J.W., Fallshore, M. & Fiore, S.M. (1995) Epilogue: putting insight into perspective. In *The Nature of Insight*, Eds. R.J. Sternberg & J.E. Davidson. Cambridge, MA: MIT Press, pp. 559–587.

Schwartz, R.C. (1998a) Symptomatology and insight in schizophrenia. *Psychological Reports*, 82, 227–233.

Schwartz, R.C. (1998b) Insight and illness in chronic schizophrenia. *Comprehensive Psychiatry*, 39, 249–254.

Schwartz, R.C. (2001) Self-awareness in schizophrenia: its relationship to depressive symptomatology and broad psychiatric impairments. *Journal of Nervous and Mental Disease*, 189, 401–403.

Schwartz, R.C. & Petersen, S. (1999) The relationship between insight and suicidality among patients with schizophrenia. *Journal of Nervous and Mental Disease*, 187, 376–378.

Segal, H. (1962) The curative factors in psychoanalysis. *International Journal of Psychoanalysis*, 43, 212–217.

Segal, H. (1991) Psychoanalyse et thérapeutique. *Revue Francoise de Psychoanalyse*, 55, 365–376.

Seifert, C.M., Meyer, D.E., Davidson, N., Patalano, A.L. & Yaniv, I. (1995) Demystification of cognitive insight: opportunistic assimilation and the prepared-mind perspective. In *The Nature of Insight*, Eds. R.J. Sternberg & J.E. Davidson. Cambridge, MA: MIT Press, pp. 65–124.

Seltzer, B., Vasterling, J.J. & Buswell, A. (1995a) Awareness of deficit in Alzheimer's disease: association with psychiatric symptoms and other disease variables. *Journal of Clinical Geropsychology*, 1, 79–87.

Seltzer, B., Vasterling, J.J., Hale, M.A. & Khurana, R. (1995b) Unawareness of memory deficit in Alzheimer's disease: relation to mood and other disease variables. *Neuropsychiatry, Neuropsychology and Behavioral Neurology*, 8, 176–181.

Seltzer, B., Vasterling, J.J., Yoder, J. & Thompson, K.A. (1997) Awareness of deficit in Alzheimer's disease: relation to caregiver burden. *The Gerontologist*, 37, 20–24.

Sevush, S. (1999) Relationship between denial of memory deficit and dementia severity in Alzheimer's disease. *Neuropsychiatry, Neuropsychology and Behavioral Neurology*, 12, 88–94.

Sevush, S. & Leve, N. (1993) Denial of memory deficit in Alzheimer's disease. *American Journal of Psychiatry*, 150, 748–751.

Sevy, S., Nathanson, K., Visweswaraiah, H. & Amador, X. (2004) The relationship between insight and symptoms in schizophrenia. *Comprehensive Psychiatry*, 45, 16–19.

Shaw, T.C. (1909) The clinical value of consciousness in disease. *Journal of Mental Science*, 55, 401–410.

Shengold, L. (1981) Insight as metaphor. In *The Psychoanalytic Study of the Child*, Vol. 36, Eds. A.J. Solnit, R.S. Eissler, A. Freud, M. Kris & P.B. Neubauer. New Haven: Yale University Press, pp. 289–305.

Sherer, M., Bergloff, P., Boake, C., High, W. & Levin, E. (1998a) The awareness questionnaire: factor analysis structure and internal consistency. *Brain Injury*, 12, 63–68.

Sherer, M., Boake, C., Levin, E., Silver, B.V., Ringholz, G. & High, W.M. (1998b) Characteristics of impaired awareness after traumatic brain injury. *Journal of the International Neuropsychological Society*, 4, 380–387.

Sherer, M., Hart, T. & Nick, T.G. (2003a) Measurement of impaired self-awareness after traumatic brain injury: a comparison of the patient competency rating scale and the awareness questionnaire. *Brain Injury*, 17, 25–37.

Sherer, M., Hart, T., Nick, T.G., Whyte, J., Thompson, R.N. & Yablon, S.A. (2003b) Early impaired self-awareness after traumatic brain injury. *Archives of Physical Medicine and Rehabilitation*, 84, 168–176.

Shimamura, A.P. (1986) Priming effects in amnesia: evidence for a dissociable memory function. *Quarterly Journal of Experimental Psychology*, 38A, 619–644.

Shimamura, A.P. (1994) The neuropsychology of metacognition. In *Metacognition. Knowing about Knowing*, Eds. J. Metcalfe & A.P. Shimamura. Cambridge, MA: MIT Press, pp. 253–276.

Shimamura, A.P. & Squire, L.R. (1986) Memory and metamemory: a study of the feeling-of-knowing phenomenon in amnesic patients. *Journal of Experimental Psychology: Learning, Memory and Cognition*, 12, 452–460.

Shimamura, A.P., Salmon, D.P., Squire, L.R. & Butters, N. (1987) Memory dysfunction and word priming in dementia and amnesia. *Behavioral Neuroscience*, 101, 347–351.

Small, I.F., Messina, J.A. & Small, J.G. (1964) The meaning of hospitalization: a comparison of attitudes of medical and psychiatric patients. *Journal of Nervous and Mental Disease*, 139, 575–580.

Small, J.G., Small, I.F. & Hayden, M.P. (1965) Prognosis and changes in attitude. *Journal of Nervous and Mental Disease*, 140, 215–217.

Small, M. & Ellis, S. (1996) Denial of hemiplegia: an investigation into the theories of causation. *European Neurology*, 36, 353–363.

Smith, C.A., Henderson, V.W., McCleary, C.A., Murdock, G.A. & Buckwalter, J.G. (2000) Anosognosia and Alzheimer's disease: the role of depressive symptoms in mediating impaired insight. *Journal of Clinical and Experimental Neuropsychology*, 22, 437–444.

Smith, S.M. (1995) Getting into and out of mental ruts: a theory of fixation, incubation and insight. In *The Nature of Insight*, Eds. R.J. Sternberg & J.E. Davidson. Cambridge, MA: MIT Press, pp. 229–251.

Smith, T.E., Hull, J.W. & Santos, L. (1998) The relationship between symptoms and insight in schizophrenia: a longitudinal perspective. *Schizophrenia Research*, 33, 63–67.

Smith, T.E., Hull, J.W., Goodman, M., Hedayat-Harris, A., Willson, D.F., Israel, L.M. & Munich, R.L. (1999) The relative influences of symptoms, insight and neurocognition on social adjustment in schizophrenia and schizoaffective disorder. *Journal of Nervous and Mental Disease*, 187, 102–108.

Smith, T.E., Hull, J.W., Israel, L.M. & Willson, D.F. (2000) Insight, symptoms and neurocognition in schizophrenia and schizoaffective disorder. *Schizophrenia Bulletin*, 26, 193–200.

Snaith, R.P., Constantopoulos, A.A., Jardine, M.Y. & McGuffin, P. (1978) A clinical scale for the self-assessment of irritability. *British Journal of Psychiatry*, 132, 164–171.

Snow, A.L., Norris, M.P., Doody, R., Molinari, V.A., Orengo, C.A. & Kunik, M.E. (2004) Dementia deficits scale. Rating self-awareness of deficits. *Alzheimer Disease and Associated Disorders*, 18, 22–31.

Snow, A.L., Kunik, M.E., Molinari, V.A., Orengo, C.A., Doody, R., Graham, D.P. & Norris, M.P. (2005) Accuracy of self–reported depression in persons with dementia. *Journal of the American Geriatrics Society*, 53, 389–396.

Société Médico-Psychologique (1866) Discussion sur la folie raisonnante, *Annales Médico-Psychologiques*, 7, 382–431.

Société Médico-Psychologique (1869/1870) Discussion sur les aliénés avec conscience. *Annales Médico-Psychologiques*, 3, 100–109, 110–130, 264–293, 304–310, 466–486.

Soskis, D.A. & Bowers, M.B. (1969) The schizophrenic experience. A follow-up study of attitude and posthospital adjustment. *Journal of Nervous and Mental Disease*, 149, 443–449.

Souchay, C., Isingrini, M. & Gil, R. (2002) Alzheimer's disease and feeling-of-knowing in episodic memory. *Neuropsychologia*, 40, 2386–2396.

Spoerl, H.D. (1936) Faculties versus traits: Gall's solution. *Personality and Character*, 4, 216–231.

Starkstein, S.E., Fedoroff, J.P., Price, T.R., Leiguarda, R. & Robinson, R.G. (1992) Anosognosia in patients with cerebrovascular lesions. A study of causative factors. *Stroke*, 23, 1446–1453.

Starkstein, S.E., Fedoroff, J.P., Price, T.R. & Robinson, R.G. (1993a) Denial of illness scale. A reliability and validity study. *Neuropsychiatry, Neuropsychology, and Behavioral Neurology*, 6, 93–97.

Starkstein, S.E., Fedoroff, J.P., Price, T.R., Leiguarda, R. & Robinson, R.G. (1993b) Neuropsychological deficits in patients with anosognosia. *Neuropsychiatry, Neuropsychology and Behavioral Neurology*, 6, 43–48.

Starkstein, S.E., Vázquez, S., Migliorelli, R., Tesón, A., Sabe, L. & Leiguarda, R. (1995a) A single-photon emission computed tomographic study of anosognosia in Alzheimer's disease. *Archives of Neurology*, 52, 415–420.

Starkstein, S.E., Migliorelli, R., Manes, F., Tesón, A., Petracca, G., Chemerinski, E., Sabe, L. & Leiguarda, R. (1995b) The prevalence and clinical correlates of apathy and irritability in Alzheimer's disease. *European Journal of Neurology*, 2, 540–546.

Starkstein, S.E., Sabe, L., Chemerinski, E., Jason, L. & Leiguarda, R. (1996) Two domains of anosognosia in Alzheimer's disease. *Journal of Neurology, Neurosurgery and Psychiatry*, 61, 485–490.

Starkstein, S.E., Chemerinski, E., Sabe, L., Kuzis, G., Petracca, G., Tesón, A. & Leiguarda, R. (1997a) Prospective longitudinal study of depression and anosognosia in Alzheimer's disease *British Journal of Psychiatry*, 171, 47–52.

Starkstein, S.E., Sabe, L., Cuerva, A.G., Kuzis, G. & Leiguarda, R. (1997b) Anosognosia and procedural learning in Alzheimer's disease. *Neuropsychiatry, Neuropsychology and Behavioral Neurology*, 10, 96–101.

Startup, M. (1996) Insight and cognitive deficits in schizophrenia: evidence for a curvilinear relationship. *Psychological Medicine*, 26, 1277–1281.

Startup, M. (1997) Awareness of own and others' schizophrenic illness. *Schizophrenia Research*, 26, 203–211.

Steiner, J. (1994) Patient-centered and analyst-centered interpretations: some implications of containment and countertransference. *Psychoanalytic Inquiry*, 14, 406–422.

Stengel, E. & Steele, G.D.F. (1946) Unawareness of physical disability (anosognosia). *Journal of Mental Science*, 92, 379–388.

Sternbach, O. (1989) Problems of insight in psychoanalysis. *Modern Psychoanalysis*, 14, 163–170.

Sternberg, R.J. & Davidson, J.E. (Eds) (1995) *The Nature of Insight*. London: MIT Press.

Strachey, J. (1934) The nature of the therapeutic action of psycho-analysis. *International Journal of Psychoanalysis*, 15, 127–159.

Stuss, D.T. (1991) Disturbance of self-awareness after frontal system damage. In *Awareness of Deficit After Brain Injury*, Eds. G.P. Prigatano & D.L. Schacter. Oxford: Oxford University Press, pp. 63–83.

Stuss, D.T. & Benson, D.F. (1986) *The Frontal Lobes*. New York: Raven Press.

Sunderland, A., Harris, J.E. & Baddeley, A.D. (1983) Do laboratory tests predict everyday memory? A neuropsychological study. *Journal of Verbal Learning and Verbal Behavior*, 22, 341–357.

Sunderland, A., Harris, J.E. & Gleave, J. (1984) Memory failures in everyday life following severe head injury. *Journal of Clinical Neuropsychology*, 6, 127–142.

Swanson, C.L., Freudenreich, O., McEvoy, J.P., Nelson, L., Kamaraju, L. & Wilson, W.H. (1995) Insight in schizophrenia and mania. *Journal of Nervous and Mental Disease*, 183, 752–755.

Takai, A., Uematsu, M., Ueki, H., Sone, K. & Kaiya, H. (1992) Insight and its related factors in chronic schizophrenic patients: a preliminary study. *European Journal of Psychiatry*, 6, 159–170.

Taylor, K.E. & Perkins, R.E. (1991) Identity and coping with mental illness in long-stay psychiatric rehabilitation. *British Journal of Clinical Psychology*, 30, 73–85.

Teri, L. & Wagner, A.W. (1991) Assessment of depression in patients with Alzheimer's disease: concordance among informants. *Psychology and Aging*, 6, 280–285.

Theml, T. & Romero, B. (2001) Selbstbeurteilung von Aufmerksamkeitsdefiziten bei Alzheimer-Kranken mit sehr leichter Demenz. *Zeitschrift für Neuropsychologie*, 12, 151–159.

Thompson, K.N., McGorry, P.D. & Harrigan, S.M. (2001) Reduced awareness of illness in first-episode psychosis. *Comprehensive Psychiatry*, 42, 498–503.

Tolor, A. & Reznikoff, M. (1960) A new approach to insight: a preliminary report. *Journal of Nervous and Mental Disease*, 130, 286–296.

Townsend, J.M. (1975) Cultural conceptions and mental illness: a controlled comparison of Germany and America. *Journal of Nervous and Mental Disease*, 160, 409–421.

Tranel, D. & Damasio, A.R. (1988) Non-conscious face recognition in patients with face agnosia. *Behavioural Brain Research*, 30, 235–249.

Trélat, U. (1861) *La Folie Lucide*. Paris: Adrien Delahaye.

Troisi, A., Pasini, A., Gori, G., Sorbi, T., Baroni, A. & Ciani, N. (1996) Clinical predictors of somatic and psychological symptoms of depression in Alzheimer's disease. *International Journal of Geriatric Psychiatry*, 11, 23–27.

Trosset, M.W. & Kaszniak, A.W. (1996) Measures of deficit unawareness for predicted performance experiments. *Journal of the International Neuropsychological Society*, 2, 315–322.

Upthegrove, R., Oyebode, F., George, M. & Haque, M.S. (2002) Insight, social knowledge and working memory in schizophrenia. *Psychopathology*, 35, 341–346.

Valenstein, A.F. (1981) Insight as an embedded concept in the early historical phase of psychoanalysis. In *The Psychoanalytic Study of the Child*, Vol. 36, Eds. A.J. Solnit, R.S. Eissler, A. Freud, M. Kris & P.B. Neubauer. New Haven: Yale University Press, pp. 307–315.

Van Putten, T., Crumpton, E. & Yale, C. (1976) Drug refusal in schizophrenia and the wish to be crazy. *Archives of General Psychiatry*, 33, 1443–1446.

Vasterling, J.J., Seltzer, B., Foss, J.W. & Vanderbrook, V. (1995) Unawareness of deficit in Alzheimer's disease. Domain-specific differences and disease correlates. *Neuropsychiatry, Neuropsychology and Behavioral Neurology*, 8, 26–32.

Vasterling, J.J., Seltzer, B. & Watrous, W.E. (1997) Longitudinal assessment of deficit unawareness in Alzheimer's disease. *Neuropsychiatry, Neuropsychology, and Behavioral Neurology*, 10, 197–202.

Vaz, F.J., Casado, M., Salcedo, M.S. & Béjar, A. (1994) Psicopatología y conciencia de enfermedad durante la fase aguda de la esquizofrenia. *Revista de Psiquiatria de la Facultad de Medicina de Barcelona*, 21, 66–74.

Vaz, F.J., Béjar, A. & Casado, M. (2002) Insight, psychopathology and interpersonal relationships in schizophrenia. *Schizophrenia Bulletin*, 28, 311–317.

Velmans, M. (Ed.) (1996) *The Science of Consciousness*. London: Routledge.

Verhey, F.R.J., Rozendaal, N., Ponds, R.W.H.M. & Jolles, J. (1993) Dementia, awareness and depression. *International Journal of Geriatric Psychiatry*, 8, 851–856.

Verhey, F.R.J., Ponds, R.W.H.M., Rozendaal, N. & Jolles, J. (1995) Depression, insight and personality changes in Alzheimer's disease and vascular dementia. *Journal of Geriatric Psychiatry and Neurology*, 8, 23–27.

Vilkki, J. (1985) Amnesic syndromes after surgery of anterior communicating artery aneurysms. *Cortex*, 21, 431–444.

Vogel, A., Hasselbalch, S.G., Gade, A., Ziebell, M. & Waldemar, G. (2005) Cognitive and functional neuroimaging correlates for anosognosia in mild cognitive impairment and Alzheimer's disease. *International Journal of Geriatric Psychiatry*, 20, 238–246.

Voruganti, L.N.P., Heslegrave, R.J. & Awad, A.G. (1997) Neurocognitive correlates of positive and negative syndromes in schizophrenia. *Canadian Journal of Psychiatry*, 42, 1066–1071.

Vuilleumier, P. (2000) Anosognosia. In *Behavior and Mood Disorders in Focal Brain Lesions*, Eds. J. Bogousslavsky & J.L. Cummings. Cambridge, UK: Cambridge University Press, pp. 465–519

Wagner, M.T., Spangenberg, K.B., Bachman, D.L. & O'Connell, P. (1997) Unawareness of cognitive deficit in Alzheimer disease and related dementias. *Alzheimer Disease and Associated Disorders*, 11, 125–131.

Wallace, C.A. & Bogner, J. (2000) Awareness of deficits: emotional implications for persons with brain injury and their significant others. *Brain Injury*, 14, 549–562.

Wallerstein, R.S. (1983) Some thoughts about insight and psychoanalysis. *Israel Journal of Psychiatry and Related Sciences*, 20, 33–43.

Warrington, E.K. & Weiskrantz, L. (1968) New method of testing long-term retention with special reference to amnesic patients. *Nature*, 217, 972–974.

Warrington, E.K. & Weiskrantz, L. (1974) The effect of prior learning on subsequent retention in amnesic patients. *Neuropsychologia*, 12, 419–428.

Warrington, E.K. & Weiskrantz, L. (1982) Amnesia: a disconnection syndrome? *Neuropsychologia*, 20, 233–248.

Watson, R.T. & Heilman, K.M. (1979) Thalamic neglect. *Neurology*, 29, 690–694.

Wciórka, J. (1988) A clinical typology of schizophrenic patients' attitudes towards their illness. *Psychopathology*, 21, 259–266.

Weiler, M.A., Fleisher, M.M. & McArthur-Campbell, D. (2000) Insight and symptom change in schizophrenia and other disorders. *Schizophrenia Research*, 45, 29–36.

Weinstein, E.A. (1991) Anosognosia and denial of illness. In *Awareness of Deficit After Brain Injury*, Eds. G.P. Prigatano & D.L. Schacter. Oxford: Oxford University Press, pp. 240–257.

Weinstein, E.A. & Kahn, R.L. (1955) *Denial of Illness: Symbolic and Physiological Aspects*. Springfield: Charles C. Thomas.

Weinstein, E.A., Friedland, R.P. & Wagner, E.E. (1994) Denial/unawareness of impairment and symbolic behavior in Alzheimer's disease. *Neuropsychiatry, Neuropsychology and Behavioral Neurology*, 7, 176–184.

Weisberg, R.W. (1992) Metacognition and insight during problem solving: comment on Metcalfe. *Journal of Experimental Psychology: Learning, Memory and Cognition*, 18, 426–431.

Weisberg, R.W. (1995) Prolegomena to theories of insight in problem solving: a taxonomy of problems. In *The Nature of Insight*, Eds. R.J. Sternberg & J.E. Davidson. Cambridge, MA: MIT Press, pp. 157–196.

Weisberg, R.W. & Alba, J.W. (1982) Problem solving is not like perception: more on Gestalt theory. *Journal of Experimental Psychology: General*, 111, 326–330.

Weiskrantz, L. (1988) Some contributions of neuropsychology of vision and memory to the problem of consciousness. In *Consciousness in Contemporary Science*, Eds. A.J. Marcel & E. Bisiach. Oxford: Oxford University Press, pp. 183–199.

Weiskrantz, L. (1990) *Blindsight. A Case Study and Implications*. Oxford: Oxford University Press.

Wertheimer, M. (1945/1961) *Productive Thinking*, Ed. M. Wertheimer, enlarged edition. London: Tavistock Publications.

White, R., Bebbington, P., Pearson, J., Johnson, S. & Ellis, D. (2000) The social context of insight in schizophrenia. *Social Psychiatry and Psychiatric Epidemiology*, 35, 500–507.

Whitman, J.R. & Duffey, R.F. (1961) The relationship between type of therapy received and a patient's perception of his illness. *Journal of Nervous and Mental Disease*, 133, 288–292.

Willingham, D.B. & Preuss, L. (1995) The death of implicit memory. *Psyche*, 2(15), http://psyche.cs.monash.edu.au/v2/psyche-2-15-willingham.html

Wilson, M. (1998) Otherness within: aspects of insight in psychoanalysis. *Psychoanalytic Quarterly*, 67, 54–77.

Wilson, T.D. & Dunn, E.W. (2004) Self-knowledge: its limits, value, and potential for improvement. *Annual Review of Psychology*, 55, 493–518.

Wing, J.K., Cooper, J.E. & Sartorius, N. (1974) *Measurement and Classification of Psychiatric Symptoms*. Cambridge, UK: Cambridge University Press.

World Health Organization (1973) *Report of the International Pilot Study of Schizophrenia*. Geneva: WHO.

World Health Organization (1992) *The ICD-10 Classification of Mental and Behavioural Disorders*. Geneva: WHO.

Wundt, W. (1886) *Éléments de Psychologie Physiologique*, Trans. É. Rouvier, 1880, 2nd edn. Paris: Félix Alcan.

Yen, C-F., Chen, C-S., Yeh, M-L., Yang, S-J., Ke, J-H. & Yen, J-Y. (2003) Changes in insight in manic episodes and influencing factors. *Comprehensive Psychiatry*, 44, 404–408.

Young, D.A., Davila, R. & Scher, H. (1993) Unawareness of illness and neuropsychological performance in chronic schizophrenia. *Schizophrenia Research*, 10, 117–124.

Young, D.A., Zakzanis, K.K., Bailey, C., Davila, R., Griese, J., Sartory, G. & Thom, A. (1998) Further parameters of insight and neuropsychological deficit in schizophrenia and other chronic mental disease. *Journal of Nervous and Mental Disease*, 186, 44–50.

Zanetti, O., Vallotti, B., Frisoni, G.B., Geroldi, C., Bianchetti, A., Pasqualetti, P. & Trabucchi, M. (1999) Insight in dementia: when does it occur? Evidence for a nonlinear relationship between insight and cognitive status. *Journal of Gerontology Series B – Psychological Sciences & Social Sciences*, 54, 100–106.

Zilboorg, G. (1952) The emotional problem and the therapeutic role of insight. *Psychoanalytic Quarterly*, 21, 1–24.

Index

Printed in the United States
by Baker & Taylor Publisher Services

Printed in the United States
by Baker & Taylor Publisher Services